JBReview

PREPARING FOR THE OCCUPATIONAL THERAPY NATIONAL BOARD EXAM

45 DAYS AND COUNTING

EDITED BY

Rosanne DiZazzo-Miller, DrOT, OTR

Assistant Professor
Department of Health Care Sciences, Occupational Therapy Program
Wayne State University
Detroit, Michigan

Joseph M. Pellerito Jr., PhD, OTR, CDI

Associate Professor and Director of the Driving Simulation Research Laboratory (DSRL)
Department of Health Care Sciences, Occupational Therapy Program
Wayne State University
Detroit, Michigan

JONES AND BARTLETT PUBLISHERS
Sudbury, Massachusetts
BOSTON   TORONTO   LONDON   SINGAPORE

World Headquarters
Jones and Bartlett Publishers
40 Tall Pine Drive
Sudbury, MA 01776
978-443-5000
info@jbpub.com
www.jbpub.com

Jones and Bartlett Publishers
Canada
6339 Ormindale Way
Mississauga, Ontario L5V 1J2
Canada

Jones and Bartlett Publishers
International
Barb House, Barb Mews
London W6 7PA
United Kingdom

Jones and Bartlett's books and products are available through most bookstores and online booksellers. To contact Jones and Bartlett Publishers directly, call 800-832-0034, fax 978-443-8000, or visit our website, www.jbpub.com.

Substantial discounts on bulk quantities of Jones and Bartlett's publications are available to corporations, professional associations, and other qualified organizations. For details and specific discount information, contact the special sales department at Jones and Bartlett via the above contact information or send an email to specialsales@jbpub.com.

Copyright © 2011 by Jones and Bartlett Publishers, LLC

All rights reserved. No part of the material protected by this copyright may be reproduced or utilized in any form, electronic or mechanical, including photocopying, recording, or by any information storage and retrieval system, without written permission from the copyright owner.

The authors, editors, and publisher have made every effort to provide accurate information. However, they are not responsible for errors, omissions, or for any outcomes related to the use of the contents of this book and take no responsibility for the use of the products and procedures described. Treatments and side effects described in this book may not be applicable to all people; likewise, some people may require a dose or experience a side effect that is not described herein. Drugs and medical devices are discussed that may have limited availability controlled by the Food and Drug Administration (FDA) for use only in a research study or clinical trial. Research, clinical practice, and government regulations often change the accepted standard in this field. When consideration is being given to use of any drug in the clinical setting, the health care provider or reader is responsible for determining FDA status of the drug, reading the package insert, and reviewing prescribing information for the most up-to-date recommendations on dose, precautions, and contraindications, and determining the appropriate usage for the product. This is especially important in the case of drugs that are new or seldom used.

Production Credits
Publisher: David Cella
Acquisitions Editor: Kristine Jones
Associate Editor: Maro Gartside
Editorial Assistant: Teresa Reilly
Senior Production Editor: Renée Sekerak
Production Assistant: Jill Morton
Marketing Manager: Grace Richards
Manufacturing and Inventory Control Supervisor: Amy Bacus
Composition: Datastream Content Solutions, LLC, Composition and Publishing Services
Cover and Title Page Design: Kristin E. Parker
Cover Image: © Photodisc
Chapter Opener Image: Vitaly M/ShutterStock, Inc.
Printing and Binding: Courier Stoughton
Cover Printing: Courier Stoughton

Library of Congress Cataloging-in-Publication Data

Preparing for the occupational therapy national board exam : 45 days and counting / [edited] by Rosanne DiZazzo-Miller and Joseph M. Pellerito Jr.
    p. ; cm.
  Includes bibliographical references and index.
  ISBN-13: 978-0-7637-5768-7
  ISBN-10: 0-7637-5768-3
  1. Occupational therapy—Examinations, questions, etc. 2. Occupational therapists—Licenses—United States—Examinations—Study guides. I. DiZazzo-Miller, Rosanne. II. Pellerito, Joseph Michael.
  [DNLM: 1. Occupational Therapy—Examination Questions. WB 18.2 P9268 2010]
  RM735.32.P74 2010
  615.8′515076—dc22
                                     2009035579

6048
Printed in the United States of America
13 12 11 10 09   10 9 8 7 6 5 4 3 2 1

Dedication

"I can do all things through Him who strengthens me." Philippians 4:23

To Carey, the love of my life, my unwavering pillar of strength and indomitable support.

To Joseph Alan, Victoria Rose, and Michael Anthony, my three pieces of Heaven on Earth.

To my parents, Rosina and Vittorio, for their courage to live the great American dream, so that their children would inherit lives of liberty and happiness.

To Josie and JoAnne for teaching me everything a little sister needs to know.

Thank you from the bottom of my heart for your unfaltering love and support.

This book is also inspired by and dedicated to all occupational therapy students who endured neuro, gross anatomy, groups, and goniometry. Cheers to coming this far and best of luck to you as you begin your journey as an occupational therapist.

Rosanne DiZazzo-Miller

To Laura Lynn for being my heart, my hope, and my love.

To Lillian Alexandra (C'mon Lil!) for bringing light and beauty into my life. You have always been my girl, and always will be.

To Joseph III (Juh!) for being the best son in the whole wide world.

To Ivy Noel (Er's on her scooter, she's running wild!) for being our miracle baby and little dancer, and making my heart leap for joy.

Joseph M. Pellerito Jr.

Brief Contents

Welcome to *Preparing for the Occupational Therapy National Board Exam: 45 Days and Counting!* This examination review book is designed to strengthen your learning skills and strategies to assist you in preparing to take the NBCOT OTR examination. This book is divided into nine sections and 25 chapters throughout the 45-day learning cycle. The sections and chapters are reflected in the following Table of Contents.

SECTION III

Therapeutic Interventions: Physical Disabilities (Days 7–15) 113

The chapters in this section include outlines, references, and work sheets on physical disability impairments, and interventions.

Chapter 7

Neurologic Impairments 115

Gerry Conti

Chapter 8

Musculoskeletal Impairments 129

Gerry Conti

Chapter 9

Musculoskeletal Assessments and Interventions 149

Gerry Conti

Chapter 10

Hand Rehabilitation and Surgical Conditions 183

Kurt Krueger

SECTION IV

Assessment of Occupational Functioning: Mental Health (Day 16) 205

The chapter in this section includes an outline with references and work sheets on client-centered assessments, interviews, and commonly used mental health evaluation tools.

Chapter 11

Assessments and Evaluations of Mental Health Conditions 207

Regina Parnell, Doreen Head, and Sophia Kimmons

SECTION V

Therapeutic Interventions: Mental Health (Days 17–19) 213

The chapters in this section include outlines, with references, and work sheets on mental health interventions, including group dynamics and therapeutic media.

Chapter 12

Psychiatric Interventions 215

Regina Parnell, Doreen Head, and Sophia Kimmons

Chapter 13

Intervention-Group Dynamics 227

Sophia Kimmons, Doreen Head, and Regina Parnell

SECTION VI

Therapeutic Specialized Pediatric Assessments and Interventions (Days 20–25) 249

The chapters in this section include outlines with references and work sheets on assessments commonly used in pediatric occupational therapy.

Chapter 14

Pediatric Conditions 251

Nancy Vandewiele Milligan

Chapter 15

Specialized Pediatric Assessments 277

Robin Mercer and Beth Angst

Chapter 16

Specialized Pediatric Interventions 299

Beth Angst and Robin Mercer

Contents

Contents

Contents

Chapter 19

Wheelchair Seating and Mobility   385

Chapter 20

Promoting Meaningful Occupations Through Assistive Technology, Home Accessibility, Driver Rehabilitation, and Community Mobility   397

SECTION VIII

Documentation, Management, Insurance, and Working with a Certified Occupational Therapy Assistant (COTA) (Days 32–35)   417

Chapter 21

Documentation of Occupational Therapy Practice   419

Chapter 22

Occupational Therapy Management and Business Fundamentals   425

Chapter 23

Insurance and Occupational Therapy Reimbursement   441

Chapter 24

Working with an Occupational Therapy Assistant   459

SECTION IX
Wrapping Up the Review (Days 36–45)   465

Chapter 25

Ten Days and Counting   467

Index   **471**

Foreword

"Never regard study as a duty, but as the enviable opportunity to learn to know the liberating influence of beauty in the realm of the spirit for your own personal joy and to the profit of the community to which your later work belongs."

Einstein

This examination review book is a great start for anyone preparing for the NBCOT certification exam. I remember studying for my occupational therapy certification examination. I was living in Hawaii and had an overwhelming urge to go to the beach when I should have been studying. I didn't know what to do or where to start to study for the exam. I felt like I was in over my head. The most difficult step for me was "getting started," followed by "what do I do now?" What I needed was this examination review book.

Preparing for the Occupational Therapy National Board Exam: 45 Days and Counting provides more than a bank of multiple-choice questions or occupational therapy facts and figures. The authors give readers an invaluable blueprint to guide them through the study process for the examination that grants entry into the occupational therapy profession. The overarching organizational structure that this book provides certainly would have lowered my study stress level. Not only does *45 Days and Counting* give readers a plan of action for studying, it also presents a review of critical information using the latest terminology. Most importantly, the authors provide readers with opportunities to process questions and apply step-by-step clinical reasoning skills to case studies—skills readers will find particularly helpful for the "new" certification.

In our contemporary world, readers will find the supplemental materials in the CD-ROM invaluable. Practicing on computers can only make readers feel more comfortable about the whole process.

So, start following this plan and applying what you know to how you think about the world. Your future in the occupational therapy profession is *45 Days and Counting. . . .*

Barbara L. Kornblau, JD, OTR/L, FAOTA, ABDA, DAAPM, CDMS, CCM
Dean, School of Health Professions and Studies
University of Michigan–Flint
Past President of the American Occupational Therapy Association

Acknowledgments

As I (Rosanne) reflect on this journey, I would like to acknowledge and thank all the kind souls who have contributed their time directly or indirectly to this project.

My wonderful husband, Carey, my very own Mr. Incredible, who learned, lived, and sang the words to "Mr. Mom" by Lonestar from time to time, while successfully managing his own business and simultaneously covering the roles of light-saber-wielding Jedi Knight, Barbie doll fashionista, and baby food chef extraordinaire. During this busy time my precious angels, Joseph, Victoria, and Michael, were content falling asleep against my shoulders, on my lap, and under my laptop during long nights of edits and emails. Perhaps my 3-year-old daughter gave me the best perspective when we sat down for a tea party in her room and she took my BlackBerry and put it in the hallway after politely informing me, "Mama, no phones allowed at my tea party." They have taught me the true meaning and purpose of life. I don't quite know how to put into words my sincere gratitude to my incredible parents for dedicating literally every minute of their lives to their children and grandchildren. Your never-ending support and encouragement have shaped my life in ways you will never know. Mom and Dad, your advice (with your strong Italian influence) rings true every time, "Worka hard, be careful witha your words, and mora careful witha who you trust!" Thank you to my sisters, Josie and JoAnne, my trustworthy "Plan B," who have been able to pick up and care for their niece and nephews at the drop of a dime. I simply would not have been able to get through this without the love and support of you all. Please know how much you will always mean to me. I would also like to express my sincere appreciation to my co-editor, Joseph M. Pellerito Jr. . . . My paisano! Reflecting back on this process, I am amazed at how much I have grown as a professional. I learned so much working on this project, but more so working with you. You have been a consummate mentor and good friend. Thank you for helping me grow in our profession! May God bless you all.

I (Joseph) also would like to extend my heartfelt gratitude and thanks to the following people who have been, and continue to be, an important source of strength, support, and inspiration in my life: Laura Lynn, my wife and best friend; Lily, Joey, and Ivy, my children who were sent from God above; Janet Pellerito, the woman who taught me the meaning of perseverance; and my friend and colleague, Rosanne DiZazzo-Miller. I am grateful for having had the opportunity to work with her on this project and will always cherish and appreciate her work ethic, sense of humor, and intellect. She is a fantastic writer, editor, and scholar! Finally, I would like to acknowledge the one true God almighty; He is the author and source of all knowledge.

We (Rosanne and Joseph) also would like to thank all those special people that helped us complete the constellation of tasks that were involved in successfully completing this book. Thank you to the alumni who participated in our focus group and shared their exam stories with us, which contributed to the spirit of this book. To the contributors who provided their expertise and content for each chapter, thank you for your invaluable time and energy. Thanks to all the reviewers who dedicated their time analyzing their assigned chapters and providing invaluable feedback with this process. Thanks to the authors of the multiple step case study questions, who answered our 11th-hour request and contributed significantly to this project. Finally, we appreciate Fredrick Pociask, our brilliant colleague and friend who helped us remember to laugh throughout this arduous process. He has provided direction on this project with his expertise in teaching and learning . . . A wise one he is.

We are so blessed to work for such a supportive institution as Wayne State University and the Eugene Applebaum College of Pharmacy & Health Sciences along with its extraordinarily supportive administrators, including President Jay Noren, Dean Lloyd Young, and Associate Dean Howard Normile, as well as the Department of Health Sciences Chair Dr. Thomas Birk. Special thanks to Melissa Kuster for her editorial consultations. Finally, thank you to all the professionals at Jones and Bartlett Publishers, especially David Cella, publisher, Maro Gartside, associate editor, Teresa Reilly, editorial assistant, and Jill Morton, production assistant. Their collegiality, prompt and helpful feedback, and steadfast support throughout the entire duration of this project are greatly appreciated.

With love and gratitude,
Rosanne and Joseph

About the Editors

Rosanne DiZazzo-Miller, DrOT, OTR was born in 1975 in Southfield, Michigan. She received her bachelor's degree from Adrian College, Adrian, Michigan; her master's degree in occupational therapy from Eastern Michigan University, Ypsilanti, Michigan; and her doctoral degree from Nova Southeastern University, Fort Lauderdale, Florida. Having entered academe in 2003, she serves on the faculty at Wayne State University (WSU) in Detroit, Michigan, as well as the part-time faculty in the Occupational Therapy Assistant Program at Wayne County Community College, also in Detroit. Prior to assuming the role of assistant professor, she worked in clinical practice in neurological rehabilitation for clients of all ages with traumatic brain and spinal cord injuries. Throughout her years of experience she served as pediatric team leader for a summer program that focuses on adolescents with traumatic brain injuries, and provided expert witness testimony. She is currently involved in assistive technology consultation for clients with brain and spinal cord injuries, and she is working in collaboration with the Alzheimer's Association of Michigan to provide training for caregivers of people with dementia-related health conditions through a Faculty Research Award Program in the Eugene Applebaum College of Pharmacy and Health Sciences at WSU. Her research interests include various modes of instructional learning delivery and outcomes research. She has presented at the state and national levels. She is a member of the American Occupational Therapy Association and has served on various committees for the Michigan Occupational Therapy Association. Rosanne was awarded the 2008 Eugene Applebaum College of Pharmacy and Health Sciences Excellence in Teaching Award for full-time faculty.

Joseph M. Pellerito Jr., PhD, OTR, CDI was born in 1961 in Detroit, Michigan, and grew up in and around the Motor City. He graduated from Western Michigan University's Honors College in 1984 with a baccalaureate of science (BS) degree in occupational therapy, completed a master of science (MS) degree in rehabilitation technology at Johns Hopkins University in 1994, and a PhD degree at Wayne State University (WSU) in Detroit. Dr. Pellerito is an associate professor and director of the Driving Simulation Research Laboratory (DSRL) in the Eugene Applebaum College of Pharmacy and Health Sciences at WSU in Detroit. He holds a research associate position at the Institute of Gerontology, also at WSU. His scholarship and research interests focus on driver rehabilitation and community mobility. He is participating in several funded research projects that seek to advance knowledge about and understanding of the impact of cell phone use on driver distractibility, driving after stroke and acquired brain injury, the impact of over-the-counter medications on driver performance and driving retirement and its impact on the quality of life among elderly citizens living in and around urban centers within the United States. Dr. Pellerito published the first textbooks on driver rehabilitation and community mobility and driving retirement. He has published numerous other books and articles in journals and online, and speaks on topics of interest locally, throughout Michigan, nationally, and internationally (Canada).

Contributors

Beth Angst, OTR
Senior Occupational Therapist
Children's Hospital of Michigan
Detroit, Michigan

Part-Time Faculty, Occupational Therapy Assistant Program
Wayne County Community College District
Detroit, Michigan

Kimberlee Bond, MOT, OTR/L, ATP
Senior Occupational Therapist, Inpatient Spinal Cord Unit
Rehabilitation Institute of Michigan
Detroit, Michigan

Gerry Conti, PhD, OTR
Assistant Professor, Occupational Therapy Program
Wayne State University
Detroit, Michigan

Doreen Head, PhD, OTR
Program Director and Assistant Professor, Occupational Therapy Program
Wayne State University
Detroit, Michigan

Sophia Kimmons, OTR
Senior Occupational Therapist, Department of Psychiatry and Behavioral Neurosciences
Detroit Receiving Hospital
Detroit, Michigan

Part-Time Faculty, Occupational Therapy Assistant Program
Wayne County Community College District
Detroit, Michigan

Sue Koziatek, MS, OTR
Occupational Therapist, Department of Support and Related Services
Macomb Intermediate School District
Clinton Township, Michigan

Part-Time Faculty, Occupational Therapy Program
Wayne State University
Detroit, Michigan

Contributors

Kurt Krueger, OTR, CHT
Clinical Specialist
Michigan Hand and Sports Rehabilitation Center
Dearborn, Michigan

Deborah Loftus, MOT, OTR
Occupational Therapist
Agility Health
Flatrock, Michigan

Life Skills Community Rehabilitation and Associates
Chelsea, Michigan

Catherine Lysack, PhD, OT(C)
Deputy Director, Institute of Gerontology
Professor, Occupational Therapy and Gerontology
Wayne State University
Detroit, Michigan

Robin Mercer, MHS, OTR
Occupational Therapist, POHI Outreach Department
Wayne Westland Schools
Westland, Michigan

Jon Nettie, MPT
Coordinator, Return-to-Work Services
Rehabilitation Institute of Michigan
Detroit, Michigan

Regina Parnell, PhD, OTR
Master of Occupational Therapy Program Coordinator, Level I Fieldwork Coordinator
Assistant Professor, Occupational Therapy Program
Wayne State University
Detroit, Michigan

Fredrick D. Pociask, PhD, PT, OCS, FAAOMPT
Assistant Professor, Physical Therapy Program
Wayne State University
Detroit, Michigan

Lettie M. Redley, MS, OTR
Assistant Program Director, Occupational Therapy Program
Wayne County Community College District
Detroit, Michigan

Anne T. Riddering, OTR/L, CLVT, COMS
Director of Rehabilitation, Visual Rehabilitation and Research Center of Michigan
Henry Ford Health System
Livonia, Michigan

Susan Ann Talley, DPT, MA
Program Director and Assistant Professor, Physical Therapy Program
Wayne State University
Detroit, Michigan

Diane Thomson, MS, OTR/L, ATP
Senior Occupational Therapist, Inpatient Physical Medicine and Rehabilitation Unit
Rehabilitation Institute of Michigan
Detroit, Michigan

Nancy Vandewiele Milligan, PhD, OTR
Academic Fieldwork Coordinator and Assistant Professor, Occupational Therapy Program
Wayne State University
Detroit, Michigan

CASE STUDY CONTRIBUTORS

Jane Pomper DeHart, MA, OTR/L
Vice President of Operations
Midwest Medical System Work-Safe Occupational Health
Detroit, Michigan

Sue Koziatek, MS, OTR
Occupational Therapist, Department of Support and Related Services
Macomb Intermediate School District
Clinton Township, Michigan

Part-Time Faculty, Occupational Therapy Program
Wayne State University
Detroit, Michigan

Deborah Loftus, MOT, OTR
Occupational Therapist
Agility Health
Flatrock, Michigan

Life Skills Community Rehabilitation and Associates
Chelsea, Michigan

Claudia Morreale, MS, OTR, CLT
Occupational Therapist, Rehabilitation Services
St. John Health System
Macomb, Michigan

Denise Nitta, OTR
Senior Clinician
Rehabilitation Institute of Michigan
Detroit, Michigan

Reviewers

Diane E. Adamo, PhD, OTR
Assistant Professor, Physical Therapy Program
Adjunct Assistant Professor, Institute of Gerontology
Wayne State University
Detroit, Michigan

Mary Kay Currie, OT, BCPR
Multidisciplinary Supervisor
Rehabilitation Institute of Michigan and Harper University Hospital
Detroit Medical Center
Detroit, Michigan

John T. Connelly, MSOL, OTR/L
Instructor and Fieldwork Coordinator
Gannon University
Erie, Pennsylvania

Cristy Daniel, MS, OTR/L
Assistant Professor and Academic Fieldwork Coordinator
College of Saint Mary
Omaha, Nebraska

Jane Pomper DeHart, MA, OTR/L
Vice President of Operations
Midwest Medical System Work-Safe Occupational Health
Detroit, Michigan

Barbara Funk, MS, OTR, CHT
Senior Occupational Therapist and Coordinator, Lymphedema Program
Rehabilitation Institute of Michigan–Novi
Novi, Michigan

Bernadette Hattjar, DrOT, MED, OTR/L, CWCE
Assistant Professor
Gannon University
Erie, Pennsylvania

Sophia Kimmons, OTR
Senior Occupational Therapist, Department of Psychiatry and Behavioral Neurosciences
Detroit Receiving Hospital
Detroit, Michigan

Part-Time Faculty, Occupational Therapy Assistant Program
Wayne County Community College District
Detroit, Michigan

Sue Koziatek, MS, OTR
Occupational Therapist, Department of Support and Related Services
Macomb Intermediate School District
Clinton Township, Michigan

Part-Time Faculty, Occupational Therapy Program
Wayne State University
Detroit, Michigan

Deborah Loftus, MOT, OTR
Occupational Therapist
Agility Health
Flatrock, Michigan

Life Skills Community Rehabilitation and Associates
Chelsea, Michigan

Denise Nitta, OTR
Senior Clinician
Rehabilitation Institute of Michigan
Detroit, Michigan

Pamela Poteete, OTR
Supervisor, Rehabilitation Services
William Beaumont Hospital
Troy, Michigan

Preethy Samuels, PhD, OTR
Research Associate, Developmental Disabilities Institute
Adjunct Faculty Member, Occupational Therapy Program
Wayne State University
Detroit, Michigan

Christi Vicino, MA, OTA/C
OTA Program Director
Grossmont College
El Cajon, California

Callie Watson, OTD, OT
Program Director of Occupational Therapy
College of Saint Mary
Omaha, Nebraska

Preparing for the NBCOT Examination (Day 1)

Getting Started

*Rosanne DiZazzo-Miller, Fredrick D. Pociask,
Joseph M. Pellerito Jr., and Sue Koziatek*

INTRODUCTION

Welcome to Day 1 of your study guide. Today we will cover Chapters 1, 2, and 3. In this chapter you will review a brief introduction to your study guide in addition to learning where to locate resources pertaining to your upcoming examination.

 Preparing for the Occupational Therapy National Board Exam: 45 Days and Counting is unlike any examination book currently available to occupational therapy students. Through research utilizing a focus group model, we learned what students preparing for this examination need and want to optimize their success.

GUIDEBOOK AT-A-GLANCE

The main theme of this book utilizes chapter outlines on subject matter that is learned throughout occupational therapy curricula using a lexicon (i.e., special vocabulary) taken from the Occupational Therapy Practice Framework. Each chapter is divided into subjects taught throughout occupational therapy curricula in the United States. From those subjects, outlines are provided as a study guide for you to begin the 45-day journey and, at the end, feel prepared and ready to take the National Board for Certification in Occupational Therapy, Inc. (NBCOT) examination. Although this book is structured to complete your studies within 45 days, it is important that you have a sense of confidence and security, which will result from your test preparation, before scheduling a date to take the examination. When you complete (or come close to completing) the 45 days of test preparation, you will have a better idea of when you should schedule your examination. The typical application turnaround time after you send your transcripts to NBCOT is approximately 1 week before receiving your Authorization to Test (ATT) letter. After you receive your letter, you can typically schedule your exam right away.

 Additionally, corresponding workbook pages throughout each chapter, along with specific references and page numbers used throughout occupational therapy curricula throughout the United States, enable additional exploration of content that students find challenging or unfamiliar. At the end of each chapter, answers to case studies or specific work sheets can be found.

 The CD-ROM accompanying this text consists of two interactive practice examinations in addition to various supplemental materials. The questions cover content as specified in the study outlines in the chapters and are appropriately distributed using the NBCOT domain areas, which can be located at http://www.nbcot.org/webarticles/anmviewer.asp?a=257. Each exam question provides a rationale for correct answers along with references for you to research. Furthermore, practice test results can be calculated to provide you with specific domain area percentage scores so you will know what areas you need to spend more time on.

OUTLINE

1. **CD-ROM Supplemental Resource Materials**
   a. Answer sheets to various learning aids (e.g., work sheets)
   b. Complete and referenced handouts to supplement your existing course material or to address gaps in knowledge
   c. Reference and resource lists with working Internet links
   d. Unique instructional materials that provide the learner with a creative means by which to learn and discover the content (e.g., case studies and clinical instruments)
   e. 600 practice examination questions that can be taken to simulate the actual exam
   f. Multiple-step case studies
2. **Examination preparation and practice**
   a. Using the Supplemental CD-ROM
   b. Running the CD-ROM
      i. Place the CD-ROM in the CD-ROM drive and close the tray.
      ii. The CD-ROM will autorun (autorun must be enabled).
      iii. If autorun is not enabled on your computer, use Windows Explorer and open Autorun.exe, which is located in the root directory of this CD-ROM.
      iv. After the CD-ROM opens, please click on the Read First tabs for complete instructions about using the Resource CD-ROM.

Each week you are asked to answer the following questions:*

1. **What?**
   What have I accomplished?
   What have I learned?
2. **So what?**
   What difference did it make?
   Why should I do it?
   How is it important?
   How do I feel about it?
3. **Now what?**
   What's next?
   Where do we go from here?

*__Note:__ *This journaling section, courtesy of Live Wire Media, is provided using a three-question reflective learning approach with which students learn individual areas to focus on and prioritize. Research suggests that reflection "illuminates what has been experienced by [one's] self . . . providing a basis for future action" (Raelin, 2001, p. 11).*

Evidence-based practice (EBP) will guide the formation of each chapter outline and work sheet, and the CD-ROM will contain a section for EBP article citations or links to further research in a particular area of study. Furthermore, references used throughout this exam review book feature robust levels of evidence to provide the student with the most current and accurate information available.

The student's health and wellness is another theme addressed throughout this book. Wellness tips and the opportunity for self-assessment reinforce healthy lifestyle choices that are conducive to success. Every week you will be asked to perform a self-assessment in the areas of sleep, nutrition, exercise, and stress. This will be completed using the Stress Vulnerability Scale. You should consider getting at least 1 to 2 *weeks* of restorative or quality sleep (i.e., 8 hours of uninterrupted sleep per day) leading up to the exam. These activities will serve as a reminder of the importance of taking care of yourself and are meant to reinforce key traits (e.g., flexibility, organization, and person-centeredness) that will enable you to become a productive and effective occupational therapist. Additionally, you will be directed to the NBCOT Web site where you can download the OT Tool, which will assist in the formulation of a personalized study plan to help keep you on track throughout this important process. This not only provides a focus, but it will inevitably guide the identification of your strengths, weaknesses, and personal challenges.

Test-taking strategies and things to do prior to, and directly after, the exam are presented in the following two chapters, with a focus on adult learning and test-taking strategies.

Now, it is time to switch on your computer and visit the NBCOT Web site at http://www. nbcot.org/. You will once again be directed to this Web site after taking the NBCOT examination in Chapter 25.

1. **National Board for Certification in Occupational Therapy, Inc. (NBCOT)**
   a. Make certain to visit http://www.nbcot.org to access and utilize the following documents listed under Exam Candidates:
      i. Frequently Asked Questions
      ii. Candidate Information
         I. Information presented here specifically focuses on the examination handbook and application, in addition to special testing accommodations, code of conduct, and official score transfer request forms.
      iii. International Candidates
         I. All forms and handbooks related to internationally educated occupational therapists and graduates are located here.
      iv. Online Examination Application and Online Application Status Check
         I. Here you will set up your account with NBCOT online to apply for the exam.
      v. Candidate Forms
         I. This section includes credential verification forms, confirmation of registration, eligibility, official and duplicate score transfer request, and reissue of authorization to test.
         II. The Special Accommodations Handbook and Application link is located in this section.
      vi. Examination Preparation Tools
         I. In this section be sure to download the free NBCOT Examination Readiness Tools (OTR Tool). This tool identifies candidates' strengths and weaknesses using a Likert-type survey throughout all four domain areas that are presented in the exam.
      vii. Score Reports
         I. Examination score reporting is explained here, along with links for the scoring calendar and steps for reapplying for the exam.
      viii. Getting Licensed
         I. Here you will find information explaining the difference between state licensure and NBCOT certification. Follow the link provided to search for your state regulatory board for any further inquiries you may have.
      ix. Useful Links
         I. Included in this list of resources is the Prometric testing center Web site, where you can find testing centers throughout the country.
      x. Clinical Simulation Test Questions
         I. A short clinical simulation tutorial can be found on the Exam Candidates Welcome page (National Board for Certification in Occupational Therapy, 2009). You can access this information at http://www.nbcot.org/simulation/web_static_sim/index.html.
      xi. Lastly, make sure to click on the Executive Summary for the Practice Analysis Study at http://www.nbcot.org/webarticles/articlefiles/PA_OTR_DTKS_2008.pdf, and download the *Executive Summary of the Practice Analysis Study for the Occupational Therapist Registered OTR*. This will identify all areas covered on the exam along with a chart of the domain areas with each percentage covered in the

exam. For example, after taking the OTR Tool and finding the domain area(s) you need to focus on, locate that domain area in the chart provided in the Practice Analysis so you know what percentage of the exam you might struggle with. The answer to this question will help structure your study skills to focus on specific areas.

2. **Focus Group Transcript Results**

   a. Before planning of this examination guidebook began, we called on our alumni to attend a videotaped focus group to provide us insight that we could implement into our book and pass along to future graduates. The results were as follows, beginning with themes and ending with specific questions:

   i. Preparation

      I. Prepare for approximately 6 weeks at a minimum, and spend some time alone and some time together in small groups.

      II. Take tests repeatedly.

      III. Don't focus on studying what you already know.

   ii. Materials for preparation

      I. NBCOT materials are popular and similar to exam questions.

      II. Other materials were too vague and concrete, with only one-step questions.

      III. The national review course was helpful but overwhelming.

      IV. Other materials were not helpful for critical thinking.

      V. The rationale for correct answers is very important.

   iii. Summary

      I. Combine diagnosis with treatment in multistep questions.

      II. Learn how to dissect questions.

   iv. Test environment

      I. The environment was anxiety provoking.

      II. The room was cold.

   v. Helpful hints

      I. Most focus group students took off weekends from studying.

      II. Make sure you focus on SCI levels of function related to levels of injury and relevant equipment!

      III. Watch your caffeine intake.

      IV. Go to the bathroom halfway through the test, even if you don't need to go.

      V. Take the clock off the computer screen if it is anxiety provoking.

      VI. Visit the site the day before and walk in to get a feel for the environment.

      VII. Dress in comfortable layers.

      VIII. Don't study the night before.

      IX. Sleep 8 hours the night before.

      X. Choose a time to take the exam that fits your personality.

      XI. Volunteer at a site that you don't feel enough exposure to.

   vi. If a retake is needed visit http://www.nbcot.org/WebArticles/articlefiles/139-2005_retake_cert_exam_brochure.pdf where you can download *Steps for Re-Applying to Take the NBCOT Certification Examination for Candidates.*

The following are some specific questions that were answered by the students in the focus group:

Q: Are the questions presented one at a time?

A: Yes

Q: Can you mark them and go back to them, and how does that work?

A: Yes, after you complete the questions, a list comes up of questions you marked to look at again.

Q: After you answer, can you change the answer later, even after you click on a selection?

A: Yes

Q: What is the best piece of advice you can give a student who is preparing to answer the questions on this examination?

A: Eliminate two answers first from the four presented, and then reread the question to make sure your answer fits exactly what the question asks!

Q: Give your best description of your testing area or environment.

A: There were rows of computers with cubicle dividers, and you can wear headphones to block out sounds. Other people are writing different tests (e.g., SAT). The test room consisted of approximately 30 individuals.

Q: What are you allowed to bring into the testing center?

A: They give you a blank sheet of paper and a pen. You cannot bring water, but you can take a break and leave for water or the bathroom. There were lockers where we had to leave our purses, etc., outside the testing room.

Q: Identify any mnemonics or charts that were helpful during your study preparation.

A: The charts and handouts with a short summary of infant and child reflexes/patterns really helped (e.g., Moro, Babinski, ATNR, STNR). Also, a synopsis of the most common splints was very helpful. It helped to have a page at a glance, with a picture of each splint and a short description, including the name and use for each. In addition, reviewing the Brunnstrum, MMT, Ranchos, Glasgow Coma Scale, and ROM norms/scales was very useful. Any kind of handout or page at a glance is helpful to reinforce the information into memory.

Q: Is there anything else you can remember about the exam and what was and was not allowed?

A: Be able to use clinical reasoning skills in terms of reading a treatment scenario and deciding on the best option. There were always two answers that were definitely wrong and two that seemed to be correct. I remember always having to narrow down out of the two which was the *better* choice.

Q: Did you learn about how to take the test through a tutorial or as you went?

A: There was a tutorial at the beginning of the test with examples, and it did not take up any examination time.

Q: Please provide any additional comments regarding what you found helpful in preparing to take the exam.

A: The most helpful thing for me was to repeatedly take practice exams. I would go back and study the areas on the practice tests that I got wrong. I also spent a lot of time studying the basics and making sure those were embedded in my memory as a knowledge base for any type of question they might throw at me. Know the various scales, norms, reflexes, most common splints, contraindications for certain diagnoses, etc. Spend time studying with a few friends, quizzing one another and discussing why an answer was wrong or right. It helped a lot to have feedback within a small group.

3. Multiple-Step Case Study Example

The new clinical simulation test question requires you to process, integrate, and apply your knowledge to the different domain areas related to a case study. Again, please be sure to visit http://www.nbcot.org, navigate to the Exam Candidates page, and click on the tutorial in the third paragraph. Let's walk through an example:

An OT working in a school setting is asked by a classroom teacher to screen a 7-year-old second grade student. The teacher is concerned that the student is still not able to form letters legibly when printing, even with a model, and even though the teacher has been practicing with the student daily and the student's mother has also been practicing with the student at home. The student cannot color thoroughly or stay in the lines. The student still scribbles colors, fills in only approximately 50% of any picture, and uses only one or two colors. The student cannot cut out simple shapes without chopping them up and drops the paper or scissors several times during the task. The student is currently certified speech and language impaired and is believed to have normal intelligence, according to the classroom teacher.

Part I

The OT receives parental permission through the classroom teacher to screen this student during her next visit to the school. What should be included in the screening process so the OT can decide if the student should be referred for an initial evaluation?

From the list below, choose the correct answer(s):

A. Ask the teacher for work samples of the student's coloring, cutting, pasting, and printing.
B. Observe the student during a reading group.
C. Observe the student in class during an art activity that combines coloring, cutting, and pasting, or work with the student individually to observe these skills.
D. Work with the student individually and have the student copy basic shapes, including lines, circles, crosses, squares, Xs, and triangles to see if the student has mastered all basic shapes.
E. Ask the teacher what the student's academic strengths and weaknesses are.
F. Observe the student at recess.
G. Ask the student to trace or copy the upper- and lowercase letters of the alphabet and numbers 1–10.
H. Observe and record the student's pencil grip.
I. Review the student's school records.
J. Observe the student during snack and lunch times.
K. Talk to the speech therapist to see what difficulties the student has regarding speech skills.

The correct answers include the following:

A. Ask the teacher for work samples of the student's coloring, cutting, pasting, and printing. This is correct because the therapist can compare the work the student does in a one-on-one screening with the student's work in the classroom environment.
C. Observe the student in class during an art activity that combines coloring, cutting, and pasting, or work with the student individually to observe these skills. This is correct because the therapist needs to observe the student either performing these activities in the classroom or individually working with the student for a brief screening to start developing a hypothesis of why this student is struggling with classroom fine motor tasks. The therapist can observe praxis as well as eye–hand coordination, range of motion, grasp, attention, and persistence simultaneously.
D. Work with the student individually and have the student copy basic shapes, including lines, circles, crosses, squares, Xs, and triangles to see if the student has mastered all basic shapes. This is correct because visual motor skills for copying designs are most highly correlated with handwriting legibility and preparedness, so if the student's handwriting problems are caused by visual motor skill impairments, design copying skills should appear to be delayed.
G. Ask the student to trace or copy the upper- and lowercase letters of the alphabet and numbers 1–10. This is correct because the therapist needs to observe the student while printing to see how the student forms letters and to observe the student's pencil pressure and pencil grip, etc., to identify possible causes for the handwriting difficulty.
H. Observe and record the student's pencil grip. This is important in a screening because handwriting difficulties is one of the teacher's main complaints.

The following answers are incorrect:

B. Observe the student during a reading group. Reading skills are not a concern of the teacher, so they do not need to be addressed at this time.

E. Ask the teacher what the student's academic strengths and weaknesses are. Strengths and weaknesses do not need to be identified during the screening process to determine if the student should be evaluated.

F. Observe the student at recess. Because this is not a concern of the teacher, it is not something that needs to be observed during the screening process.

I. Review the student's school records. This is not necessary for screening; it should be done for an evaluation.

J. Observe the student during snack and lunch times. This observation is not necessary for screening.

K. Talk to the speech therapist to see what difficulties the student has regarding speech skills. This is not necessary for screening but is important if it progresses to an evaluation.

Let's move on to the next step in the occupational therapy process. Using the same information as previously provided, answer the following question:

Part II

Following the screening the OT decides to approve a referral for a comprehensive OT evaluation. Which assessment tools(s) should the OT use as part of the initial evaluation process?

From the following list, choose the correct answer(s):

A. Pediatric Evaluation of Disability Inventory (PEDI)

B. Grip and pinch strength test

C. Beery-Buktenica Developmental Test of Visual–Motor Integration (Beery VMI)

D. Gross Motor Function Measure (GMFM)

E. The Motor Free Test of Visual Perception Test, Third Edition (MVPT-3)

F. Sensory Profile

G. Bruininks-Oseretsky Test of Motor Proficiency, Second Edition (BOT-2)

H. Evaluation Tool of Children's Handwriting-Manuscript (ETCH-M)

I. Vineland Adaptive Behaviors Scales

J. Functional Independence Measure for Children (WeeFIM)

The correct answers include the following:

C. The Beery VMI is important because research has shown that scores from this test are most highly correlated with poor handwriting.

G. The BOT-2 is recognized as the most valid and reliable standardized test that most highly correlates with fine motor skill deficits in children and teenagers.

H. ETCH-M is correct because it is a handwriting assessment that covers all but the long endurance writing component that experts recommend be tested when evaluating a student's handwriting skills.

The rest of the choices are incorrect because they do not target the areas identified by the teacher as the primary problem areas. Therefore, although they may provide beneficial information to the therapist, they are not the most efficient tools to assess the areas identified as the main problems.

Part III

Based on the results of the student's evaluation, which of the following recommendations should the OT make to the Individualized Education Program team for goals that will help improve the student's educational fine motor, visual motor, and printing skills?

From the list below, choose the correct answer(s):

A. The student will copy all lowercase cursive letters legibly 80% of the time.

B. The student will read text accurately from left to right at the appropriate grade level 80% of the time.

    C. The student will copy all manuscript lowercase and uppercase letters legibly with correct orientation 80% or more of the time.

    D. The student will organize math problems legibly on graph paper 80% or more of the time.

    E. The student will cut out simple and complex shapes within 0.25 inches of the line with good bilateral coordination.

    F. The student will complete classroom written work legibly 80% of the time when allowed to copy dictated answers.

    G. The student will type all long multisentence writing assignments with minimal verbal and physical assistance.

The correct answers include the following:

    C. The student will copy all manuscript lowercase and uppercase letters legibly with correct orientation 80% or more of the time. This answer is correct because one of the main problems identified by the teacher is that the student is not able to form his or her letters correctly, even with a model.

    E. The student will cut out simple and complex shapes within 0.25 inches of the line with good bilateral coordination. This is an important goal because for being in the second grade, the student was greatly delayed for cutting skills. The therapist would hope to improve the student's cutting skills to an appropriate functional level for the student's grade.

    F. The student will complete classroom written work legibly 80% of the time when allowed to copy dictated answers. This choice is correct because the therapist would hope that within 1 year of treatment the student would not only learn how to print letters legibly, but hopefully words and simple sentences too, because the student is already in second grade and would be required to answer in sentences for many classroom written work assignments.

The rest of the answers are incorrect because the goals are set too high. The cursive goal would not be pursued until the student's printing skills are functional, the student is in at least third grade, or the student receives intervention for printing skills for at least a year because progress was not sufficient. The copying left to right goal is not necessary yet because that was not described as a concern by the teacher in the initial screening request, so the student's copying skills may be adequate. The typing goal is not needed yet because the student would just be beginning printing intervention skills, and most teachers and parents prefer to try to develop printing skills for at least a year before giving up and teaching word processing skills, especially at age 7 years.

Part IV

Based on the student's Individualized Education Program's goals, the OT will try to improve motor planning of visual motor, fine motor, and printing skills. What specific intervention activities should the OT include to meet these goals?

From the list below, choose the correct answer(s):

    A. Play on the playground equipment, with emphasis on swings.

    B. Practice cutting out simple shapes from card stock that are outlined with a bright marker to highlight the cutting line.

    C. Have the student do a hidden picture puzzle.

    D. Have the student do a few pages in the first-grade level of Handwriting Without Tears workbook after practicing letter formation on the chalkboard with verbal cues.

    E. Do rainbow writing with a vibrating pen or chalk while tracing letters.

    F. Have the student go through an obstacle course containing a tunnel, scooter boards, hopscotch, monkey bars, slide, and minitramp.

G. Try different pencil grips, short pencils, and repositioning the student's thumb and fingers into a mature pencil grip while writing on a vertical surface.

The correct answers include the following:

B. Practice cutting out simple shapes from card stock that are outlined with a bright marker to highlight the cutting line. This would help the student see the lines, and if the lines are larger, the student will be more likely to be successful cutting on or near the lines. The types of shapes and complexity should follow the developmental approach, so the easiest shapes are given first and progress to the most difficult shapes; for example, lines, curves, circles, squares, triangles, and other basic shapes.

D. Have the student do a few pages in the first-grade level of Handwriting Without Tears workbook after practicing letter formation on the chalkboard with verbal cues. This is a very good multisensory handwriting remediation program with good research support, and it is an excellent tool to use when remediating handwriting skills.

E. Do rainbow writing with a vibrating pen or chalk while tracing letters. These are appropriate interventions for handwriting remediation. The vibrating pen helps with motor planning because vibration uses a different neurological pathway than the tactile and proprioceptive systems. Rainbow writing helps with making repetition of the same motor plan more interesting, thus enhancing attention to task and motor memory.

G. Try different pencil grips, short pencils, and repositioning the student's thumb and fingers into a mature pencil grip while writing on a vertical surface. This is appropriate for a remediation technique when the student does not have a mature pencil grip. Short pencils help inhibit primitive pencil grips and facilitate a tripod, a more mature pencil grip.

The rest of the activities do not target the particular skills outlined in the goals as specifically as these activities do. The perceptual activities are not needed for this student's goals. The obstacle course activities, although they are good for overall motor planning, are not necessarily needed if the student's motor planning difficulties are limited to visual and fine motor skills. Playing on the swings to stimulate maturation of the vestibular system does not directly affect visual motor and fine motor skills and therefore may not help the therapist reach the student's goals in the most efficient manner possible.

How did you do? Keep in mind that there are three clinical simulation test questions on the exam. This provides an example of how to progress through a multiple-step case study. After each section of this book, make sure you can answer questions in this manner, moving from screening and assessment into implementation and intervention. We offer further multiple-step clinical scenarios on the CD-ROM that is included with this book.

FINAL THOUGHTS

The following outline provides some keys to success as you progress through your 45-day journey:

1. **Know your facts.**
   a. Review, study, and become familiar with the facts presented; that is what this entire book is about!
2. **Learn how to answer questions strategically.**
   a. Keep in mind that the exam questions will contain a lot of information. You will need to focus on some of the information, but other information will not be relevant to the final question being asked. *Remember to read each question statement one last time before selecting your answer.* Don't get tripped up on answer options that make sense for only

certain parts of the question. Make sure the answer you select addresses the central theme of the question being asked.

3. **Take at least two practice exams on a computer, and remember to time yourself to try to simulate the actual testing environment.**

   a. Get used to taking practice exams while being timed. Experience what answering *one question per minute* feels like in an environment where you hear people typing, fidgeting in their seats, and getting up to go to the restroom. Only bring items that are allowed in the testing environment. Complete at least two practice tests in this environment. You will find it very different than taking an exam at your leisure in your pajamas while munching on a snack!

4. **At the 2009 American Occupational Therapy Association Annual Conference in Texas, the NBCOT reported that test takers who took the full 10-minute tutorials during the exam performed better than students who did not. There are two tutorials, neither of which count against your exam time. Now . . . let's get started!**

REFERENCES

National Board for Certification in Occupational Therapy, Inc. (2009). *Welcome, exam candidates.* Retrieved March 27, 2009, from http://www.nbcot.org/

Raelin, J. A. (2001). Public reflection as the basis of learning. *Management Learning, 32*(1), 11–30.

Exhibit 1-1 Stress Vulnerability Scale

In modern society, most of us can't avoid stress. But we can learn to behave in ways that lessen its effects. Researchers have identified a number of factors that affect one's vulnerability to stress—among them are eating and sleeping habits, caffeine and alcohol intake, and how we express our emotions. The following questionnaire is designed to help you discover your vulnerability quotient and to pinpoint trouble spots. Rate each item from 1 (always) to 5 (never), according to how much of the time the statement is true of you. Be sure to mark each item, even if it does not apply to you—for example, if you don't smoke, circle 1 next to item six.

		Always		Sometimes		Never	
1.	I eat at least one hot, balanced meal a day.	1	2	(3)	4	5	✳
2.	I get 7–8 hours of sleep at least four nights a week.	1	(2)	3	4	5	
3.	I give and receive affection regularly.	(1)	2	3	4	5	
4.	I have at least one relative within 50 miles on whom I can rely.	1	2	3	4	(5)	✳
5.	I exercise to the point of perspiration at least twice a week.	1	2	(3)	4	5	✳
6.	I limit myself to less than half a pack of cigarettes a day.	(1)	2	3	4	5	
7.	I take fewer than five alcohol drinks a week.	1	2	(3)	4	5	✳
8.	I am the appropriate weight for my height.	1	(2)	3	4	5	
9.	I have an income adequate to meet basic expenses.	(1)	2	3	4	5	
10.	I get strength from my religious beliefs.	1	(2)	3	4	5	
11.	I regularly attend club or social activities.	(1)	2	3	4	5	
12.	I have a network of friends and acquaintances.	(1)	2	3	4	5	
13.	I have one or more friends to confide in about personal matters.	(1)	2	3	4	5	
14.	I am in good health (including eyesight, hearing, and teeth).	1	2	(3)	4	5	✳
15.	I am able to speak openly about my feelings when angry or worried.	1	2	(3)	4	5	✳
16.	I have regular conversations with the people I live with about domestic problems—for example, chores and money.	1	(2)	3	4	5	
17.	I do something for fun at least once a week.	(1)	2	3	4	5	
18.	I am able to organize my time effectively.	1	(2)	3	4	5	
19.	I drink fewer than three cups of coffee (or other caffeine-rich drinks) a day.	(1)	2	3	4	5	
20.	I take some quiet time for myself during the day.	1	(2)	3	4	5	

(continues)

Exhibit 1-1 Stress Vulnerability Scale *(continued)*

Scoring Instructions: To calculate your score, add up the figures and subtract 20.

$$40 - 20 = 20$$

Score Interpretation:
A score below 10 indicates excellent resistance to stress.
A score over 30 indicates some vulnerability to stress.
A score over 50 indicates serious vulnerability to stress.

Self-Care Plan: Notice that nearly all the items describe situations and behaviors over which you have a great deal of control. Review the items on which you scored three or higher. List those items in your self-care plan. Concentrate first on those that are easiest to change—for example, eating a hot, balanced meal daily and having fun at least once a week—before tackling those that seem difficult.

Source: Exhibit courtesy Copyright 2009 Stress Directions, Inc., Lyle H. Miller and Alma Dell Smith, Boston, MA
www.stressdirections.com

Exhibit 1-2 Stress Busters

Tips and Techniques for Managing Stress and Introducing Relaxation into Your Life

What Is Stress?

Stress is the physiological and psychological response of the body to some sort of threat to our safety, self-esteem, or well-being. Stressors can be physical (e.g., illness), social (e.g., a relationship breakup or other loss), circumstantial (e.g., a poor exam grade or moving), or psychological (e.g., low self-esteem or worry). Often, transitions or changes, such as a new semester or new job, can bring on stress.

We are all under stress every day. A certain amount of stress helps us all to function better, keep ourselves safe from harm, and get things done during the day. Too much stress, however, can lead to physical illness, difficulty concentrating, or feelings of sadness or isolation.

Did You Know . . .

Most college campuses and communities have counseling and psychological services available for students and community residents at low cost. If the stress you experience interferes meaningfully with your ability to work, study, engage in positive social interactions, or feel okay, having an individual assessment and counseling for stress reduction and relaxation may be helpful. In a supportive environment, clients learn new stress reduction techniques and create an individualized plan to manage stress.

What Are the Symptoms of Stress?

Everyone responds to stress in different ways. What might be stressful for one person may be another person's hobby. In a similar way, everyone reacts differently to stress. Common stress reactions include:

- Muscle tension or soreness in the back and shoulders
- Stomach troubles or digestive distress
- Difficulty falling asleep or waking early
- Increased heart rate or difficulty breathing
- Fatigue or exhaustion
- Lack of interest or boredom
- Engaging in destructive behaviors (e.g., drinking too much alcohol, overeating)
- Inability to concentrate
- Avoidance or fear of people, places, or tasks

In addition, stress can lead to more serious problems, such as depression, anxiety, hypertension, and other illnesses. These symptoms may also be caused by medical or psychological conditions other than stress.

Remember, chronic stress can have long-term effects on health and well-being, so if your symptoms are severe or prolonged, get outside support. If stress becomes too much to manage on your own, schedule a visit to see a qualified healthcare provider.

Questions to Ask Yourself About Your Stress

- What are the primary sources of stress in my life?
- What are the signs and symptoms in my body that let me know I'm stressed?
- What have I done that worked in the past to manage my stress?
- What can I do to integrate more relaxation into my daily routine?
- What do I want to do today to resolve my stress and work toward relaxation?

Effective Ways to Manage Your Stress

- Think about possible causes of your stress and be active in reducing stress. Small shifts in your thinking, behaviors, or breathing can make a very big difference.
- Avoid stress-producing situations. Although it is not always possible, many stressful situations can be avoided. Watch for places where you can avoid inviting stress; seek out places to relax.
- Engage in some regular exercise, which has been shown to alleviate the impact of stress. Choose an assortment of tension-building and tension-releasing exercises; remember that even small doses help! Take a quick walk, stretch in your office, even simple stretches help!
- Examine if the way that you are thinking about your life (e.g., perfectionist thinking) is adding to or decreasing your stress. Are there other ways to think about the situation that are less stress inducing? Are there positive thoughts you could integrate into your daily thinking?

(continues)

Exhibit 1-2 Stress Busters *(continued)*

- Engage in activities that you enjoy and that give you an outlet for thinking about other things besides your stress.
- Increase your social connections . . . find other people who can relate to your experience. Do stress-busting activities together! Talk about the stressor and your plan to resolve your stress!
- Take good care of your body . . . eat well, get enough sleep, and *avoid* alcohol and drugs, which can increase stress.
- Use self-relaxation techniques like deep breathing, muscle relaxation, and visualizing successes or relaxing places (provided later).
- Download soothing music or music that makes you smile, and listen to it when you are feeling stressed.
- Search for meditation podcasts that are specific to your needs (e.g., pregnancy meditation, reducing test-taking anxiety). Many podcasts are available online and free!
- Consider writing a list of your stresses, including ways to address those stresses. Sometimes even the act of writing the list can ease worry. Start checking items off your list!
- Find your own optimal stress relievers. Is it changing your thoughts? A physical activity? A social occasion? Look for the healthy ways that help you to feel less stressed and do them!

From the Expert!

In his research, Stanford professor and expert on stress Dr. Robert Sapolsky has identified four important components of reducing stress, which include:

1. Predictive information, such as a sign that the stress is going to be increasing (e.g., knowing a test date). That awareness gives us more control over our stress reactions.
2. Finding an outlet for dealing with stress (e.g., exercise, meditation, deep breathing).
3. Having a positive outlook or belief that life is going to get better, rather than get worse.
4. Having friends. Social support from others is an important component in keeping stress levels down.

Some Relaxation Techniques to Get You Started

- Try deep breathing exercises. Lie or sit in a comfortable position with your muscles relaxed, and take a few deep breaths. With your hand on your belly, feel your belly rise and fall as you inhale and exhale. Work toward breathing in to a slow count to five. 1 . . . 2 . . . 3 . . . 4 . . . 5 . . . Exhale slowly. Rely on this technique when you start to feel stressed.

- When your body feels tense, take 3 minutes to sit or lie down quietly and focus on calming all of the muscle groups in your body. Begin with the muscles in your feet and slowly work your way up your body. Relax your legs, back muscles, chest, arms, hands, cheeks, and forehead. You may wish to focus on areas that feel tense or where you are experiencing pain. Breathe air into those areas. Relaxing all of the major muscle groups will help your whole body feel at ease.

- If you are anticipating a stressful event, such as taking an exam or a difficult social interaction, take a few moments to visualize the event going well. See yourself experiencing success. Envision the details of what you might say or do that will result in positive outcomes. If negative thoughts or images occur, take a deep breath and refocus on the positive. Invite a successful outcome through visualization!

- After doing some breathing and muscle relaxation, or just taking time to rest, take a moment to calm your thoughts and visualize a peaceful place in your mind, either a place you have been or would like to go. Allow your body to relax more and your mind to calm. Take just 10 minutes! Recognize that you can go to that peaceful place in your mind and feel relief from life's stressors whenever you need a break!

Source: Exhibit courtesy of Shannon Casey-Cannon, PhD, Alliant International University.

Table 1-1 Study Guide Calendar

Day 1	Day 2	Day 3	Day 4	Day 5
Chapters 1, 2, & 3	Chapter 4	Continue Chapter 4	Chapter 5	Continue Chapter 5 Stress scale & reflection
Day 6 Chapter 6	**Day 7** Chapter 7	**Day 8** Continue Chapter 7	**Day 9** Chapter 8	**Day 10** Continue Chapter 8 Stress scale & reflection
Day 11 Chapter 9	**Day 12** Continue Chapter 9	**Day 13** Continue Chapter 9	**Day 14** Chapter 10	**Day 15** Continue Chapter 10 Stress scale & reflection
Day 16 Chapter 11	**Day 17** Chapter 12	**Day 18** Continue Chapter 12	**Day 19** Chapter 13	**Day 20** Chapter 14 Stress scale & reflection
Day 21 Chapter 15	**Day 22** Continue Chapter 15	**Day 23** Chapter 16	**Day 24** Continue Chapter 16	**Day 25** Chapter 17 Stress scale & reflection
Day 26 Chapter 18	**Day 27** Continue Chapter 18	**Day 28** Chapter 19	**Day 29** Continue Chapter 19	**Day 30** Chapter 20 Stress scale & reflection
Day 31 Continue Chapter 20	**Day 32** Chapter 21	**Day 33** Chapter 22	**Day 34** Chapter 23	**Day 35** Chapter 24 Stress scale & reflection
Day 36 Chapter 25	**Day 37** Take Exam 1	**Day 38** Exam 1 Review	**Day 39** Exam 1 Review	**Day 40** Take Exam 2 Stress scale & reflection
Day 41 Exam 2 Review	**Day 42** Exam 2 Review	**Day 43** Review areas of difficulty and Q&A	**Day 44** Continue review until confident with results and REST!	**Day 45** Downtime!

Learning as an Adult and Cognitive Factors in Learning

Fredrick D. Pociask, Rosanne DiZazzo-Miller, and Joseph M. Pellerito Jr.

INTRODUCTION

If you're reading this page, you probably have completed or will soon complete an occupational therapy curriculum and will soon embark on a rewarding and challenging career as an occupational therapist and healthcare provider. The transition between an academic and professional career is truly an exciting point in one's professional development, and for the typical graduate, emotions may range from exuberance and extreme personal satisfaction to uncertainty and anxiousness over a pending national board examination. It is the intent of this chapter and this book to help the reader hold on to the extreme personal satisfaction that comes with completing a challenging academic program and to help manage any uncertainty and anxiousness that is so often typical for a new graduate who is facing a board examination.

This chapter has two sections. Section 1 introduces principles and concepts of lifelong learning, which includes a discussion of learning as an adult, the key differences between entry-level and adult learners, what we know about successful learners, and key determinants of student success and failure. Section 2 introduces cognitive factors in learning and understanding, which include memory and retention, strengths and limitations of working long-term memory, the importance of monitoring comprehension, and helpful cognitive learning strategies. The information in this chapter is intentionally presented in sufficient detail and with supporting evidence because comprehension and adoption of productive learning behaviors are only fostered by understanding and perceived usefulness.

SECTION 1: LIFELONG LEARNING

It should be evident for individuals who are leaving the folds of an academic institution and embarking on lifelong careers as healthcare professionals that the transition from an academic to a professional career does not signify an end to formal learning. In contrast, graduation day simply signifies the official shift of ownership and responsibility for lifelong learning to the new graduate, a responsibility that will undoubtedly affect both professional opportunities and define professional reputations. The following paragraphs will discuss lifelong learning as an adult and discuss factors that can help account for student success.

Key Terms

Active learning	Learners take an active role in their own learning and are in part responsible for learning outcomes.
Attention	"Arousal and intention in the brain that influence an individual's learning processes. Without active, dynamic, and selective attending of environmental stimuli, it follows that meaning generation cannot occur" (Lee, Lim, & Grabowski, 2007, p. 112).
Human cognitive architecture	The manner in which structures and functions required for human cognitive processes are organized (Sweller, 2007, p. 370).
Knowledge generation	"Generation of understanding through developing relationships between and among ideas" (Lee, et al., 2007, p. 112).
Long-term memory	Component of the information-processing model of cognition that stores all knowledge and skills in hierarchical networks.
Meaning making	"The process of connecting new information with prior knowledge, affected by one's intention, motivation, and strategies employed" (Lee, et al., 2007, p. 112).
Memory	The mental faculty of retaining and recalling past experiences (Seel, 2007, p. 40).
Motivation	"The choice people make as to what experiences or goals they will approach or avoid and the degree of effort they will exert in that respect" (Crookes & Schmidt, 1991, p. 481).
Problem solving	"A process of understanding the discrepancy between current and goal states of a problem, generating and testing hypotheses for the causes of the problem, devising solutions to the problem, and executing the solution to satisfy the goal state of the problem" (Hung, Jonassen, & Liu, 2007, p. 486).
Self-concept	An individual's total picture of him- or herself (e.g., self-definition in societal roles, beliefs, feelings and values) that is typically focused on societal and personal norms.
Self-efficacy	An individual's belief that he or she can attain his or her goals or accomplish an identified task or tasks.
Self-regulation	Active participation in one's own learning process in terms of behavior, motivation, and metacognition in one's own learning process.
Sensory memory	A component of the information-processing model of cognition that describes the initial input of information (such as vision or hearing) (Lohr & Gall, 2007, p. 80).
Working memory (i.e., once referred to as short-term memory)	The structure that processes information coming from either the environment or long-term memory and that transfers learned information for storage in long-term memory (Sweller, 2007, p. 370).

Lifelong Learning as an Adult

Although there are numerous philosophies, theorists, theories, and models supporting adult learning, there is good consensus on the characteristics that make up the deliberative adult learner. Adult learning characteristics also comprise the emotional, psychological, and intellectual aspect of an individual and minimally include the following traits and behaviors (Knowles, Holton, & Swanson, 1998; Merriam & Caffarella, 1999; Snowman & Biehler, 2006):

- Experience: The adult learner utilizes prior knowledge and experience as a vehicle for future learning, readily incorporates new knowledge into similar prior learning, and appreciates the application of knowledge in the context of real-life problems.
- Self-concept: The adult learner moves away from self-concept based on dependency and toward a self-concept based on self-direction and personal independence.
- Communication: Adult learners become increasingly able to effectively express and exchange feelings, thoughts, opinions, and information through verbal and nonverbal modes of communication and varied forms of media.
- Orientation to learning: Adult learners increasingly move away from a subject-centered orientation toward knowledge that will be applied at some future point in time to a problem-specific application of knowledge in the context of real-world problems.
- Motivation to learn: Motivation toward learning shifts away from extrinsic incentives, such as course grades, and becomes increasingly directed toward intrinsic incentives, such as the completion of defined goals and tasks in the fulfillment of social and professional responsibilities.
- Responsibility: Adult learners are capable of reflective reasoning. They analyze knowledge, personal behaviors, and interactions on an ongoing basis; incorporate constructive feedback; and adapt knowledge, behaviors, and interactions to reflect ethical societal standards and values.
- Intrapersonal and interpersonal skills: Adult learners increasingly develop the ability to work independently and cooperatively with others and across varied circumstances and issues that affect the common well-being and one's own well-being in relationship to the world around them.
- Critical inquiry and reasoning: Adult learners increasingly develop the ability to examine and utilize reasoning and decision-making strategies to select, apply, and evaluate evidence in the context of real-world problems.

Although many characteristics of the model adult learner can be identified in adult learning philosophy and theory, we can certainly agree that seeking to achieve the previously described attributes would be a worthwhile endeavor. Now that we know important characteristics of an adult learner, let's make a simple comparison between college-level learning characteristics and adult learning characteristics, as depicted in **Table 2-1** (Knowles, et al., 1998; Merriam & Caffarella, 1999; Snowman & Biehler, 2006).

Now that we've identified key characteristics of the adult learner and compared them to typical college-level learning, it should be apparent that the attributes identified in the right column of Table 2-1 are well-aligned with lifelong professional development and achievement. Relative to the task at hand (i.e., successful completion of the NBCOT), and in terms of common obstacles to learning and achievement, some of the greatest barriers to learning arise from discrepancies between learner behavior and expectations and authentic real-world expectations and anticipated outcomes. In practical terms, holding on to entry-level or college-level behaviors and expectations while preparing for the NBCOT would be expected to hinder preparedness and potentially limit achievement and confidence. The following paragraphs will describe why adult learning behaviors are well aligned with learner achievement, so regardless of where you fall on the spectrum of entry-level to adult learning behaviors, it's officially time to jump aboard the adult learning bandwagon.

What We Know About Successful Self-Directed Learners

Over the years, much effort has been directed toward understanding the complexity of the learning process and to identify the determinants or attributes that account for student success and failure (Carroll, 1989; Flippo & Caverly, 2008; Morrison, Ross, & Kemp, 2006; Rachal, Daigle, & Rachal, 2007; Spector, Merrill, Merriënboer, & Driscoll, 2007). Although it is obvious that there are many fixed factors that we cannot change in preparation for an examination, such as intelligence quotient (IQ),

Table 2-1 Comparison of College-Level Learning and Learning as an Adult

	College-Level Learning	Learning as an Adult
Instructor	The instructor is the source of knowledge, decides what is important and what will be learned	If present, the instructor is a facilitator or resource, and learners evaluate needs based on real-world goals and problems and decide what is important to be learned
Learning	Passive learners and individual work Accept learning experience and knowledge at face value	Active learners, teamwork, and collaboration Validate learning experience and knowledge based on experiences and usefulness
Content	Homogeneous and stable content Content learned in the abstract	Diverse and dynamic content Content learned in context
Organization	Learning is organized by subject and content area	Learning is organized around personal experiences, context, and problem solving
Orientation	Acquiring entry-level competencies	Acquiring real-world problem-solving competencies
Utility	Developing subject matter attitudes, knowledge, and fundamental skill sets	Developing lifelong learning attitudes, expertise, and advanced skill sets

there are a number of adaptable factors or variables that will, in part, determine your successfulness on the NBCOT, as specifically introduced and discussed as follows (**Table 2-2**):

- Understanding of task requirements: Developing a thorough understanding of NBCOT task requirements should be one of your first objectives. For example, very important task considerations include what is the structure and complexity of the examination, how is the examination administered, when is the examination administered, how do you schedule the examination, what documentation needs to be completed by your university before you can schedule an examination date, when do you report on the day of the examination, can you find a testing center without getting lost, and what do you do if you need to reschedule. Additionally, a thorough understanding of task requirements will set your mind at ease and avoid any unnecessary panic attacks the day before the examination.

- Ability to comprehend and follow instructions: The ability to comprehend and follow instructions begins with the understanding of task requirements and continues throughout the examination preparation process. Because the brunt of the preparation for the NBCOT will be through self-directed learning and preparatory lectures and/or courses, it is important to keep a running list of items that need clarification, principles and concepts you do not fully understand, and even simple task requirements that are not clear. Whether the need for further comprehension is related to the quality of information or gaps in knowledge, you'll need to take deliberate action to seek help from resources such as your textbooks, journals, former professors, peers, clinical mentors, and/or the American Occupational Therapy Association (AOTA).

- Basic aptitudes and general abilities: Regardless of fixed factors, such as intelligence quotient, basic aptitudes and general abilities can have a big affect on student success. These factors can encompass very manageable aptitudes and abilities, such as basic computer skills, library skills, and project management skills, to more challenging factors, such as verbal ability. Chapter 3 will offer much advice in terms of study tips, skills, and strategies, but it will be up to the self-directed learner to identify any weaknesses in general abilities and tackle them early on in the examination preparation process.

- Time saved by prior learning: Time saved by prior learning can be a substantial determinant in terms of student success or failure. Regrettably, courses that foster the use of rote recall strategies and fail to ask the learner to recall or apply knowledge beyond the examination or course conclusion have left many learners at a disadvantage. In simple terms, forgetting and relearning can be cognitively taxing and will place additional constraints on available time and resources. This said, regardless of the degree of prior learning you are able to access when you begin preparing for the NBCOT, you'll need to use productive learning strategies to make sure the information gained on day one is still retained on day 45 (i.e., without forgetting and relearning).

- Time allocated to learning: The learner's decision to allocate suitable time to a given learning task is a very important consideration when preparing for the NBCOT. In very simple terms, the time needed should clearly match the time allowed, and sufficient flexibility should be maintained in project management to address additional and unforeseen demands placed on your available time. In terms of examination preparation, if you find that you are frustrated or anxious because you cannot complete scheduled learning objectives in the time that you allowed for a given task, you are simply telling yourself that you have not allowed adequate time for the task.

- Academically engaged time: All learners probably realize that there can be small-to-colossal gaps between time allocated to a learning task and the amount of time actually devoted to learning with understanding. This said, academically engaged time is the time spent fully attending to a given learning task to meet prespecified learning objectives. For example, if a learner has scheduled a 2-hour block of time to achieve a specific study objective and spends half of the time sorting and organizing materials to be learned, sending and receiving text messages, setting up a study playlist on the iPod, and allowing a friend to interrupt, academic engagement was, at best, 50%. From a more practical perception, remaining academically engaged during scheduled study periods would be expected to reduce undue frustration and anxiety levels, allow achievement of study objectives, and potentially open up free time to do activities that you enjoy.

- Environmental characteristics: Recommendations on how to control study environments will be discussed in Chapter 3; however, factors such as a distraction-free environment, location, time of day, and even temperature and lighting can affect study efficiency and effectiveness.

- Quality and organization of instruction: The clarity and adequacy of the instructional material to be learned can have a significant impact on student success. Because preparation for the NBCOT will be predominantly self-directed learning, it will be important to identify and organize quality instructional materials in the initial stages of preparation and to note any gaps that will need to be filled through supplemental resources. The use of this NBCOT preparation text in combination with your course materials, course texts, acquired literature, and the supplemental resources contained on the companion CD-ROM should be more than sufficient for the task at hand.

Now that we've introduced some very important determinants of student success or failure, let's take a step back and identify the determinants that are fully or predominantly under the direct control of the learner, those that are partially controlled by the learner, and those for which the learner will have no control in preparation for the NBCOT.

In reflection, and in context of NBCOT preparation, it should be apparent that attributes under direct learner control include (1) understanding of task requirements, (2) ability to comprehend and follow instructions, (3) basic aptitudes and general abilities, (4) time saved by prior learning, (5) time allocated to learning, and (6) academically engaged time. In fairness, (7) environmental characteristics and (8) quality and organization of instruction are under partial to full learner control, and none of the attributes are outside of direct or partial learner control. In the grand scheme of things, this is great news because as a self-directed adult learner you will have considerable direct control over some of the most important determinants that will contribute to your success on the NBCOT.

Common Obstacles to Learning

Now that we've discussed characteristics of the adult learner and determinants of learning that are readily modified to achieve successful outcomes, we can discuss common obstacles that can impede

Table 2-2 Attributes Under Direct Learner Control

Determinant of Success or Failure	Learner Control	Partial Learner Control	No Learner Control
1. Understanding of task requirements	☐	☐	☐
2. Ability to comprehend and follow instructions	☐	☐	☐
3. Basic aptitudes and general abilities	☐	☐	☐
4. Time saved by prior learning	☐	☐	☐
5. Time allocated to learning	☐	☐	☐
6. Academically engaged time	☐	☐	☐
7. Environmental characteristics	☐	☐	☐
8. Quality and organization of instruction	☐	☐	☐

learning and performance. It is our hope that knowledge of these obstacles in combination with sound reflective reasoning will help the reader to avoid many learning obstacle pitfalls.

- Attitude obstacles: Attitude obstacles include making excuses, procrastination, decision avoidance, avoiding seeking help, task avoidance, approach-avoidance conflict behavior (i.e., the fear of something a person desires), lack of commitment or excessive commitment, requiring unattainable perfection, and lack of positive feedback and reinforcement. Although some learners may overlook or underestimate the impact of attitude obstacles, we should take a momentary pause to acknowledge that attitude obstacles can have a significant impact on both learning and performance under many circumstances (Anderson, 2003; Elliot, 1999; Elliot & Covington, 2001; Ferrari, Johnson, & McCown, 1995; Levinger, 1957; Owens, 2001; Ryan, Pintrich, & Midgley, 2001; Steel, 2007).

- Academic self-handicapping: An excellent example of obstacle of attitude is cleverly coined "academic self-handicapping" and is described as "creating impediments to successful performance on tasks that the individual considers important" (Urdan & Midgley, 2001, p. 116). Academic self-handicapping (1) is a conscious decision to pursue a behavior or establish an excuse before or alongside anticipated achievement activity, not after, (2) occurs prior to important situations where the probability of success is uncertain or in doubt, and (3) occurs as a consequence of both specific actions and lack of action (Thomas & Gadbois, 2007; Urdan, 2004). Academic self-handicapping is noted in higher- and lower-level performing college students. Common examples of academic self-handicapping include procrastination, excuses, overinvolvement in nonacademic activities, and choosing socializing in place of examination preparation (Hall, 2000; Urdan, 2004). The psychology behind academic self-handicapping is complex, but the cognitive affective and motivational factors driving academic self-handicapping are most likely a manifestation of avoidance motives driven by a fear of failure or fear of feeling less capable in the eyes of others (Urdan & Midgley, 2001). Additionally, high-self-esteem learners may use self-handicapping to enhance success, and low-self-esteem learners may use self-handicapping to construct plausible explanations for failure (Tice, 1991). Regardless of your circumstances and motivation, academic self-handicapping and the NBCOT do not make a good combination.

  Let's take a ridiculously unscientific quiz to see if you may be an academic self-handicapper (see **Table 2-3**).

  Well, seeing as this is a ridiculously unscientific quiz, there are no passing or failing scores. However, if you found yourself answering yes to one or more questions without an authentic explanation, you may, in fact, be an academic self-handicapper. The good news is that because academic self-handicapping frequently occurs before an anticipated important event

Table 2-3 Academic Self-Handicapper Quiz

	Yes	No
I typically put off preparing for an examination until the last minute.	☐	☐
I typically put off completing homework until the last minute.	☐	☐
I allow my friends to distract me from paying attention in class.	☐	☐
I allow my friends to distract me from examination preparation.	☐	☐
When I do poorly on an exam it's typically because I didn't try.	☐	☐
When I do poorly on an exam it's typically because I'm involved in many activities and have numerous commitments.	☐	☐
I tend to procrastinate or I have been labeled as a procrastinator by those who know me best.	☐	☐
I've been known to socialize the night before an examination even though I am not fully prepared.	☐	☐
I know I could have gotten better grades in certain courses if I just spent the time studying.	☐	☐
I have difficulty performing well on exams because of lack of sleep.	☐	☐
I often tell my friends that I don't expect to do well on an examination for reasons such as illness and excessive commitment.	☐	☐
When I do poorly on an examination or homework assignment, I always have a good excuse for the poor performance.	☐	☐
I downplay examination and assignment performance because I feel like my friends and classmates will think of me as stupid if I do poorly.	☐	☐

(e.g., NBCOT), applicable individuals can seek to avoid these impediments to successful performance.

- Lack of professional skills obstacles: Unlike attitude obstacles, lack of professional skills obstacles does not reflect a conscious or counterproductive behavior; rather, it reflects general ability deficits, such as planning, goal setting, project management, technical skills (e.g., using a computer or conducting an online literature search), or writing skills. Lack of professional skills obstacles additionally includes soft skill sets, such as lack of professional networking and peer interactions and lack of professional contacts.
- External obstacles: External obstacles are usually unrelated to either attitudes or professional skill sets and may reflect highly personal, subjective, and multifactorial experiences. Examples of external obstacles can include the death of a loved one, chronic illness within a family, and financial hardships.

SECTION 2: COGNITIVE FACTORS IN LEARNING WITH UNDERSTANDING

Have you ever completed a challenging 2- or 3-hour lecture composed of predominantly new material and felt like all of the important details and concepts quickly blurred into nothing more than the gist or general picture of the lecture? Additionally, have you ever left a learning experience with a solid framework for the lecture material only to find that by the time you go to study you have forgotten most details and are forced to relearn what was forgotten? If you answered yes to either or both questions, the good news is that you're 100% normal, and although there is no bad news, the implications are that we must recognize these limitations of our cognitive architecture and actively seek to overcome them. The following pages will discuss factors that have considerable impact on learning with both understanding and retention.

Memory and Retention

The previously mentioned 3-hour lecture or forgetting-and-relearning scenario should sound familiar to most readers simply because human working memory is not capable of processing and effectively storing a 3-hour lecture in long-term memory, especially if the information is both novel and cognitively demanding (Sweller & Chandler, 1994). Although human working memory is certainly amazing because it is able to temporarily store and manipulate information related to higher-level cognitive behaviors, such as understanding and reasoning, it presents with an unexpected limitation in that it can only process a few elements of information at any given time (Baddeley, 1992a; Becker & Morris, 1999). Miller (1956) established that working memory can only manage about seven elements of information at a time. This notion or acknowledgment of the number of elements a learner's working memory capacity can effectively manage has endearingly developed into the phrase "the magical number seven, plus or minus two" (Miller, 1956). In practical terms, human working memory is surprisingly prone to errors as the learning task becomes more complex, and under typical circumstances it can hold on to information only for a matter of seconds without rehearsal (Anderson, Reder, & Lebiere, 1996; Baddeley, 1992a; Miller, 1956; Shiffrin & Nosofsky, 1994). This is why we tend to appreciate the "gist" or essence of a learning experience, such as the previously described 3-hour lecture, as opposed to remembering everything.

Let's take a little break to demonstrate capacity limitations of working memory. Please solve the following questions solely in your head or working memory and without the use of any external aids, such as pen and paper; the answers are explained later, so please don't read ahead.

- Question one: What is the four-digit number in which the first digit is one-third the second, the third is the sum of the first and second, and the last is three times the second?
- Question two (from Cooper, 1998): Determine if either of the following statements could be true.
  1. My father's brother's grandfather is my grandfather's brother's son.
  2. My father's brother's grandfather is my grandfather's brother's father.

For the typical individual, trying to solve either or both questions without the use of external memory aids, such as paper and pen, would have likely exceeded the processing capacity of working memory. To explain, in situations involving serial processing of four or five independent items, little or no overlap exists between information, and the demands placed on working memory are low. Additionally, understanding or recall of one piece of information will have little or no bearing on the understanding or recall of another information element, and the learning task will not typically become difficult unless the number of independent elements is very high. For example, remembering the carpal bones is relatively simple because there are only eight bones, and forgetting the name of one bone will have no impact on the ability to recall the others (i.e., serial processing). Remembering all the bones in the human body is similar in that the items are unrelated; however, the high number of bones will make the task a bit more difficult. In contrast, the preceding questions require that all information be maintained in working memory and manipulated simultaneously to properly solve the problems (i.e., parallel processing). Incidentally, the answer to question one is 1349; the answer to the first part of question two is false, and the answer to the second part of question two is true.

Understanding Sensory, Working, and Long-Term Memory

To manage complex cognitive tasks, individuals must be able to access large amounts of information. Long-term memory effectively stores all of our knowledge (content, skills, and strategies) on a permanent basis, with the ability to recall this information being somewhat more variable (Baddeley, 1992b; Ericsson & Kintsch, 1995). Furthermore, information may only be stored in long-term memory after first being processed by working memory; the activation of long-term memory can only occur by bringing the desired elements into working memory. It is additionally noted that knowledge elements that are activated with high regularity are activated automatically with little to no effort (Ericsson & Kintsch, 1995; Sweller & Chandler, 1994). **Figure 2-1**, which describes the relationships between sensory, working, and long-term memory, is depicted on the next page.

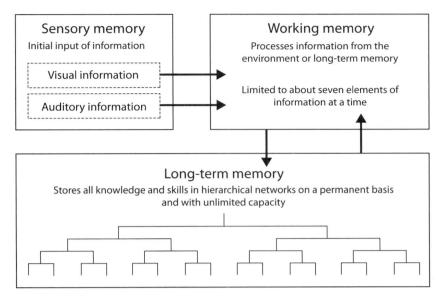

Figure 2-1 Memory Diagram.

Within the constraints of the strengths and limitations of human memory, learning requires a change in the schematic structures of long-term memory (Cooper & Sweller, 1987). Schemata are cognitive constructs that allow an individual to treat multiple elements of information as a single element in terms of imposed working memory demands. Schemata are additionally hierarchical in nature and are usually made up of many interrelated elements, which include both the cognitive representation of the problem and the problem solution. Given that a schema can be managed in working memory as a single element, increased working memory can be left open to address the problem state at hand. A second and equally essential aspect of schemata is the principle of automation. Automation allows for the processing of a schema in an automated fashion in further reducing imposed demands on working memory (Cooper & Sweller, 1987; Sweller, 1999).

For example, a skilled driver of an automobile will identify the many elements associated with the task of driving a car as a single schema in working memory, which, in addition to being automated, imposes few to no cognitive demands on working memory. In contrast, a novice medical student examining a patient for the first time may be presented with considerable information. Assuming a lack of an adequate schema, important information will likely be dropped from working memory, and few cognitive resources (if any) will likely be available to diagnose the patient's condition.

What Is Learning?

Defining or describing learning may seem straightforward at first glance (e.g., the accumulation of knowledge), but it is somewhat difficult without first coming to agreement on the functions and outcomes of learning. The process of learning is often associated with relatively short-term classroom or university experiences, and the products of learning are often described in terms of credit hours and grades. In contrast to this perception is the idea that learning is fundamental and essential to individual and professional development, which encompasses the need for individuals to actively accept responsibility for their own learning and actively strive to develop themselves through the course of their lifetime. Robert Mayer (1982, p. 1040) offers a definition for learning that is well aligned with an adult learning perspective, which states "Learning is a relatively permanent change in a person's knowledge or behavior due to experience." This definition has three components, which describe that (1) the duration of changes is long-term as opposed to short-term, (2) change entails the restructuring of the learner's cognitive architecture and/or the learner's behaviors, and (3) the catalyst for change is the learner's experience in the environment (Mayer, 1982). We will use Mayer's definition for learning because it matches quite well with our discussions on adult learning and memory.

What Is Metacognition?

In addition to being a very cool-sounding word that you can use to impress your friends and family, metacognition is a very important concept for the adult learner and will certainly have great bearing on successful NBCOT preparation. This said, metacognition simply means thinking about thinking and learning, or knowing how to learn (Winn, 2003). Metacognition consists of two separate processes that occur simultaneously: (1) monitoring progress as you learn and (2) making necessary changes and adapting learning strategies when needed to achieve optimal learning outcomes (Winn, W. & Snyder, D., 1996). **Figure 2-2** represents the minimal necessary skills needed to monitor comprehension of learning, which would additionally include factors such as motivation, attention, self-regulation, goal setting, and project management.

The development of metacognitive self-monitoring skills will play a critical role in the development of active and self-regulated learning behaviors, but it is highly unlikely that the skill set will develop if left to chance (Butler & Winne, 1995; Stone, 2000). It has been shown that novice learners do not evaluate content comprehension or work quality, fail to examine problems in depth, and fail to analyze effectiveness and correct errors as they learn (Ertmer & Newby, 1996).

In contrast, high metacognitive self-monitors are aware of when they need to check for errors, understand why they fail to comprehend, know how to redirect their efforts, and are more likely to use feedback from earlier testing experiences to further develop metacognitive skills and alter metacognitive self-judgments, as compared to novice learners (Ertmer & Newby, 1996; Lin-Agler, Moore, & Zabrucky, 2004).

What Do We Know in a Nutshell in Case You Forgot?

1. Information about the world enters working memory through sensory information (e.g., vision, hearing, touch).
2. There are monumental information processing and manipulation differences between the information entering working memory via the senses and information entering working memory via long-term memory.
3. Working memory is greatly limited in both capacity and duration, and these limitations can impede learning.

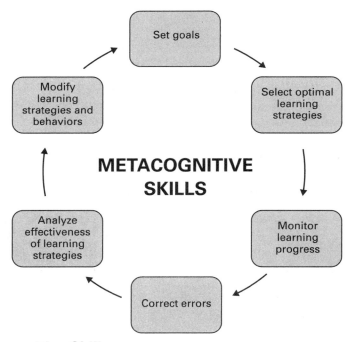

Figure 2-2 Metacognitive Skills.

4. If the capacity of working memory is exceeded while processing information, some or all of the information will be lost.

5. The efficiency of memory is strongly linked to how we direct our attention. Lack of attention devoted to academic tasks will be expected to decrease learning efficiency and effectiveness to some degree.

6. The robust nature of long-term memory is a function of schemata that allow an individual to treat multiple chunks of information as a single element in terms of imposed demands placed on working memory.

7. Continued review and repetition will reinforce neural connections to information stored in long-term memory.

8. Knowledge that is activated with high regularity is activated automatically with little to no effort.

9. Learning will be more efficient and effective if learning tasks are matched to the strengths and limitations of working and long-term memory.

What Does All of This Mean in Terms of NBCOT Preparation?

Learning Requires Comprehension. Recalling information that you do not understand is highly unlikely. Monitor comprehension by building reflection points into your examination preparation. If information is not getting through or not making sense, adjust comprehension or modify applicable conditional factors accordingly. Conditional factors, such as sleep, nutrition, attention, motivation, anxiety, strategy selection, and study environments, can greatly affect learning recall and retention.

Learning Requires Relationships, Organization, and Structure. It is very difficult to recall random knowledge as compared to knowledge that is organized with some structure or in some pattern. Avoid line item or bullet point, book page, and flash card learning for complex principles and concepts because they are not efficient or effective means for learning with understanding.

- Generate understanding by developing relationships between and among ideas.
- Actively associate or connect, and then add new information with, related prior knowledge to progressively construct robust schemata.
- Redefine new information in the context of practical real-world problems that can be solved using the knowledge being studied, or ask yourself how you will use the knowledge being studied in the clinic.
- Link new information to relevant personal experiences and/or historic events to enhance long-term memory storage and retention.

Learning Is Layered. Broad concepts can be remembered more easily than details, and if the broad concept is learned and anchored in memory first, details tend to readily fall into place. Conversely, it is much more difficult to learn and retain details if you do not understand how they fit into the big picture.

Learning Requires Review and Repetition. Avoid learning–forgetting–relearning pitfalls by using multiple learning strategies, such as concept maps and imagery (as covered in Chapter 3), combined with continued review and repetition to reinforce neural connections to information stored in long-term memory.

Learning Is Closely Linked to Metacognition Self-Monitoring. Take control over the cognitive processes engaged in learning by actively thinking about thinking and learning. Monitor retention by thinking about how you think and learn: (1) set goals, (2) select learning strategies that best match the content to be learned and learn how to redirect cognitive efforts, (3) correct errors while you learn and understand why you fail to comprehend when it occurs, (4) analyze the effectiveness of your learning strategies after you complete a learning task, and (5) modify your learning strategies and behaviors when needed, and make certain to use feedback from earlier academic experiences.

Learning Is Problem Solving. Learning is "a process of understanding the discrepancy between current and goal states of a problem, generating and testing hypotheses for the causes of the problem, devising solutions to the problem, and executing the solution to satisfy the goal state of the problem" (Hung, et al., 2007, p. 486).

REFERENCES

Anderson, C. J. (2003). The psychology of doing nothing: Forms of decision avoidance result. *Psychological Bulletin, 129*(1), 139–167.

Anderson, J. R., Reder, L. M., & Lebiere, C. (1996). Working memory: Activation limitations on retrieval. *Cognitive Psychology, 30*(3), 221-256.

Baddeley, A. (1992a). Working memory. *Science, 255*(5044), 556–559.

Baddeley, A. (1992b). Working memory: The interface between memory and cognition. *Journal of Cognitive Neuroscience, 4*(3), 281–288.

Becker, J. T., & Morris, R. G. (1999). Working memory(s). *Brain & Cognition, 41*(1), 1–8.

Butler, D. L., & Winne, P. H. (1995). Feedback and self-regulated learning: A theoretical synthesis. *Review of Educational Research, 65*(3), 245–281.

Carroll, J. B. (1989). The Carroll model: A 25-year retrospective and prospective view. *Educational Researcher, 18*(1), 26–31.

Cooper, G. (1998). *Research into cognitive load theory and instructional design at UNSW.* Retrieved July 30, 2009 from http://www.springerlink.com/content/vj4917q523256673/

Cooper, G., & Sweller, J. (1987). Effects of schema acquisition and rule automation on mathematical problem-solving transfer. *Journal of Educational Psychology, 79*(4), 347–362.

Crookes, G., & Schmidt, R. W. (1991). Motivation: Reopening the research agenda. *Language Learning 41,* 469–512.

Elliot, A. J. (1999). Approach and avoidance motivation and achievement goals. *Educational Psychologist, 34*(3), 169–189.

Elliot, A. J., & Covington, M. V. (2001). Approach and avoidance motivation. *Educational Psychology Review, 13*(2), 73–92.

Ericsson, K. A., & Kintsch, W. (1995). Long-term working memory. *Psychological Review, 102*(2), 211–245.

Ertmer, P. A., & Newby, T. J. (1996). The expert learner: Strategic, self-regulated, and reflective. *Instructional Science, 24,* 1–24.

Ferrari, J. R., Johnson, J., & McCown, W. G. (1995). *Procrastination and task avoidance: Theory, research, and treatment.* New York: Plenum Press.

Flippo, R. F., & Caverly, D. C. (2008). *Handbook of college reading and study strategy research* (2nd ed.). New York: Routledge.

Hall, T. R. (2000). *Self-handicapping: An evaluation and comparison of honors and traditional college students' utilization.* Retrieved February 24, 2009, from http://clearinghouse.missouriwestern.edu/manuscripts/151.php

Hung, W., Jonassen, D. H., & Liu, R. (2007). Problem-based learning. In J. M. Spector, M. D. Merrill, J. V. Merriënboer & M. P. Driscoll (Eds.), *Handbook of research on educational communications and technology* (3rd ed., pp. 485–505). New York: Taylor & Francis.

Knowles, M. S., Holton, E., & Swanson, R. A. (1998). *The adult learner: The definitive classic in adult education and human resource development* (5th ed.). Houston, TX: Gulf.

Lee, H. W., Lim, K. Y., & Grabowski, B. L. (2007). Generative learning: Principles and implications for making meaning. In J. M. Spector, M. D. Merrill, J. v. Merriënboer & M. P. Driscoll (Eds.), *Handbook of research on educational communications and technology* (3rd ed., pp. 111–124). New York: Taylor & Francis.

Levinger, G. (1957). Kurt Lewin's approach to conflict and its resolution: A review with some extensions. *The Journal of Conflict Resolution, 1*(4), 329–339.

Lin-Agler, L. M., Moore, D., & Zabrucky, K. M. (2004). Effects of personality on metacognitive self-assessments. *College Student Journal, 38*(3), 453.

Lohr, L. L., & Gall, J. E. (2007). Representation strategies. In J. M. Spector, M. D. Merrill, J.J. G. Van Merriënboer & M. P. Driscoll (Eds.), *Handbook of research on educational communications and technology* (3rd ed., pp. 85–96). New York: Taylor & Francis.

Mayer, R. E. (1982). Learning. In H. E. Mitzel, J. H. Best, W. Rabinowitz & A. E. R. Association (Eds.), *Encyclopedia of educational research* (5th ed., pp. 1040–1058). New York: Free Press.

Merriam, S. B., & Caffarella, R. S. (1999). *Learning in adulthood: A comprehensive guide* (2nd ed.). San Francisco: Jossey-Bass.

Miller, G. A. (1956). The magical number seven, plus or minus two: Some limits on our capacity for processing information. *Psychology Review, 63,* 81–97.

Morrison, G. R., Ross, S. M., & Kemp, J. E. (2006). *Designing effective instruction* (5th ed.). San Francisco, CA: Jossey-Bass.

Owens, R. G. (2001). So perfect it's positively harmful? Reflections on the adaptiveness and maladaptiveness of positive and negative perfectionism. *Educational Psychology Review, 13*(2), 157–175.

Rachal, K. C., Daigle, S., & Rachal, W. S. (2007). Learning problems reported by college students: Are they using learning strategies? *Journal of Instructional Psychology, 34*(4), 191–199.

Ryan, A. M., Pintrich, P. R., & Midgley, C. (2001). Avoiding seeking help in the classroom: Who and why? *Educational Psychology Review, 13*(2), 93–114.

Seel, N. M. (2007). Empirical perspectives on memory and motivation. In J. M. Spector, M. D. Merrill, J. van Merriënboer & M. P. Driscoll (Eds.), *Handbook of research on educational communications and technology* (3rd ed., pp. 39–54). New York: Taylor & Francis.

Shiffrin, R. M., & Nosofsky, R. M. (1994). Seven Plus or Minus Two: A Commentary on Capacity Limitations. *Psychological Review, 101*(2), 357–361.

Snowman, J., & Biehler, R. F. (2006). *Psychology applied to teaching* (11th ed.). Boston: Houghton Mifflin.

Spector, J. M., Merrill, M. D., Van Merriënboer, J. J. G. , & Driscoll, M. P. (Eds.). (2007). *Handbook of research on educational communications and technology* (3rd ed.). New York: Taylor & Francis.

Steel, P. (2007). The nature of procrastination: A meta-analytic and theoretical review of quintessential self-regulatory failure. *Psychological Bulletin, 133*(1), 65–94.

Stone, N. J. (2000). Exploring the relationship between calibration and self-regulated learning. *Educational Psychology Review, 12*(14), 437–475.

Sweller, J. (1999). *Instructional design in technical areas.* Camberwell, Australia: ACER Press.

Sweller, J. (2007). Human cognitive architecture. In J. M. Spector, M. D. Merrill, J. J. G. VanMerriënboer & M. P. Driscoll (Eds.), *Handbook of research on educational communications and technology* (3rd ed., pp. 369–381). New York: Taylor & Francis.

Sweller, J., & Chandler, P. (1994). Why some material is difficult to learn. *Cognition and Instruction, 12*(3), 185–233.

Thomas, C. R., & Gadbois, S. A. (2007). Academic self-handicapping: The role of self-concept clarity and students' learning strategies. *British Journal of Educational Psychology, 77*(1), 101–119.

Tice, D. M. (1991). Esteem protection or enhancement? Self-handicapping motives and attributions differ by trait self-esteem. *Journal of Personality and Social Psychology, 60*(5), 711–725.

Urdan, T. (2004). Predictors of academic self-handicapping and achievement: Examining achievement goals, classroom goal structures, and culture. *Journal of Educational Psychology, 96*(2), 251–264.

Urdan, T., & Midgley, C. (2001). Academic self-handicapping: What we know, what more there is to learn. *Educational Psychology Review, 13*(2), 115–139.

Winn, W. (2003). Cognitive perspectives in psychology. In D. H. Jonassen (Ed.), *Handbook of research for educational communications and technology* (pp. 112–142). New York: Lawrence Erlbaum Associates.

Winn, W., & Snyder, D. (1996). Cognitive perspectives in psychology. In D. H. Jonassen (Ed.), *Handbook of research for educational communications and technology.* (pp. 112–142). New York: Simon & Schuster Macmillan.

Study Tips, Skills, Methods, and Strategies

Fredrick D. Pociask, Joseph M. Pellerito Jr., and Rosanne DiZazzo-Miller

CHAPTER

3

INTRODUCTION

This chapter introduces important learning tips, skills, methods, and strategies, which include project and time management, collecting and organizing study resources, study environment management and study methods, and test-taking strategies. The chapter is organized in a logical fashion using easy-to-locate headings, and the individual sections contain brief introductions, easy-to-read bullet lists, and examples when necessary.

Keep an open mind as you explore this chapter because as learners we often know what we like and what we want but not necessarily what we need in terms of optimal learning outcomes. For this reason, try to stick with objective measures of performance when evaluating a given learning tip, method, or strategy, such as completion of study goals in a timely fashion and performance of NBCOT sample test items. It may be the case that the strategies and methods that are most helpful are the ones that require active engagement, motivation, and perseverance to adopt and stick with. Conversely, it will be wise to drop a particular tip, strategy, or method if it proves to be of little benefit when objectively scrutinized. The benefits of successful study habits include:

- Productive study habits typically result in improved self-confidence and improved self-concept.
- Productive study habits can readily translate to productive lifelong learning as an adult.
- Productive study habits typically result in learning with understanding and academic engagement, as opposed to rote recall and forgetting.
- Productive study habits can equate to a decrease in frustration and procrastination.
- Productive study habits allow for more free time spent doing things you enjoy.
- Productive study habits lend themselves to improved knowledge acquisition retention and may facilitate improved problem-solving skills.

STUDY TIPS

Maintain Focus, Endurance, and Motivation

- Focus on the endgame, which is successful completion of the NBCOT and beginning a career as a healthcare professional. Use imagery to clearly picture yourself achieving this goal.
- Focus on the task at hand instead of perseverating on the monumental task of preparing for the entire exam. This strategy is additionally true for individual tasks. For example, if you have 50 pages to study, go forward one page at a time, and you will be done before you know it.
- Maintain healthy dietary habits and a consistent eating schedule.

- Have a few healthy snacks and water available for study periods.
- Maintain normal and healthy sleep patterns and a consistent sleep schedule.
- Take short 10- to 15-minute breaks during long study sessions, or even consider a 15-minute power nap to help maintain concentration and focus.
- Maintain physical health and personal appearance.
- Manage stress and anxiety.
- Schedule time for relaxation and social interactions.
- Establish clear study goals.
- Avoid procrastination and stay on task while studying.
- Change topics every couple of hours to add some variety to your study plan.
- Create study incentives, such as calling a friend, watching a television show, or exercise. Additionally, give yourself small rewards upon completion of primary study tasks.

Maintain and Bolster Self-Confidence

- Establish and maintain a realistic exam preparation schedule. Successfully completing study tasks in a timely fashion is an excellent strategy for maintaining self-confidence.
- Use positive words or attributions to describe desired behaviors, such as "I can do this" as opposed to "I cannot do this."
- After you complete a given task, make sure to acknowledge the accomplishment before moving on to the next task.
- Avoid negative people, study groups, and study environments . . . period.

Actively Monitor Learning and Comprehension

- Schedule time to reflect on your learning progress and make certain to keep track of what works, what doesn't work, and what needs to be tweaked.
- Use self-questioning, self-testing, peer discussions, prior examinations and feedback, and NBCOT preparatory questions to objectively evaluate learning.
- Use a notepad or similar tool to keep track of self-generated or peer feedback, important terminology, or any helpful information that needs to be recorded for later use.

Facilitate Productive Collaborative Learning

Metacognitive strategies for group learning include collaborative goal setting and scheduling, selecting optimal learning strategies with emphasis on individual and group fairness, monitoring your progress, analyzing your effectiveness and efficiency, and modifying your learning strategies and behaviors as necessary. Attention given to the following will help facilitate optimal collaborative learning:

- Establish meeting schedules and ground rules while forming groups or at the beginning of the initial meeting. Everyone involved should agree that you are forming a study group and not a social club.
- Keep the group to a manageable size, and keep the number of groups that you participate in to a manageable size.
- Select group members that you can readily work with and that have a solid track record for preparedness and punctuality.
- Establish your unproductive study group exit strategy on day one. Clearly state that you will not be able to participate in the study group if the group does not stay on task or fails to complete established study objectives. Select a qualified group leader if individuals in the group have difficulty staying on task.
- Remember that primary reasons for forming the group are knowledge sharing, collaboration, and dissemination. Identify combined resources and a means for collection and dissemination early on.
- Preparing and disseminating assignments before meetings will likely be more productive in that meeting time and can be used to seek clarification, discuss, debate, and further anchor knowledge and long-term memory.

- Remember that collaborative learning does not necessarily mean face-to-face learning. Take advantage of academic course management sites, email, blogs, or even your Facebook page if it helps to achieve a collaborative learning goal.

Choose Study Companions and Study Groups Wisely

The study companions and groups that you collaborate with in preparation for the NBCOT will most likely affect your examination preparedness. If you associate with motivated, goal- and task-oriented, and overall well-rounded and positive colleagues, this will likely carry over into your self-confidence and preparedness. In contrast, if your collaborative learning experiences are plagued by more socializing and negative self-talk than examination preparation, it's time to break up and move on, but don't be sad because you can still be friends.

STUDY SKILLS

Project and Time Management

Project and time management will be very important factors in terms of NBCOT preparation and preparedness. The following project and time management factors will be grouped together for the purposes of this chapter and will be further discussed in subsequent sections:

- Goal setting
- Scheduling and planning time for studying, which includes the following:
  - Creating prioritized to-do lists
  - Establishing a study routine
  - Making use of free time
  - Scheduling regular reviews
  - Scheduling relaxation time
  - Identifying start and stop points or dates
- Collecting and organizing study resources

Goal Setting and Scheduling

- Establish straightforward long-term goals and time frames before writing short-term goals. These goals should identify major start and stop points or dates, such as the final date for collecting and organizing study materials, the date you will begin studying, and the date of the examination.
- Short-term goals will typically span no more than 1 to 4 weeks based on your organization style, they should be kept simple and concise, and they should reflect specific study objectives and specific completion dates. For example, "Construct a study aid for all peripheral nerve compression neuropathies by Friday, May 5."
- Break the exam preparation down into smaller and manageable tasks that can be readily accomplished in the time allotted.
- Reevaluate goals and time frames on a daily to weekly basis based on attainment of study objectives. Remember that the objective is learning with understanding and retention as opposed to poor learning outcomes and/or forgetting and relearning.
- Keep short-term goals and time frames challenging, but they should be realistic and consistent with the long-term goals and major start and stop points or dates.
- Take a few minutes to review and summarize your study objectives before beginning a study session or collaborative learning experience.
- Numerous short-term goals may be better managed by the use of daily and weekly prioritized to-do lists.
- Keep your short-term goals and to-do list in a highly visible location or multiple visible locations.
- Consider using a computer program or equivalent electronic resource specifically designed for project management, and make certain to back up frequently.
- Acknowledge the success of a given task because this will give you motivation to continue studying.

Collecting and Organizing Study Resources

Learners will predominantly have NBCOT study resources available as a function of completing an accredited OT program. The wild cards will likely be the organization and ease of access to previous curricular materials and identifying and filling gaps in available resources. If you have an organization scheme that has served you well, you can jump to the next section; otherwise, following these guidelines will be helpful in collecting and organizing study resources.

- Identify and physically locate existing curricular resources, with specific emphasis placed on textbooks, course notes, and key assigned readings.
- Course notes are ideally managed using three-ring binders organized by course name, content area, or study domain, and the side of each binder should be clearly labeled for quick access. Supplemental resources, such as photocopied journal articles and text chapters, can be organized in a similar fashion. If necessary, labeled tabs can be used to add additional levels of organization to existing course materials.
- Electronic resources (e.g., PDF) can be organized using folders and directories to match the organization of hard copy materials.
- Avoid the use of unsubstantiated and non-peer-reviewed references. For example, Wikipedia is not the ultimate source of all knowledge and is, in fact, riddled with errors and unsubstantiated facts. For an examination such as the NBCOT, you'll want to stick with resources such as instructor recommended texts, peer-reviewed journals (e.g., *American Journal of Occupational Therapy*), and similar MEDLINE-accessible references.
- Store all materials in a safe location and in an organized fashion as previously suggested. If applicable, make certain your friends, family, and children know that there'll be hell to pay if they even think about messing with your stuff. If at all possible, your safe storage location should be your preferred study environment as described later.
- Identify supplemental resources that are presently of unidentified value and place them in a nearby location to be used only if necessary.
- If your curriculum required the use of literature on the Web, create a single document or Web folder with all URLs clearly labeled and in one place.
- After you've completed the previous steps, additional management of study resources should be based on short-term objectives and study goals. For example, if you plan to spend next week studying anatomy, you should pull your anatomy text and course notes from compiled resources and return them when you are finished.
- In terms of project management, only seek supplemental resources based on identified gaps, and avoid the traps of constantly reorganizing, sorting, and resorting materials because this typically has little to do with studying and learning with understanding.

Important Considerations for Electronic Resources

If your institution uses an electronic learning management system (LMS), such as Blackboard or Moodle, make certain to download and save applicable course material because your access to campus learning management systems will typically expire upon or shortly after graduation. Additionally, programs such as Blackboard Backpack can be used to capture all courses and content in a few clicks of a button and with similar organization to actual Blackboard sites (provided that the course site is enabled). Lastly, because existing electronic resources, as well as those that you will generate in preparation for the examination, can be easily backed up, backups should be performed on a regular basis and stored at two different locations.

Study Environment Management

Remember that what you like and want may not necessarily be what you need in terms of study times, study locations, and environmental factors. Pay close attention to your completion of study objectives and tasks, or lack of successful completion, and match your environmental factors to what works.

- Select optimal study times: Identify your best time of day to study, and try to arrange work and play around optimal study time. Optimal study times should reflect when you are most alert and when you make your greatest achievements toward your daily learning objectives, not simply when you like to study.

- Select optimal study locations: Identify the best location to study, and if applicable arrange work and play around access to your optimal study environment. Optimal study locations may range from a quiet library to a local coffee shop. Additionally, determine if you prefer to use the same study location whenever you sit down to study (typically recommended) or if you prefer some variety in your study locations.
- Control environmental factors: The following factors will help facilitate an optimal study environment:
  ◦ Remove unnecessary distractions from the study environment, such as cell phones, audio-visual devices, friends, and family members. It's okay to tell mom and dad that you need peace and quiet so that you can pass the examination, get a job, and properly support them in their older years.
  ◦ Determine the ideal lighting for your study environment. Low to moderate levels of indirect natural light are considered best for reading, followed by equivalent levels of indirect full-spectrum incandescent lighting, with equivalent levels of full-spectrum fluorescent lighting typically following last on the list (Dunn, 1985; Hathaway, Hargreaves, Thompson, & Novitsky, 1992).
  ◦ Determine the ideal temperature for your study environment. Room temperatures between 68° and 72° Fahrenheit (20° to 22° Celsius) are said to be best for learning and comprehension. Higher and lower temperatures have been shown to result in decreased performance and increased error rates (Canter, 1976; Harner, 1974; Herrington, 1952; Manning & Olsen, 1965).
  ◦ Determine the ideal noise for your study environment, which may range from dead silence to quiet white noise or soft instrumental music.
  ◦ Other environmental factors include humidity, air flow, drafts, room color, work space ergonomics, clutter, odors, or any other environmental factor that proves to be an annoyance or detrimental to concentration.

Understand Content Areas and Performance Expectations

Table 3-1 was adapted from Morrison, Ross, and Kemp (2006), and it can be used to easily define content area and level of performance or to quickly give meaning to an existing examination or study question.

Table 3-1 Content Area and Level of Performance

Content	Performance	
	Recall Memorization for later recall or simple association	*Application* Application of information to an abstract or actual case
Fact A statement that associates one item with another	Simple associations between names, objects, symbols, locations, etc.	There is no such thing as application of a fact
Concept Concepts are categories we use for simplifying the world; a grouping of similar objects	What are the characteristics of . . .	Compare and contrast . . .
Principle or rule A principle or rule expresses a relationship between concepts, cause and effect, explanations and predictions	What happens when . . .	Explain why . . .

(continues)

Table 3-1 Content Area and Level of Performance *(continued)*

Content	Performance	
	Recall *Memorization for later recall or simple association*	*Application* *Application of information to an abstract or actual case*
Procedure A procedure is a sequence of steps one follows to achieve a goal	List the steps . . .	Demonstrate the steps . . .
Interpersonal This category describes verbal and nonverbal interaction between two or more people	List the steps . . .	Demonstrate how to . . .
Attitude Objectives that seek to change or modify a learner's attitude are classified in this category	State the behaviors . . .	Demonstrate the behaviors . . .

STUDY METHODS AND STRATEGIES

This section will present reading, recall, and learning comprehension methods and strategies with brief descriptions for use when applicable (Cooper, Tindall-Ford, Chandler, & Sweller, 2001; Flippo & Caverly, 2008; Gagné, 2005; Hung, Jonassen, & Liu, 2007; Leahy & Sweller, 2005; Lee, Lim, & Grabowski, 2007; Morrison, 2006; Reigeluth & Moore, 1999; Shepard & Jensen, 2002; Spector, Merrill, Merriënboer, & Driscoll, 2007; Tennyson & Dijkstra, 1997). As always, please try to match the method or strategy to the content to be learned and level of performance expectation. For example, prereading should be helpful for any new information or information that you did not grasp the first time it was read, an acronym or mnemonic would be a good memorization strategy for recalling carpal bones, and mental rehearsal or imagery would be a good match for learning complex concepts and abstractions.

Reading Comprehension Methods and Strategies

Prereading (Skim Before You Read)

1. Review the title and recall previous knowledge about the subject or content.
2. Review the subheadings and recognize the organizational structure of the content to be read.
3. Ask yourself what type of information is being presented.
4. Ask yourself what you expect to learn.

Read Critically

Critical reading reflects the ability to analyze, evaluate, and synthesize what one reads, which minimally includes identifying relationships in linking new information with prior knowledge. Some suggestions for critical reading are as follows:

- Begin with prereading.
- Highlight, underline, and take notes as needed.
- Generate a terminology list as needed.
- Identify the purpose and central claims.
- Identify the source and credibility of the publication.
- Identify the author and his or her credentials and qualifications.

Table 3-2 Primary Ideas and Important Points

of most importance	a key feature	the primary characteristic
above all	a central issue	especially relevant
the principal item	the chief complaint	the primary distinguishing factor
of particular value	always document	the most distinctive symptom

- Identify the context and intended audience.
- Distinguish the kinds of reasoning employed.
- Examine and evaluate the evidence.
- Identify strengths, weaknesses, and validity.
- Identify possible alternative conclusions.
- Write up notes immediately after reading.

Identify Emphasis Words

Pay close attention for words that signify primary ideas and important points as shown in **Table 3-2**.

Taking Notes from a Textbook

1. Begin with prereading as previously described.
2. Read the chapter or chapter section without taking notes and with the sole purpose of maintaining an understanding of the material.
3. Review the chapter or chapter section for a second time and locate the main ideas, emphasis words, and important points.
4. Paraphrase the information in your own words and without the use of the text. This step can be broken up into cognitively obtainable chunks, and the text can be used for review as long as you avoid copying directly from the text.
5. Now use the paraphrased ideas to generate the actual note pages, and again, do not copy any information directly from the textbook.

The SQ3R Method of Reading

The SQ3R method of reading is intended for individual study but can be applied to groups.

- **S**urvey: Scan the titles, headings, pictures, and chapter summaries before you read.
- **Q**uestion: Formulate questions before you read, such as, what are the key topics in this section or chapter?
- **R**ead: Read for comprehension by locating concepts and facts and by synthesizing and writing key information in the margins.
- **R**ecite: Verbally restate the main principles and concepts and summarize the reading in your own words.
- **R**eview: Actively review and reflect on the main principles and concepts, and then anticipate and write down probable exam questions.

The KWL Method of Reading

The KWL method of reading and tabled format presented in **Table 3-3** is intended as a learning exercise for study groups or classroom use and is composed of three stages: (1) what we **K**now, (2) what we **W**ant to know, and (3) what we **L**earned.

Comprehension Strategies

- Outline: Outlines are a quick and effective means to organize main and subsidiary ideas for any subject, which is well matched to both simple and complex relationships and hierarchies.

Table 3-3 KWL Method of Reading

what we **K**now	what we **W**ant to know	what we **L**earned

- Graphic organizer, mind map, and concept map: These tools are pictorial or graphic representations of concepts, knowledge, or ideas. Graphic organizers are similar to an outline and show the organization and structure of concepts, as well as the relationships between concepts.
- Question answering: Answer preinstructional questions from textbooks, mock examination questions, and questions posed during study groups, to name a few.
- Question generation: Formulate questions during prereading or during any applicable stage of learning.
- Summarization: Summarize text passages or applicable learning based on keywords, eliminate redundant and unnecessary information and information that does not satisfy study objectives, and always summarize in your own words.
- Mental imagery: Create a mental visual image of a procedure or concept.
- Teaching (if you truly know it, you should be able to teach it): Teach something you believe you know to yourself using active imagery, or teach it to a mentor or a colleague in a study group. It's a very quick litmus test for knowing if you've mastered applicable content, and it will facilitate background processing to fill in the blanks and further anchor content in long-term memory. This strategy is helpful with broad concepts and principles that are cognitively demanding.
- Case studies: Use case studies to integrate knowledge in the context of realistic or real-life scenarios.
- Cooperative learning: Use any of the preceding comprehension strategies and small groups.
- Combine comprehension strategies: Try to combine any or all of the preceding strategies individually or in small groups, with an emphasis on connecting principles and concepts, visualizing solutions to problem states, generating and answering questions, determining importance, and synthesis.

Memorization Methods and Strategies

Mnemonics

A mnemonic is a common memory aid used to facilitate retrieval in which each letter identifies or suggests what the learner wishes to remember. A mnemonic does not stand for a name, title, or phrase, and is typically recommended for up to 20 items. For example:

Cubital fossa contents from lateral to medial: "**R**eally **N**eed **B**rownies **T**o **B**e **A**t **M**y **N**icest."

- **R**adial **N**erve
- **B**iceps **T**endon
- **B**rachial **A**rtery
- **M**edian **N**erve

Acronyms

Acronyms are similar to mnemonics with the exception that acronyms stand for an actual name, title, or phrase. For example:

- **ADL**
  - **A**ctivities of
  - **D**aily
  - **L**iving

- **FOGS** (method for mental status assessment)
  - **F**amily story of memory loss
  - **O**rientation
  - **G**eneral information
  - **S**pelling

Flash Cards

Flash cards are perhaps the most classic rote-recall memory aid known to the healthcare science student. Flash cards are ideal for a serial recall task where the number of items is relatively high and the text density on each flash card is relatively low. Flash cards are worth mentioning in this section because they are frequently and erroneously used with complex principles and concepts, for which they are poorly suited.

Vocabulary List

Keep a hard copy or electronic medical dictionary close at hand. When you come across a term that you do not know or are uncertain about, look it up, and make certain that you understand the use of the term in the context in which it is was used. Lastly, add all referenced terms to a running terminology list to be used for quick access and ongoing study. A simple bulleted list maintained as an electronic document is recommended.

The Method of Loci

The method of loci (i.e., locations) is a classic memory aid, is typically recommended for lists up to 20 items, and is perhaps best suited for visual and kinesthetic learners. In this technique the learner vividly imagines him- or herself in a fixed position or walking a fixed path within a very familiar environment. For example, imagine walking into your study area and picturing the examination equipment that is required for cranial nerve examination evaluation laid out on your filing cabinet and desk.

Chaining

Chaining is a memory aid in which the learner creates a story in which each word that must be remembered acts as a cue for the next word or idea that needs to be recalled. For example, a learner trying to remember signs and symptoms that indicate the need for a neurological examination may create a story such as, "My weakness led to asymmetries, which then caused my gait to become altered and unsteady, and this definitely raised some concerns for safety, which were probably appropriate because I neglected to see the wall as I ran into it, but it didn't hurt because I do not have any feeling in that arm," and so on.

Tips and Strategies for Taking Multiple-Choice Examinations

Test-Taking Strategies

- Read all testing directions carefully before beginning the examination.
- Remember that there is no such thing as a really obvious correct answer on a well-written multiple-choice examination.
- Read the question completely and concisely and then try to answer the question without reviewing the responses.
- Read the question completely and concisely and then read all responses in a similar manner. If you believe that you identified the correct response along the way, make a quick mental note and then *read all responses completely and concisely one more time before recording your response.*
- Read the question completely and concisely and then treat each option as a true or false question. This strategy is particularly helpful when you must identify the best response among several correct choices (i.e., choose the most correct or most true).
- Eliminate responses that you know are incorrect before marking the correct answer.

- Pay very close attention to the wording of the question and identify conditional phrases, such as "all of the following are correct except," or "which of the following interventions is most appropriate."
- Do not add or delete information from a question or bend a response to match knowledge that you know.
- Do not use answer pattern strategies when taking a randomized, computer-based examination.
- If the opportunity presents itself, use information found in other test questions to answer difficult questions.
- Keep track of time throughout the examination without obsessing about the remaining time. Keep in mind you will have approximately one minute to answer each of the 170 multiple choice questions, with seventy minutes remaining to answer three sets of clinical simulation test questions.
- The best way to prepare for multiple-choice examinations is to practice taking multiple-choice examinations that best match the actual examination content, format, and testing environment.
- Do not guess unless absolutely necessary.

Changing an Answer to a Multiple-Choice Question

Please always remember that changing an answer to a multiple-choice question and guessing on the multiple-choice question are not the same. Additionally, advice that tells students never to change their first response on a multiple-choice examination under certain conditions is one of the most-noted testing myths or urban legends in higher education. Specifically, the majority of time an answer is changed, it is changed from the incorrect to the correct answer, and most students who change their answers improve their test scores (Bauer, Kopp, & Fischer, 2007; Fischer, Herrmann, & Kopp, 2005; Benjamin, Cavell, & Shallenberger, 1984). For example:

- Change an answer if you made a mistake or misread the question.
- Change an answer if you find information found in other test questions that indicates your first choice was incorrect.
- Change an answer if you had no objective basis for your initial response.

Tips for Guessing on Multiple-Choice Questions

- Guessing an answer is only of value when there is no penalty for guessing.
- The first rule of guessing is to rely on your knowledge before guessing.
- The second rule of guessing is to rely on your knowledge before guessing.
- Identify the wrong answers before attempting to guess the correct answer.
- A response that repeats keywords that are in the stem is likely to be correct.
- A positive answer is more likely to be correct as compared to a negative answer.
- In some circumstances, the longest and most complicated response is correct.
- If two answers are in direct opposition, one of them is likely to be the correct answer.
- If two answers convey similar or relatively identical information, choose neither.
- Answers that contain words such as "always" and "never" are usually incorrect.
- Answers that contain words such as "usually or typically" are more likely to be correct.

REFERENCES

Bauer, D., Kopp, V., & Fischer, M. R. (2007). Answer changing in multiple choice assessment change that answer when in doubt—and spread the word! *BMC Medical Education, 7*(28), 1–5.

Benjamin, L. T., Cavell, T. A., & Shallenberger, W. R. (1984). Staying with initial answers on objective tests: It is a myth? *Teaching of psychology, 11*(3), 133–141.

Canter, D. V. (1976). *Environmental interaction psychological approaches to our physical surroundings.* New York: International University Press.

Cooper, G., Tindall-Ford, S., Chandler, P., & Sweller, J. (2001). Learning by imagining [Special issue]. *Journal of Experimental Psychology, 7*(1), 68–82.

Dunn, R. (1985). Light up their fives: A review of research on the effects of lighting on children's achievement and behavior. *Reading Teacher, 38*(9), 836–869.

Fischer, M. R., Herrmann, S., & Kopp, V. (2005). Answering multiple-choice questions in high-stakes medical examinations. *Medical Education, 39,* 890–894.

Flippo, R. F., & Caverly, D. C. (2008). *Handbook of college reading and study strategy research* (2nd ed.). New York: Routledge.

Gagné, R. M. (2005). *Principles of instructional design* (5th ed.). Belmont, CA: Thomson/Wadsworth.

Harner, D. P. (1974). Effects of thermal environment on learning skills. *CEFP Journal, 29*(4), 25–30.

Hathaway, W. E., Hargreaves, J. A., Thompson, G. W., & Novitsky, D. (1992). *A study into the effects of light on children of elementary school-age—A case of daylight robbery.* Edmonton, Alberta, Canada: Alberta Department of Education, Edmonton. Planning and Information Services.

Herrington, L. P. (1952). Effects of thermal environment on human action. *American School and University, 24,* 367–376.

Hung, W., Jonassen, D. H., & Liu, R. (2007). Problem-based learning. In J. M. Spector, M. D. Merrill, J. v. Merriënboer & M. P. Driscoll (Eds.), *Handbook of research on educational communications and technology* (3rd ed.). New York: Taylor & Francis.

Leahy, W., & Sweller, J. (2005). Interactions among the imagination, expertise reversal and element interactivity effects. *Journal of Experimental Psychology, 11,* 266–276.

Lee, H. W., Lim, K. Y., & Grabowski, B. L. (2007). Generative learning: Principles and implications for making meaning. In J. M. Spector, M. D. Merrill, J. v. Merriënboer & M. P. Driscoll (Eds.), *Handbook of research on educational communications and technology* (3rd ed.). New York: Taylor & Francis.

Manning, W. R., & Olsen , L. R. (1965). Air conditioning: Keystone of optimal thermal environment. *American School Board Journal, 149*(2), 22–23.

Morrison, G. R., Ross, S. M., & Kemp, J. E. (2006). *Designing effective instruction* (5th ed.). New York: Wiley.

Reigeluth, C. M., & Moore, J. (1999). Cognitive education and the cognitive domain. In C. M. Reigeluth (Ed.), *Instructional-design theories and models: A new paradigm of instructional theory* (Vol. II). Hillsdale, NJ: Lawrence Erlbaum Associates.

Shepard, K., & Jensen, G. M. (2002). *Handbook of teaching for physical therapists* (2nd ed.). Boston: Butterworth-Heinemann.

Spector, J. M., Merrill, M. D., Merriënboer, J. Vv., & Driscoll, M. P. (Eds.). (2007). *Handbook of research on educational communications and technology* (3rd ed.). New York: Taylor & Francis.

Tennyson, R. D., & Dijkstra, S. (1997). *Instructional design: International perspectives.* Mahwah, NJ: Lawrence Erlbaum Associates.

Assessment of Occupational Functioning Physical Disabilities (Days 2–6)

Assessment of Sensation, Range of Motion, Strength, and Coordination

Rosanne DiZazzo-Miller, Susan Ann Talley, Fredrick D. Pociask, and Joseph M. Pellerito Jr.

OBJECTIVES

1. Using a variety of standardized and nonstandardized tests and measures, describe how to evaluate the following:
   a. Sensation
   b. Range of motion (ROM)
   c. Strength
   d. Coordination
2. Interpret and document results from the assessment of sensation, range of motion, strength, and coordination.
3. Identify precautions and contraindications associated with the assessment of sensation, range of motion, strength, and coordination.
4. Given a case study, select and sequence appropriate tests and measures to assess sensation, range of motion, strength, and coordination.

Table 4.1 Key Terms

Sensation	
Radomski & Latham, 2008, p. 213	*Pendleton & Schultz-Krohn, 2006, p. 513*
Aesthesiometer	Chemoreceptors
Hypersensitivity/hyperesthesia	Desensitization
Kinesthesia	Habituation
Monofilament	Mechanoreceptors
Paresthesia	Neuropathy
Proprioception	Nociceptors
Stereognosis	Proprioception
Vibrometer	Sensory threshold
	Stereognosis
	Thermoreceptors

(continues)

Table 4.1 Key Terms *(continued)*

Range of Motion	
Radomski & Latham, 2008, p. 92	*Pendleton & Schultz-Krohn, 2006, p. 437*
Active range of motion	Active range of motion
Anatomical position	End feel
Contracture	Functional range of motion
Limits of motion	Goniometer
Passive range of motion	Joint measurement
Reliability	Mechanoreceptors
Standard deviation	Palpation
Tenodesis	Passive range of motion
	Range of motion
Strength	
	Pendleton & Schultz-Krohn, 2006, p. 469
Calibrate	Against gravity
Maximum voluntary contraction	Gravity minimized
Mechanical advantage	Manual muscle test
	Muscle coordination
	Muscle endurance
	Muscle grades
	Resistance
	Screening tests
	Substitutions
Coordination	
	Pendleton & Schultz-Krohn, 2006, pp. 418–419
	Adiadochokinesis
	Ataxia
	Dysarthria
	Dysmetria
	Dyssynergia
	Incoordination
	Nystagmus
	Rate, rhythm, range, direction and force of movement
	Rebound phenomenon of Holmes

INTRODUCTION

Welcome to Days 2 and 3 of your study guide. This is your first content chapter, and we wish you well on your journey. This chapter will provide you with an in-depth review of how to assess sensation, range of motion, strength, and coordination. Utilize the outlines to gather pertinent information and complete the corresponding work sheets at the end of the chapter to reinforce your understanding of principles, concepts, and application of knowledge.

OUTLINE

1. Sensation

(Pendleton & Schultz-Krohn, 2006, pp. 513–531)
(Radomski & Latham, 2008, pp. 212–233)

a. Principles of sensation testing: Sensation assessment should give the occupational therapist a clear picture of which sensations are intact, which sensations are impaired, and which sensations are absent in a given client (Pendleton & Schultz-Krohn, 2006, p. 518; Radomski and Latham, 2008, p. 219).

b. Indications

    i. Spinal nerves: An injury to a spinal nerve can result in a motor or sensory impairment or a combination of both.

        I. Anatomical pathways: There are 31 pairs of spinal nerves: 8 cervical, 12 thoracic, 5 lumbar, 5 sacral, and 1 coccygeal. Each spinal nerve is made from a dorsal root (i.e., afferent or sensory) and a ventral root (i.e., efferent or motor) from the spinal cord.

        II. Dermatome distributions: A dermatome is the section of skin that is supplied by the sensory component of a spinal nerve.

        III. Complete the Dermatomal Distribution Learning Activity, now.

    ii. Peripheral nerve: An injury to a peripheral nerve may result in a motor or sensory impairment or a combination of both.

        I. Anatomical pathways: Spinal nerves combine to form peripheral nerves, which are outside of the brain and spinal cord. The brachial and lumbar plexuses regroup these sensory neurons into the peripheral nerves. Sensory information from peripheral nerves is sent to the brain primarily through the anterolateral spinothalamic tracts (pain, temperature, and crude touch) and the posterior/dorsal column-medial lemniscus pathway (conscious proprioception, discriminatory touch, and vibration).

        II. Peripheral nerve cutaneous distribution: Sensory distributions of peripheral nerves are different from dermatomes because peripheral nerves are comprised of more than one spinal nerve.

        III. Complete the Peripheral Nerve Learning Activity, now.

    iii. Central nerve injury

        I. Anatomical considerations

            a. Sensory cortex: Sensory information from the periphery is primarily sent to the sensory cortex for interpretation. The sensation is received and organized somatotopically. More sensory cortex is utilized to process sensory input from areas with greater sensitivity, such as the fingertips and lips. A homunculus is often used to illustrate the proportions of the sensory cortex utilized by various body areas (see Pendleton & Schultz-Krohn, 2006, p. 517, Figure 22-3; Radomski & Latham, 2008, p. 216, Figure 7-1).

            b. Sensory tracts: The primary tracts that transmit conscious sensation from the periphery to the brain are the anterolateral spinothalamic tracts (pain, temperature, crude touch) and the posterior column-medial lemniscus pathway (conscious proprioception, vibration, and discriminatory touch). These pathways cross at various levels in the central nervous system. It is important for the occupational therapist to understand the level of crossing for each sensory pathway.

        II. Peripheral distributions: Injuries to the central nervous system may result in wide variations in the distribution and types of sensory loss.

    c. Types of sensory impairment

        i. Anesthesia: A complete loss of sensation.

        ii. Paresthesia: A sensation that is typically described as pins and needles, tingling, or an electric shock.

        iii. Hypersensitivity: Increased sensitivity.

        iv. Hyperalgesia: Increased pain sensation.

        v. Allodynia: A painful response to a nontissue damaging stimulus that would not be expected to evoke pain.

        vi. Diminished or inaccurate sensation: Sensation may be present but is not consistent or may be misinterpreted.

    d. Levels of sensory awareness

        i. Detection: The ability to be aware of a sensation.

        ii. Discrimination: The ability to distinguish between two or more different sensations (e.g., the ability to discriminate between sharp and dull or one and two points with vision occluded).

        iii. Quantification: The ability to perceive different intensities of sensory stimuli.

        iv. Recognition: The ability to meaningfully interpret a combination of sensations (e.g., stereognosis, which is the ability to identify an object placed in the hand with vision occluded).

    e. General procedures

        i. An excellent open source resource for sensory testing can be found at http://healthcaresciencesocw.wayne.edu/sensory/start.htm.

        ii. Be sure that the procedure used to test sensation is reliable and valid.

            I. Assure that the client understands the procedure before beginning the actual testing.

                a. Explain and demonstrate the procedure for the client with his or her eyes open and on an area of skin that has intact sensation.

                    i. Use standardized instructions.

                b. Have the client respond to the test procedures with his or her eyes open to confirm understanding.

                c. Responses may need to be varied depending upon the client's communication skills or limitations.

            II. Assure that there are no extraneous cues that the client may use to respond to the testing.

                a. Hand placement by the OT should be limited to the lateral borders of the body segment(s) to limit pressure cues.

                b. Do not let clothes, bedding, or other similar objects touch the body segment being tested.

                c. Avoid predictable patterns when testing—in terms of timing, spacing, and expected response.

            III. Minimize distractions in the environment.

            IV. Apply the stimulus in a consistent manner.

            V. All testing is done with vision occluded (e.g., eyes closed or blindfolded or by placing an object, such as a clipboard, between the patient's eyes and the area being tested).

    f. Exteroceptive senses (touch, pain, temperature)

        i. Touch: Touch can be measured in a variety of ways and at a variety of levels of discrimination. Touch sensation is important for fine motor function of the hands and for safety.

            I. Light touch: The ability to sense light touch on the skin.

                a. Equipment: Cotton ball

                b. Use a cotton ball to lightly touch the skin. Ask the patient to indicate when he or she feels the cotton ball touch the skin, such as by saying "now."

                c. Document the accuracy of the responses (e.g., percent correct). Conclude if light touch is intact, impaired, or absent.

    II. Touch–Pressure
- **a.** Equipment: Semmes-Weinstein Monofilaments (a series of nylon filaments of various thicknesses used to determine the minimal threshold for touch pressure)
- **b.** The OT determines through the testing procedure the thinnest filament at which the patient can reliably determine that he or she is being touched.
- **c.** Document the smallest size monofilament the patient can perceive at various sites. Compare to normative data.

    III. Touch localization: The ability to accurately identify the location of light touch. Highly correlated with 2-point discrimination.
- **a.** Equipment: Cotton ball; thinnest Semmes-Weinstein Monofilament the patient can perceive; a very fine tipped gel pen
- **b.** Lightly touch an area and ask the patient to point to the area that was touched.
- **c.** Document the accuracy of the responses (the distance between where the patient was touched and where he or she indicates the touch was felt).

    IV. Two-point discrimination: The minimum distance between two points where the two points can be accurately perceived by the patient.
- **a.** Equipment: Boley gauge or Disk-Criminator
- **b.** Ask the patient to identify whether he or she is being touched with one point or two points. The OT determines the minimum distance between two points that the patient can accurately perceive as two points.
- **c.** Document the minimum distance for accurate perception of two points at specific areas of the skin. Compare results to normative data.

ii. Pain (sharp–dull discrimination): Pain perception is important for protection and safety.

    I. Equipment: Safety pin (sterilized between uses) or a tongue depressor broken diagonally along its length to produce sharp edges

    II. Randomly touch the patient with the sharp or dull sides of the pin or tongue depressor.

    III. Document the accuracy of the responses (e.g., percent correct). Conclude if pain is intact, impaired, absent, or if hyperalgesia is present.

iii. Temperature (hot–cold discrimination): The ability to perceive hot and cold is important for safety, both in the environment and for the use of thermal modalities as an intervention.

    I. Equipment: Test tubes of equal sizes with cold and warm water (the difference in temperature must be significant enough to be perceived)

    II. Randomly touch the patient with the two test tubes and ask the patient to identify the stimulus as hot or cold.

    III. Document the accuracy of the responses (e.g., percent correct). Conclude if temperature sensation is intact, impaired, or absent.

g. Proprioceptive senses

i. Joint position sense (proprioception): The ability to perceive the position of a joint in space.

    I. Equipment: None

    II. Position a joint of one limb and ask the patient to imitate the position with the opposite limb.

    III. Document the accuracy of the responses. Conclude if proprioception is intact, impaired, or absent at each joint.

ii. Joint movement sense (kinesthesia): The ability to perceive the movement of a joint in space.

    I. Equipment: None

    II. Isolate movement to one joint. Ask the patient to identify the direction of movement of the joint. Use terms such as "up," "down," "in," and "out." Alternatively, for the upper limbs, move one upper limb through space and ask the patient to simultaneously mirror the movement with the opposite limb.

   III. Document the accuracy of the responses. Conclude if kinesthesia is intact, impaired, or absent at each joint.

   iii. Vibration

   I. Equipment: Tuning fork

   II. The OT strikes the tuning fork to begin the vibration and places the end of the tuning fork on a bony prominence. The patient is asked to indicate when he or she feels the vibration. The OT manually stops the tuning fork vibration and asks the patient to indicate when he or she feels the vibration stop. Common bony prominences include the mastoid, acromion, and the olecranon processes, styloid process of the radius, and the patella and the lateral malleolus.

   III. Document the accuracy of the responses. Conclude whether the perception of vibration is intact, impaired, or absent at each bony prominence tested.

h. Discriminatory sensations

   i. Stereognosis: The ability to identify an object in the hand with vision occluded.

   I. Equipment: A set of common objects or a set of geometric shapes

   II. The OT places each object in the patient's hand and asks the patient to identify the object either by naming it or pointing to a similar object (e.g., a picture of the object).

   III. Document the accuracy of the responses (e.g., percent correct). Conclude whether stereognosis is intact, impaired, or absent (astereognosis).

   ii. Graphesthesia: The ability to identify a number or letter drawn on the palm of the hand with vision occluded.

   I. Equipment: Pencil with an eraser

   II. Using the eraser end of a pencil, draw letters or numbers on the palm of the patient's hand with his or her vision occluded. Orient the bottom of the letter proximally. Ask the patient to identify the letter or number.

   III. Document the accuracy of the responses (e.g., percent correct). Conclude whether graphesthesia is intact, impaired, or absent (agraphesthesia).

i. Role of sensation in functional activities

   i. Safety: Protective sensations, such as touch, pressure, pain, and temperature, are necessary to ensure safety during performance of occupation (e.g., ADL, IADL). Impaired pain and temperature sensation may contraindicate the use of thermal modalities.

   ii. Sensory feedback for movement: Touch, pressure, and the discriminatory sensations, including proprioception and two-point discrimination, are necessary for unimpaired performance of functional activities.

   iii. Interaction with environment: Somatosensation, in addition to vision, hearing, and vestibular input, enhance an individual's ability to perceive and interact within the context of the environment. Impairment or absence of one or more sensory modalities may require the individual to learn compensatory activities.

2. Range of motion (ROM)

(Pendleton & Schultz-Krohn, 2006, pp. 437–445)
(Radomski & Latham, 2008, pp. 92–123)

a. Principles of ROM

   i. Before beginning an ROM assessment, it is important to be familiar with average ROM measurements, joint end feel, palpation sites, testing procedures, and correct limb positioning. It is important to note that there are various ways to assess ROM. Keeping this in mind, the OT must remember that although there are different methods of assessment, it is important to always test and retest using the same methods to maintain intratester reliability and validity of the examination procedure.

The validity of a measurement refers to how well the measurement represents the true value of the variable of interest. Reliability simply means the consistency or the repeatability of the measurements or whether the application of the instrument and the procedures will produce the same measurements consistently under the same conditions (i.e., intratester reliability—same examiner; intertester reliability—different examiners).

b. Indications for ROM testing

    i. It is appropriate to follow up a functional ROM screen with full goniometric assessment procedures when it is clear that limitations interfere with occupational functioning.

c. Precautions and contraindications

    i. Identifying precautions and contraindications is the most important area to review prior to any assessment. Contraindications will require the OT to exclude one or more joints from the ROM assessment. Precautions require the OT to use professional judgment about how to proceed.

d. Shoulder

    i. Flexion
    ii. Extension
    iii. Abduction
    iv. Adduction
    v. External rotation
    vi. Internal rotation
    vii. Horizontal abduction
    viii. Horizontal adduction

e. Elbow

    i. Flexion
    ii. Extension

f. Forearm

    i. Pronation
    ii. Supination

g. Wrist

    i. Flexion
    ii. Extension
    iii. Radial deviation
    iv. Ulnar deviation

h. Hand

    i. MCP, PIP, DIP flexion
    ii. MCP, PIP, DIP extension
    iii. MCP abduction
    iv. MCP adduction
    v. Thumb
        I. Flexion
        II. Extension
        III. Opposition
        IV. Abduction
        VI. Adduction

i. Hip

    i. Flexion
    ii. Extension
    iii. Abduction
    iv. Adduction
    v. External rotation
    vi. Internal rotation

   j. Knee
      i. Flexion
      ii. Extension
   k. Foot and ankle
      i. Dorsiflexion
      ii. Plantarflexion
      iii. Inversion
      iv. Eversion

3. Strength

(Pendleton & Schultz-Krohn, 2006, pp. 471–512)
(Radomski & Latham, 2008, pp. 125–172)

   a. Principles of strength testing
      i. Performing a screening test of strength develops a framework for more specific muscle strength testing using a manual muscle test (MMT).
      ii. The OT attempts to isolate muscles or a specific movement during strength testing.
         I. A client with weakness will attempt to substitute other muscles or movements when attempting the weaker movement.
         II. The OT should assure proper alignment and stabilization of body parts to minimize substitution.
         III. The OT should give specific, standardized instructions to ensure understanding by the client of the movement to be performed.
         IV. Palpate the muscle being tested to assure that it is contracting during the movement.
      iii. Positioning of the client and the body part is essential for accurate interpretation of the results.
         I. The OT should plan ahead to minimize position changes during the testing process.
         II. If a client cannot assume the standardized position, the OT will need to problem solve alternative positioning and use clinical judgment when assigning a grade to a muscle strength test. Any deviations from standard procedures should be documented in the client's record.
   b. The impact of gravity on a movement must be understood in each position on each tested movement. The two standard considerations are movements *against gravity (i.e., antigravity),* where gravity resists the movement, and movements with *gravity minimized (i.e., gravity eliminated),* where the movement is not directly resisted by gravity. Complete Manual Muscle Testing Exercise 1, now (see **Table 4-2**).
   c. Indications of strength testing
      i. Assessment of the strength of individual muscles or movements is necessary when muscle weakness is suspected in a client.
      ii. The etiology of muscle weakness can be quite varied, including, but not limited to, the following:
         I. Peripheral nerve, spinal nerve, and spinal cord injury or disease
         II. Primary muscle disease; injury
         III. Disease of upper motor neurons
         IV. Disuse, immobilization, or deconditioning
      iii. The results of a strength assessment are important to:
         I. Establish a baseline strength assessment to evaluate progress
         II. Establish a baseline strength assessment to develop an intervention program
         III. Evaluate the impact of muscle weakness on occupational performance
         IV. Identify potential risks for injury, deformity
         V. Identify the need for assistive devices
   d. Precautions and contraindications
      i. Identifying precautions and contraindications is the most important area to review prior to any assessment. Contraindications will require the OT to exclude one or

more joints from the ROM assessment. Precautions require the OT to use professional judgment about how to proceed.

    ii. An MMT is contraindicated when inflammation or pain prevents performance of the movement(s) required.

    iii. An MMT is contraindicated when there is a dislocation or unhealed fracture that will be stressed by the required movement(s).

    iv. An MMT is contraindicated if the client has a disorder that has weakened the strength of the underlying bones or joints.

    v. Precautions need to be taken when an MMT may aggravate a current condition (e.g., a subluxation of a joint, abdominal surgery, cardiovascular–pulmonary conditions, etc.).

e. Manual muscle test grading scale

    i. The typical scales used to grade an MMT of a given muscle derive the grade based on one or more of the following:

        I. The maximum contraction a client can generate in the muscle being tested

            a. Variables include gravity minimized, against gravity alone, and against manual resistance

        II. The range of motion through which a client can move a joint using the muscle being tested

        III. Clinical judgment and experience of the tester

    ii. Muscle strength, as measured by an MMT, is often graded on a 6-point scale.

        I. 0, 1, 2, 3, 4, 5

        II. 0, Trace, Poor, Fair, Good, Normal (0, T, P, F, G, N)

        III. Additional grades of (+) and (−) are used to describe strength that is between the primary grades.

    iii. The definitions of each primary grade vary. Consult your text for definitions of the (+) and (−) grades.

    iv. Study muscle grading scales and complete Manual Muscle Testing Exercise 2 (see **Table 4-3**).

f. Procedures for MMT

    i. Basic considerations for testing each movement or muscle include the following:

        I. Position the patient for the appropriate movement and gravity minimized or against gravity. To minimize position changes, often the easiest way to begin is to test all possible movements against gravity in sitting, progress to supine, side lying on one side, prone, side lying on the other side. Add movements with gravity minimized as needed.

            a. If a movement can be performed against gravity, there is no reason to test it with gravity minimized.

        II. Instruct the client on how to do the movement you want to test.

        III. Stabilize the client to minimize substitutions.

        IV. Observe the movement and palpate the muscles being tested to assure valid testing.

        V. Add resistance as appropriate. Hand placement should be precise for each test.

        VI. Retest if the client uses substitutions, deviates from the testing position, or stabilization is inadequate.

    ii. For each of the following movements, understand the positions for against gravity and gravity minimized testing, proper stabilization, muscles to palpate, and hand placements to provide resistance.

        I. Neck MMT

            a. Flexion

            b. Extension

            c. Lateral flexion right and left

II. Scapular MMT
   a. Abduction
   b. Adduction
   c. Elevation
   d. Depression
III. Shoulder MMT
   a. Flexion
   b. Extension
   c. Abduction
   d. Adduction
   e. External rotation
   f. Internal rotation
   g. Horizontal abduction
   h. Horizontal adduction
IV. Elbow MMT
   a. Flexion
   b. Extension
V.   Forearm MMT
   a. Pronation
   b. Supination
VI. Wrist MMT
   a. Flexion
   b. Extension
   c. Radial deviation
   d. Ulnar deviation
VII. Hand MMT
   a. MCP, PIP, DIP flexion
   b. MCP, PIP, DIP extension
   c. MCP abduction
   d. MCP adduction
   e. Thumb
      i.   Flexion
      ii. Extension
      iii. Opposition
      iv. Abduction
      v.   Adduction
VIII. Hip
   a. Flexion
   b. Extension
   c. Abduction
   d. Adduction
   e. Internal rotation
   f. External rotation
IX. Knee
   a. Flexion
   b. Extension
X.   Foot and ankle
   a. Dorsiflexion
   b. Plantarflexion
   c. Inversion
   d. Eversion

4. Coordination

(Pendleton & Schultz-Krohn, 2006, pp. 421, 994)
(Radomski & Latham, 2008, p. 1140)

   a. Principles of coordination: It is important to note that in terms of coordination and hand function, the OT will use a variety of tests to provide a complete analysis.

   b. Indications: It is appropriate for the OT to assess coordination when the client is unable to accurately control movement. Examples of uncoordinated movement include errors in timing, sequencing, direction, accuracy, speed, force, and smoothness.

   c. Signs of uncoordinated movement
     i. Ataxia
     ii. Dysdiadochokinesis
     iii. Dysmetria
     iv. Dyssynergia
     v. Dysarthria
     vi. Tremor (e.g., intention or nonintention)
     vii. Athetosis
     viii. Ballistic movements
     ix. Dystonia

   d. Dexterity and hand function tests: There are a variety of standardized fine and gross motor dexterity tests available to the OT that are valid and reliable. It is, however, more telling to engage the client in a functional activity that is both meaningful and purposeful, in which case the OT can use observation skills to assess the client and apply his or her challenges directly to the client's life tasks.
     i. 9-Hole Peg
     ii. Box and Block
     iii. Purdue Pegboard
     iv. Minnesota Rate of Manipulation
     v. Jebsen Test of Hand Function
     vi. TEMPA

WORK SHEETS

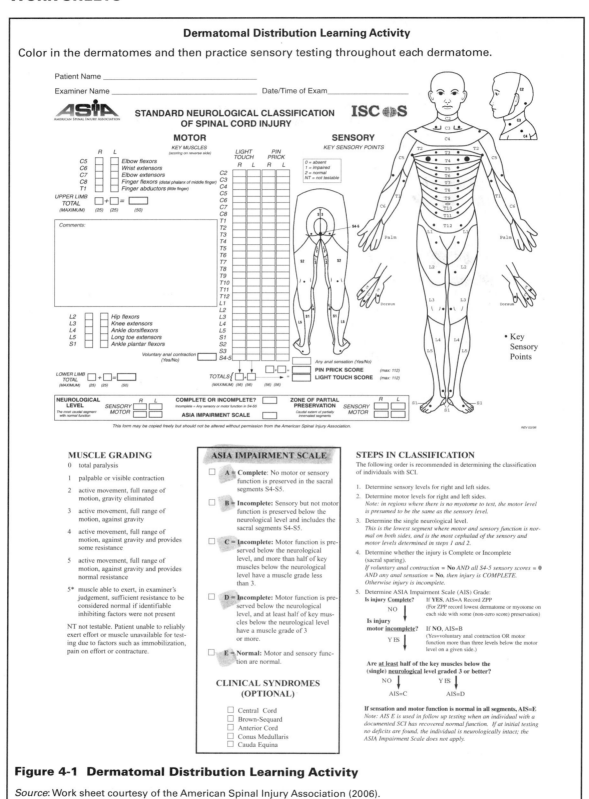

Figure 4-1 Dermatomal Distribution Learning Activity

Source: Work sheet courtesy of the American Spinal Injury Association (2006).

Peripheral Nerve Learning Activity

Color in the following peripheral nerve distributions and then practice completing all peripheral nerve testing for each nerve distribution.

Upper Extremities

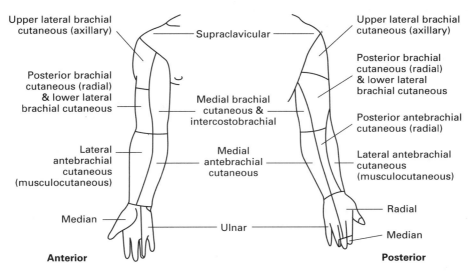

Figure 4-2 Upper Extremities.

Source: Figure courtesy of The Merck Manual of Diagnosis and Therapy, Edition 18, p. 1754, edited by Mark H. Beers. Copyright 2006 by Merck & Co., Inc., Whitehouse Station, NJ. Available at http://www.merck.com/mmpe. Accessed (February 26, 2009). Please visit all of the Merck Manuals free online at www.MerckManuals.com

Lower Extremities

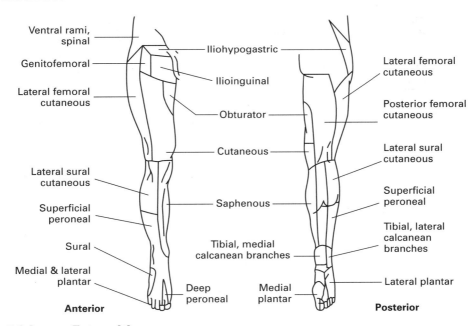

Figure 4-3 Lower Extremities.

Source: Figure reprinted with permission from The Merck Manual of Diagnosis and Therapy, Edition 18, p. 1754, edited by Mark H. Beers. Copyright 2006 by Merck & Co., Inc., Whitehouse Station, NJ. Available at http://www.merck.com/mmpe. Accessed (February 26, 2009). Please visit all of the Merck Manuals free online at www.MerckManuals.com

Manual Muscle Testing Exercise 1

Complete the following table, indicating which muscles or movements are performed *against gravity* and which are performed with *gravity minimized* in each position.

Table 4-2 Manual Muscle Testing Exercise 1

Position	Joint	Movement(s) *Against Gravity*	Movement(s) with *Gravity Minimized*
Sitting	Neck		
	Scapula		
	Shoulder		
	Elbow		
	Wrist		
	Hand		
	Hip		
	Knee		
	Ankle		
	Foot		
Position	**Joint**	**Movement(s) *Against Gravity***	**Movement(s) with *Gravity Minimized***
Supine	Neck		
	Scapula		
	Shoulder		
	Elbow		
	Wrist		
	Hand		
	Hip		
	Knee		
	Ankle		
	Foot		
Position	**Joint**	**Movement(s) *Against Gravity***	**Movement(s) with *Gravity Minimized***
Prone	Neck		
	Scapula		
	Shoulder		
	Elbow		
	Wrist		
	Hand		
	Hip		
	Knee		
	Ankle		
	Foot		
Position	**Joint**	**Movement(s) *Against Gravity***	**Movement(s) with *Gravity Minimized***
Side lying	Neck		
	Scapula		
	Shoulder		
	Elbow		
	Wrist		
	Hand		
	Hip		
	Knee		
	Ankle		
	Foot		

Manual Muscle Testing Exercise 2

(Pendleton & Schultz-Krohn, 2006, p. 475; Radomski & Latham, 2008, p. 127)

Fill in and memorize the following table.

Table 4-3 Manual Muscle Testing Exercise 2

Muscle Grade	Word/Letter Grade	Definition
0		
1		
2−		
2		
2+		
3−		
3		
3+		
4−		
4		
4+		
5		

Note: Radomski & Latham have an additional grade of 4− or Good−, which is full ROM that takes less than moderate resistance.

CASE STUDIES

Case Study 4-1. Carson is a 5-year-old client who sustained a C6 spinal cord injury secondary to a motor vehicle accident (MVA). The injury occurred to the right side of his spinal cord. The OT begins the evaluation knowing that the sensation will most likely be impaired on the left side of the body, below the level of the lesion is:

    A. Two-point discrimination
    B. Touch localization
    C. Temperature
    D. Joint motion or kinesthesia

Case Study 4-2. The OT receives orders to evaluate and treat a patient with a T2 spinal cord injury (SCI). What will be the focus of the sensory testing?

    A. Peripheral nerve distribution
    B. Dermatomal distribution
    C. Central nervous distribution

Case Study 4-3. The OT receives orders to evaluate and treat a 72-year-old male with left hemiplegia secondary to a CVA. Should the OT include a peripheral nerve, dermatomal, and/or central nervous system distribution? Please explain the rationale for your response.

Case Study 4-4. A 40-year-old female with a newly acquired mild traumatic brain injury and history of diabetes mellitus is referred to the OT for evaluation and treatment. She complains of numbness throughout the thumb region of her right hand. Should the OT include a peripheral nerve distribution, dermatomal distribution, and/or central nervous system distribution? Please explain the rationale for your response.

REFERENCES

American Spinal Injury Association. (2006). *Standard neurological classification of spinal cord injury.* Retrieved November 18, 2008, from http://www.asia-spinalinjury.org/publications/2006_Classif_worksheet.pdf

Pendleton, H. M., & Schultz-Krohn, W. (Eds.). (2006). *Pedretti's occupational therapy: Practice skills for physical dysfunction* (6th ed.). St. Louis, MO: Mosby.

Radomski, M. V., & Latham, C. A. T. (Eds.). (2008). *Occupational therapy for physical dysfunction* (6th ed.). Philadelphia: Lippincott Williams & Wilkins.

CASE STUDY RATIONALE

Case Study 4-1. Correct Answer: C. Pain and temperature will be absent on the left side of the body below the level of the lesion to the right half of the spinal cord. Joint motion, touch localization, and two-point discrimination will likely remain intact.

Case Study 4-2. Correct Answer: B. Peripheral nerve distributions are used for clients who experience trauma to the peripheral nerves either by injury or disease, and central nervous system distributions occur when clients sustain head injuries or some other trauma to the brain.

Case Study 4-3. Somatosensory examination to evaluate central nervous system is indicated for Case Study 4-3. The client had a CVA, which commonly affects sensory and motor functions.

Case Study 4-4. The OT should assess for somatosensory losses in peripheral nerve distributions secondary to peripheral neuropathies associated with diabetes in addition to central nervous system distribution secondary to the traumatic brain injury.

Vision and Cognition: Assessment and Intervention

Anne T. Riddering

OBJECTIVES

1. Define the key structures of the eye and the visual pathway as well as its functions.
2. Describe key areas of the brain and its affect on vision when injured.
3. Describe the main eye diseases and injuries and their affects on vision.
4. For the following deficit areas, explain occupational therapy (OT) low vision assessment and intervention, including clinical observations, standardized tests, affect on activities of daily living (ADL), and intervention: visual acuity, visual field, contrast sensitivity, oculomotor function, and visual perceptual deficits.
5. Apply knowledge of assessment and intervention of low vision rehabilitation to clinical case scenarios.
6. Define the key functions of cognition and the deficits and intervention related to each function.
7. Apply knowledge of assessment and intervention to clinical case scenarios for individuals who are cognitively-impaired.

Table 5.1 Key Terms

Radomski & Latham, 2008, pp. 235, 261, 729, 749	*Pendleton & Schultz-Krohn, 2006, pp. 532, 573, 589*
Age-related macular degeneration	Convergence
Astigmatism	Divergence
Diabetic retinopathy	Esophoria
Fixation	Esotropia
Fovea	Exophoria
Glaucoma	Exotropia
Hyperopia	Extinction
Legal blindness	Generalization
Macula	Hyperopia

(continues)

Table 5.1 Key Terms *(continued)*

Radomski & Latham, 2008, pp. 235, 261, 729, 749	*Pendleton & Schultz-Krohn, 2006, pp. 532, 573, 589*
Myopia	Hyperphoria
Normal limits of visual field	Hypokinesia
Presbyopia	Hypometria
Retina	Hypotropia
Saccade	Impersistence
Smooth pursuits/tracking	Limb akinesia
	Motor preservation

INTRODUCTION

Welcome to Days 4 and 5 of your study guide. In this chapter you will learn about vision and cognition as it is applicable to the occupational therapist. Key areas of the brain and their impact on vision will be discussed as well as low vision assessment and intervention for the entry-level therapist. Key functions of cognition, deficits, and intervention are included.

OUTLINE

1. **Vision and function: Basics**
   a. Role of vision

   (Pendleton & Schultz-Krohn, 2006, pp. 533–534)

   i. Human interaction
      I. Vision allows us to:
         a. See facial expressions
         b. Observe nonverbal gestures
         c. See body expressions
      II. Vision aids memory and learning
   ii. Environmental interaction: Vision allows for:
      I. Adaptation of visual motor activities
      II. Speed when adapting to the environment during ADL
   iii. Safety
      I. Vision aids us with spatial relations (orientation).
      II. Vision assists us in adapting to maintain balance.
      III. Vision allows for early warning of danger.
   iv. Pleasure and enjoyment: Vision allows for:
      I. Observation of color
      II. Detection of details during ADL
   b. Vision defined

   (Radomski & Latham, 2008, pp. 729–730)

   i. Normal vision
      I. Visual acuity: 20/30 or better vision; able to read standard print
      II. Visual field: Horizontal approximately 150°; vertical approximately 120°
   ii. Low vision
      I. Visual function is severe enough to interfere with performance but allows some usable vision.
      II. The vision is no longer correctable by conventional measures, such as a change in the prescription of glasses, surgery, or medication.

    iii. Legal blindness
        I. Acuity level: 20/200 or less (best corrected vision in the best eye)
        II. Visual field: 20° or less in the best eye
    iv. Low vision professionals
        I. Eye care physicians: Evaluate and diagnose vision deficits and diseases; recommend treatment, including medication, surgery, optical changes, and assistive devices.

(Radomski & Latham, 2008, pp. 238, 729)

        a. Ophthalmologist: A medical doctor who evaluates, treats, and manages structures, functions, and diseases of the eye.
        b. Optometrist: Professional with 4 years of postgraduate training who is trained to evaluate the eye's function, diagnose disease, and correct refractive errors with glasses or contact lenses.
      II. Other practitioners involved in low vision care

(Radomski & Latham, 2008, p. 730)

        a. Occupational therapist, generalist: May train client in some general adaptations for low vision, such as increased lighting and contrast; refers to specialists for more extensive training.
        b. Occupational therapist, specialist (SCLV): Professionals who have become involved in the process of ongoing, focused, and targeted professional development in the area of low vision rehabilitation. An OT specialist may train clients in the use of residual vision to complete ADL; training includes environmental adaptation, compensatory techniques, community training, client and family training, and training with optical and nonoptical devices.
        c. Certified Low Vision Therapist (CLVT): Trains clients to use vision more effectively to complete daily activities, with and without devices.
        d. Certified Vision Rehabilitation Therapist (CVRT) (formerly rehabilitation teacher): Emphasis of training is on blind techniques, assistive technology, and device use for persons who are blind or have low vision; teaches braille.
        e. Certified Orientation and Mobility Specialist (O&M; COMS): Teaches clients in systematic, efficient techniques to remain oriented and safe when traveling using long canes, sighted guide, and dog guides.
c. Warren's visual perceptual hierarchy (listed from foundational level to more advanced levels)

(Pendleton & Schultz-Krohn, 2006, pp. 538–540, 1225)
(Radomski & Latham, 2008, pp. 235–237)
(Zoltan, 2007, p. 50)

    i. Visual perception: The complex method by which an image is seen, interpreted, and processed by the brain. The image is integrated with other sensory features and stored in one's memory so that it can be used for decision making in ADL.
    ii. Basic level skills (foundational skills)
        I. Oculomotor control: Efficient movement of the eyes in a coordinated manner allowing for perceptual stability; includes eye alignment, accommodation, convergence and divergence, saccadic eye movements, and smooth pursuit eye movements (tracking)
        II. Visual field: The entire area that the eyes are able to see; normal horizontal field (left to right) 150°; normal vertical field (superior to inferior) 120°
        III. Visual acuity: The ability of the eye to distinguish the fine details of what is seen
    iii. Intermediate-level skills

I. Attention (alert and attending): The awareness and identification of the body, the environment around one's body, and the relationship between the two; the ability to search, scan, and identify an object and filter out unnecessary details
    a. Alertness: Most basic type of attention
    b. Attending: "Allows us to determine the what and where of things in our environment" (Radomski & Latham, 2008, p. 242).
       i. Two categories

(Pendleton & Schultz-Krohn, 2006, p. 557)

         1. Selective or focal: Concerned with the visual details
         2. Ambient or peripheral: Detection in the peripheral environment and relationship to the person

II. Scanning or visual search: The ability to search the environment, focus on the most important details to interpret and identify correctly; accomplished using saccadic eye movements; scanning is a result of visual attention (see Pendleton & Schultz-Krohn, 2006, p. 540).

III. Pattern recognition: Recognition of relevant details of an object and using these specific details to discriminate an object from its background
    a. Identification of general characteristics: Shape and outline
    b. Identification of specific characteristics: Color, shaping, and texture
    c. Disorders include lack of visual discrimination.

  iv. Advanced-level skills
    I. Visual memory: One's proficiency in taking, retaining, and processing a mental picture of an object; includes storing and retrieving images from short- and long-term memory
    II. Visuo-cognition: "The ability to manipulate and integrate visual input with other sensory information to gain knowledge, solve problems, formulate plans, and make decisions" (see Pendleton & Schultz-Krohn, 2006, p. 538)
       a. Facilitates complex visual analysis; basis for academic learning (reading, writing, mathematics, etc.)
       b. Disorders include agnosia, alexia, visual closure, figure ground, and spatial relations.
       c. Mastery-level skills: Adaptation through vision occurs when one is able to filter, organize, and process information acquired through the visual system to adapt to the environment. This adaptive response requires one to use visual perceptual skills, other pertinent sensory information, and cognitive concepts throughout the integrated central nervous system (CNS) process (see Zoltan, 2007, pp. 50–51).

2. **Eye function**
  a. Extraocular muscles (6)

(Pendleton & Schultz-Krohn, 2006, p. 535)

    i. Rectus muscles (4)
       I. Medial: Function is adduction.
       II. Lateral: Function is abduction.
       III. Inferior: Function is depression.
       IV. Superior: Function is elevation.
    ii. Oblique muscles (2)
       I. Superior: Function is turning inward and down; longest, thinnest muscle.
       II. Inferior: Function is turning outward and up.
  b. Cranial nerves impacting vision

(Pendleton & Schultz-Krohn, 2006, pp. 564–565)

    i. Optic nerve (II): Tract of brain; cells originate in the retina and axon fibers group together to form the optic nerve; optic nerves travel posteriorly then cross at the optic chiasm with neurons leading to the visual cortex in the occipital lobe.

    ii. Oculomotor nerve (III)
        I. Controls four eye muscles: Medial rectus (adduction), inferior rectus (depression), superior rectus (elevation), and inferior oblique (outward and upward)
        II. Controls dilation and constriction of the pupil
        III. Controls positioning of eyelid
    iii. Trochlear nerve (IV): Controls the superior oblique muscle (inward and downward)
    iv. Trigeminal nerve (V): Ophthalmic branch supplies sensory fibers to the upper eyelid, eyeball, and skin surrounding the eyes.
    v. Abducens nerve (VI): Controls the lateral rectus muscle (abduction of the eye)
  c. Anatomy of the eye

(Jose, 1983, pp. 3–6)
(Pendleton & Schultz-Krohn, 2006, pp. 542–544)

    i. Cornea: Outermost transparent layer protecting the eye; assists in light refraction
    ii. Iris: Colored part of the eye; muscular ring that controls the amount of light that enters the eye by dilating and constricting the pupil
    iii. Lens: Biconvex structure that bends light to focus rays on the retina
    iv. Ciliary body: Muscle and fluid that aids the focusing of the lens
    v. Vitreous: Clear gel-like substance that maintains the shape of the eye
    vi. Sclera: Tough coating of the eye that protects the inner structures
    vii. Choroid: Layer between the sclera and the retina that contains the blood vessels for the eye
    viii. Retina: Multilayer, sensory structure for the eye that contains rods and cones; initiates impulses to visual cortex via the optic nerve
        I. Macula: Area of the retina that is the area of best vision
        II. Fovea: Center of the macula where the focus area of vision is located
    ix. Optic nerve: Carries the picture to the brain for interpretation
  d. Visual pathway

(Pendleton & Schultz-Krohn, 2006, pp. 534–537)
(Warren, 2008, pp. 29–30)

    i. Optic nerve: Cranial nerve II carries the visual message beginning in the retina; contains fibers from one eye.
    ii. Optic chiasm: The point at which the optic nerve fibers cross; the medial half of each eye crosses to the opposite side and travels along with the information from the other eye.
    iii. Optic tract: Carries the visual message from the optic chiasm to the thalamus of the brain; contains fibers from both eyes
    iv. Lateral geniculate nucleus (LGN) of the thalamus: Structure at which fibers of the optic tract synapse; assists the CNS to filter out input that is not needed; refines the image
    v. Visual cortex: Area of the occipital lobe in which enhancement of an image occurs before it is cortically processed

3. Areas of the brain responsible for vision
  a. Occipital lobe: Contains visual cortex; scanning; identification of objects; awareness, and discrimination
  b. Frontal lobe: Planning, problem solving, organizing, attention, appropriate behavior, and initiation of movement
  c. Parietal and temporal lobes
    i. Right parietal: Visual spatial relations
    ii. Left parietal: Understanding spoken and written language
    iii. Right temporal: Visual recognition and memory
    iv. Left temporal: Verbal memory
  d. Thalamus: Eye movement; integration of visual and cognitive information

    e. Cerebellum: Eye control and coordination

    f. Brainstem: Has the cranial nerves running through it; protective eye responses

4. **Pathologies of the eye**

    a. Refractive errors (these are not diseases!)

(Jose, 1983, pp. 5–33)
(Pendleton & Schultz-Krohn, 2006, pp. 544–545)

    i. Myopia (nearsightedness)

        I. Long eyeball, front to back

        II. Light rays entering converge to focus before they get to the retina.

        III. Near objects are clear, distant objects are blurred.

        IV. Corrected with a concave lens

    ii. Hyperopia (farsightedness)

        I. Short eyeball, front to back

        II. Light rays entering the eye get to the retina before they have converged to a point of focus (they pass the retina before converging).

        III. Corrected with a convex lens

    iii. Astigmatism

        I. Cornea is oval instead of round.

        II. Light rays converge at more than one point of focus.

    iv. Presbyopia

        I. In childhood near and distance vision is clear because the lens can change its shape to converge light rays; in adulthood (older than 40 years), people may experience blurred images, near more than distant, because lenses become stiff and the ability to focus is lost.

        II. Nearsighted people older than 40 years can see near as long as they are not wearing their distance glasses; with glasses they need a bifocal to see near, which may be clear glass.

        III. Farsighted people older than 40 years need more power for near than they do for distance.

        IV. People who may not need a bifocal are those who have one eye nearsighted and the other eye normal for distance (natural monovision), or people who are nearsighted and take their glasses off to read

    b. Diseases affecting peripheral vision

    i. Retinitis pigmentosa (RP)

        I. Visual effects: Decreased visual acuity; sensitivity to light (photophobia); constriction of the peripheral visual field; night blindness

        II. Causes: hereditary

        III. Treatment of disease: No known cure; optical aids, long cane techniques, substitution techniques, and visual rehabilitation training

        IV. Prognosis: Slow, progressive field loss that may lead to blindness

    ii. Glaucoma

        I. Acute narrow angle glaucoma (closed angle glaucoma): Acute episode

            a. Visual effects: Severe redness, pain in the eye, headache, or nausea

            b. Causes: Acute attack due to the inability of aqueous humor to drain, causing increased intraocular pressure; increased intraocular pressure causes tissue damage in retina near optic nerve

            c. Treatment of disease: Emergency surgery, either large laser hole or an incision to allow aqueous humor to drain quickly and pressure to drop

            d. Prognosis: Without surgery or if left untreated for too long, permanent damage can result, causing loss of visual acuity and field.

        II. Chronic open angle glaucoma (COAG): Chronic episode; most common type

            a. Visual effects: Decreased visual acuity and peripheral fields; light sensitivity in some cases; no pain

      b. Causes: Blockage in the drainage system (trabecular meshwork) that increases the pressure in the eye and puts pressure on the optic nerve

      c. Treatment of disease: Eye drops or several different types of drops to decrease production of aqueous humor

      d. Prognosis: Eye tissue damage is preventable with regular monitoring and treatment of intraocular pressure; decreased visual acuity or peripheral fields result if the disease is left untreated.

c. Diseases affecting central vision

(Warren, 2008, pp. 31–41)

    i. Age-related macular degeneration (ARMD or AMD)

      I. Facts

        a. Leading cause of visual impairment in older adults (60 years and older).

        b. The incidence of ARMD is likely to rise because the number of seniors is increasing.

        c. The following may contribute to higher risk: smoking, air pollution, sunlight, deficient nutrition (low in green leafy vegetables, fish, and fruit).

      II. Types

        a. Dry: Drusen deposits form in the retina, increasing in number to form scotomas (scarred areas) in the macula.

        b. Wet: Abnormal vessel growth under the retina; the vessels leak fluid, causing damage to the cells of the macula.

      III. Visual effects: Only the central vision of the macula is affected, causing scotomas (scarred areas); reduced contrast sensitivity.

      IV. Causes: Deterioration of the retinal cells in the macula and fovea

      V. Treatment

        a. Laser surgery: Cauterizes unwanted vessels but causes scarring from heat of laser.

        b. Photodynamic therapy: Uses the light of a laser reacting with an injected medicine to stop leaking; less scarring and possible slowed progression.

        c. A fair amount of research is being done to explore other options.

        d. Nutritional supplements are recommended for people who are diagnosed with wet or dry types to slow the progression of the disease.

    ii. Retinal degenerations

      I. Best disease: Autosomal dominant; usually diagnosed in childhood; affects central vision

      II. Stargardt disease: Autosomal recessive; diagnosed in childhood; affects central vision

d. Diseases affecting central vision, peripheral vision, or both

    i. Cataracts: Cloudiness of the lens of the eye

      I. Visual effects: Decreased acuity; progressively blurred vision, both central and peripheral; glare sensitivity; near vision may be better than distance vision.

      II. Causes

        a. Age related; called senile cataracts

        b. Trauma to the lens of the eye

        c. Congenital or hereditary

      III. Treatment of disease: Surgery to remove the lens and replace it with an artificial lens inside the eye or use of a prescription in glasses or contact lenses

      IV. Prognosis: Good; inability to accommodate for near vision after surgery, but this is usually correctable with glasses.

    ii. Retinopathy of prematurity (ROP; also called retrolental fibroplasia)

      I. Visual effects: Decreased visual acuity, scarring, and retinal detachment causing possible field loss or blindness

    II. Causes: Premature birth interrupts the process of developing blood vessels to the retina. Normal vessels may stop growing. The edges of the retina may not get enough oxygen and nutrients. These blood vessels constrict; new abnormal and fragile blood vessels can leak into the vitreous; can cause retinal detachment.

    III. Treatment of disease: Optical aids, glare control, long cane techniques, substitution techniques, and visual rehabilitation training

    IV. Prognosis: Secondary complications include glaucoma, increased occurrence of retinal detachment, inflammation of the uvea, increased risk for strabismus (crossed eyes), and amblyopia (lazy eye).

  iii. Albinism: Total or partial loss of pigment

    I. Visual effects: Decreased acuity, usually between 20/70 and 20/200; nystagmus (involuntary oscillation of the eyeballs); high refractive error and astigmatism; visual field effects are variable.

    II. Causes: Hereditary, underdeveloped macula of the retina

    III. Treatment of disease: Glare control, contact lens, optical aids, and training

    IV. Prognosis: Nonprogressive

  iv. Diabetic retinopathy

    I. Types

      a. Background diabetic retinopathy (BDR): Changes in the small retinal vessels; also causes macular edema

      b. Proliferative diabetic retinopathy (PDR): New, abnormal vessels grow as a replacement for the damaged vessels (neovascularization); new vessels are weak and tend to bleed, causing further damage.

        i. New vessels can leak into the vitreous, resulting in decreased vision; requires surgery to remove.

        ii. New vessels can cause traction retinal detachments.

        iii. New vessels can develop on the iris, causing neovascular glaucoma.

    II. Visual effects: Spotted areas of vision (Swiss cheese effect); fluctuations in vision based on glucose levels; decreased visual acuity, contrast sensitivity, color vision, and night vision; temporary diplopia (from neuropathy affecting CN III or VI)

    III. Causes: Systemic disease of diabetes that affects the blood vessels of the eye that supply the retina; caused by elevated and fluctuating blood glucose levels

    IV. Increased risk for cataracts, glaucoma, and retinal detachments

    V. Treatment

      a. Leaking vessels: Laser treatment stops leaking vessels, destroys new vessel growth, and prevents new vessel development.

      b. Vitreous damaged by leaking blood: Surgery called vitrectomy, which is removal of the vitreous and insertion of an artificial substance in its place

      c. Retinal detachment: Surgery

      d. Macular edema: Current research involves using the injection of a drug to stop leakage.

    VI. Prognosis: Progressive; untreated can cause blindness; important to rigorously monitor glucose daily, exercise regularly, and follow a diet to help maintain glucose level.

  v. Neurological injuries

    I. General information

      a. Deficits are caused by cerebrovascular accident (CVA), traumatic brain injury (TBI), multiple sclerosis, Parkinson disease, brain tumor, hypoxia, or surgery.

      b. Deficits and patterns of vision loss depend upon location of lesion.

    II. Deficits: Right hemisphere versus left hemisphere

      a. Right

        i. Hemi-inattention: Decreased search to left field

    ii. Visual inattention: Both visual field loss and hemi-inattention; may be referred to as visual neglect

    iii. Focus is on the whole

    iv. Visual spatial perception disorders

  b. Left

    i. Focus is on the details

    ii. Difficulty identifying objects

    iii. May miss details of an object

    iv. Apraxia more common but can be present with right hemisphere damage

III. Deficits: lobes of the brain

  a. Occipital lobe: Visual field deficits (partial to complete visual field loss), scanning deficits

  b. Frontal lobe: Fixation and saccade deficits, slowed responses in periphery, reduced speed in visual motor tasks

  c. Parietal and temporal lobes: Deficits in spatial relations, visual memory, visual discrimination, visual attention, visual field, agnosia

  d. Thalamus, cerebellum, and brainstem: Eye movement deficits (eye control and coordination), visual and cognitive processing deficits

5. Low vision intervention

  a. Visual acuity deficits

(Pendleton & Schultz-Krohn, 2006, pp. 542–547)
(Radomski & Latham, 2008, pp. 235–238, 729–732)
(Zoltan, 2007, pp. 55–59)

    i. Purpose

      I. The ability to recognize the small details of the object; good acuity allows for speed and accuracy in processing what is seen; also aids in decision making.

      II. Important to screen in older adults; complaints may seem unrelated to vision.

      III. Deficits may be due to a refractive error, a disease (disrupting the ability to process what is seen), or a disruption in the optic nerve (transmission of what is seen).

    ii. Assessment

(Pendleton & Schultz-Krohn, 2006, pp. 546–547)
(Radomski & Latham, 2008, pp. 238–239)

      I. Snellen charts: U.S. standard measurement chart; big "e" chart

        a. Understanding the numbers: Measured by a ratio of the size of a letter or symbol a client can read over the distance the client's eyes are from the chart. A person with 20/70 vision can see the same size object at 20 feet that a person with normal vision could see at 70 feet.

        b. Test the client with the best correction (wearing glasses).

        c. Test one eye at a time, then both eyes together.

        d. Test near acuity (reading distance) at 16 inches and distance acuity at approximately 20 feet.

      II. Other charts

        a. Single letter: Colenbrander chart; symbol or tumbling "e" chart for clients with aphasia, non-English speaking, etc.

        b. Continuous print (words and sentences): Colenbrander continuous print chart; MNREAD chart

      III. Scotoma considerations and impact on acuity: Scotomas, or scarred areas, form in the central vision. The pattern of vision loss can impact performance during ADL. Physicians who specialize in low vision can assess scotomas, as well as OTs who specialize in low vision.

    iii. Clinical observations and affect on ADL

       I. Near acuity deficits: Clinical observations

         a. Complaints include needing more or brighter light; print being too faint, too small, blurred, or fuzzy; difficulty reading small print.

         b. The client moves the reading material to one side of midline (horizontal or vertical) toward the eyes then away as if trying to bring the print into focus.

         c. The client changes head position often to try to locate a clear area.

         d. The client is unable to stay on a line when writing or loses track of the tip of the pen.

       II. Near acuity deficits: Affect on ADL

         a. Activities involving reading, writing, fine motor coordination (e.g., reading labels on medication or food, setting appliance dials, threading a needle, reading bills and writing checks, identifying money, pouring)

         b. Socialization and communication with others (e.g., dialing the phone, writing a letter, reading newsletters; may be embarrassed by difficulty eating, such as cutting and seasoning foods)

         c. Safety during ADL

           i. Cooking: Cutting, chopping, slicing

           ii. Accessing emergency assistance (via phone)

       III. Distance and intermediate deficits

         a. Complains of difficulty reading signs, seeing television, reading the computer monitor or sheet music, or playing cards or bingo

         b. Has difficulty navigating or driving

         c. Has difficulty seeing bowling pins or following a ball on golf course

       IV. Distance and intermediate deficits: Affect on ADL

         a. Activities involving reading, writing, fine motor coordination (e.g., reading room numbers, street signs, and store signs; seeing the television, bowling pins, or ball on golf course; difficulty driving; seeing cards on the middle of a table; playing board games; reading computer screen or seeing letters on keyboard)

         b. Socialization and communication with others (e.g., difficulty emailing, seeing food at a buffet, or reading directional or restroom signs)

         c. Safety during ADL

           i. Driving

           ii. Reading signs for emergency exit procedures

           iii. Stove and oven safety

  iv. OT intervention

(Radomski & Latham, 2008, p. 191)

       I. Access community resources

         a. Refer to an eye care practitioner when an older adult has not had his or her eyes checked and/or disease managed for 1 year; refer to low vision physician (ophthalmologist, optometrist) when client's acuity is moderately or severely impaired (moderately impaired starts at 20/70; severely impaired starts at 20/200).

         b. Library of Congress: Large-print materials and talking resources, including books, magazines, and sheet music

         c. Large-print books and audio books: Many available from local libraries or bookstores and also book clubs that individuals can join

         d. Radio reading services: Often in conjunction with university radio stations; information is read over the air, such as local and national newspapers, advertisements, and magazines

         e. Operator assistance: Available for assistance with dialing and locating a phone number; only available from some phone companies

II. Lighting

    a. When possible, increase available room lighting.

    b. Increase task lighting; explore use of different types of lighting (incandescent, fluorescent, halogen, full spectrum, natural lighting from window).

    c. For near tasks, position lighting closest to the better eye; for fine motor tasks, place light opposite writing hand to minimize shadows.

    d. Control glare; adjust blinds and window shades; yellow sunglasses may help indoors, and yellow and amber sunglasses, hats, and visors may help control glare outdoors.

III. Magnification

(Pendleton & Schultz-Krohn, 2006, p. 547)

(Radomski & Latham, 2008, p. 732)

    a. Relative size magnification: Use large-print books, clocks, checks and check registers, playing cards and board games, pill boxes, glucose monitors.

    b. Relative distance magnification: Move object closer to eyes (book closer to face or eyes and body closer to television or sign).

    c. Optical devices: Usually recommended or prescribed by low vision physicians

        i. Handheld devices

            1. Small enough to hold in hand, fit in pocket

            2. Illuminated and nonilluminated versions

            3. Must be held at specific distance to maintain focus

            4. Difficult for individuals with tremors

        ii. Stand magnifiers

            1. Set focus distance

            2. Illuminated and nonilluminated versions

            3. Not portable

            4. Easier to use for individuals with hand problems (arthritis, tremors)

        iii. Head-worn devices (including microscopic glasses, high-powered spectacles, clip-on lenses, etc.)

            1. Offers wide field of view, and hands are free for tasks

            2. Many models are portable

            3. Binocular viewing and increased reading speed for some models

            4. Must hold reading material close to eyes to maintain focus, but light is obstructed when held close

        iv. Electronic magnification devices or closed-circuit televisions (CCTV)

            1. Greatest range of magnification and largest field of view

            2. Desktop and portable color models

            3. Can change the magnification and background color and contrast

            4. Expensive

        v. Telescopic devices

            1. Mainly for spotting in the distance; some can be used at intermediate or near distance

            2. Types

                a. Monocular: Portable; difficult to use with tremors; may require manual focusing for changes in distance

                b. Binocular: Portable; lightweight; allows for wider field of view (compared to monocular); comfortable options for television, movies

                c. Bioptics: Individually fitted telescope (either monocular or binocular style) that is mounted on upper portion of glasses; individual dips head and spots objects; in some states, can be used for driving (one eye only)

b. Peripheral visual field deficits

(Pendleton & Schultz-Krohn, 2006, pp. 548–557)
(Radomski & Latham, 2008; pp. 191, 235–236, 239–240)
(Zoltan, 2007, pp. 64–69)

i. Purpose
  I. The visual field is the entire area that the eyes are able to see
    a. Center 10° is called the fovea and is responsible for identifying details.
    b. Peripheral field (all of the field except the fovea) is responsible for identification of shape and form and movement in the environment. Peripheral field aids mobility.
  II. Normal visual field: Superior 60°; inferior 75°; nasal side 60°; temporal side 100°
  III. Damage can occur to retina or along the optic pathway (location will determine the pattern of vision loss)
ii. Assessment: Perimetry (measuring the visual field)
  I. Common tests for peripheral field
    a. Confrontation testing: Gross examination of visual field in which therapist sits in front of client and asks client to focus on therapist's eyes while therapist brings in two targets from different areas in the field. Client indicates if targets are seen and where they are seen. It can also be done with two therapists; the one standing behind the client presents the targets. This is not a reliable visual field test but rather a gross assessment.
    b. Tangent screen: Black felt screen with a grid visible only to the examiner. The client, at 1 meter away, is asked to fixate on the target affixed to the center of the screen. A white target (affixed to a black wand) is moved around the screen. The client indicates when the target is seen. The client's answers of seen (and unseen) targets allows the therapist to plot out the visual field deficit.
    c. Goldmann: Manual bowl perimetry administered at office of optometrist or ophthalmologist
    d. Humphrey: Automated bowl perimetry administered at office of optometrist or ophthalmologist
  II. Common tests for the central field
    a. Damato 30-Point Campimeter: Portable test card that measures the central 30° of the visual field; included as part of the Brain Injury Visual Assessment Battery for Adults (biVABA) (see Warren, 1998).
    b. Pepper Visual Skills for Reading Test (VSRT): Functional test that indicates scotomas and their affects on function (see Watson, Whittaker, & Steciw, 1995).
    c. Scanning laser ophthalmoscope (SLO): Allows very precise imaging of the macula area but is very expensive
iii. Clinical observations and affect on ADL
  I. Clinical observations
    a. Reading: Omits letters or words; consistently loses place on one side of page or when finding next line; uses finger to maintain place on page
    b. Mobility: Watches feet when walking; has poor navigational skills and gets lost easily; avoids obstacles in familiar areas but collides or comes close to obstacles in unfamiliar areas; stays close to one side of hallway; uses finger to trail the wall to tactually guide self; difficulty or unable to navigate in crowded areas; stops walking when approaching or passing another person; refuses to take lead when ambulating, prefers to follow others
    c. Other ADL: Has poor or absent eye contact; complains of seeing one-half an image or that objects are darker on one side; difficulty judging distances; reluctant to change head position or holds head to one side; displaces writing

to one side when completing a form or drifts off line; becomes upset with others who leave items out or returns them to a different location

II. Affect on ADL

    a. Activities involving reading, writing: Due to reduced perceptual span, reading speed and accuracy reduced; frequently misses letters, difficulty reading long words; difficulty locating next line when reading or writing and may lose place when writing; superior field cuts tend to cause more difficulty with reading (near and distance), writing, and tabletop activities (cutting, chopping, stove top, cards, medication management)

    b. Activities involving mobility: Difficulty walking, may shuffle feet; frequent bumps, trips, stumbles, and falls cause client to decrease walking in unfamiliar areas; inferior field loss causes decreased balance, difficulty seeing steps, curbs, and identifying visual landmarks

    c. Socialization and communication with others: Difficulty entering a room, locating a friend in a restaurant, and locating an empty chair in a room; difficulty navigating in crowded rooms and stores; may be reluctant to use a long cane for mobility because of social stigma

    d. Safety during ADL: Because of reduced field, individual may be more at risk for falls

iv. OT intervention

    I. Access community resources

        a. Refer to an orientation and mobility specialist for training in mobility

(Warren, 2008, pp. 148, 150–152, 158)

        i. Clients with significant field loss

        ii. Clients who need to travel in special or complicated environments

            1. Crossing streets with traffic lights, multiple lanes, or traffic moving at speeds greater than 25 miles per hour

            2. Travel in areas without sidewalks

            3. Particular difficulties or needs, such as:

                a. Difficulty detecting curbs, steps, drop-offs

                b. Frequently getting lost or unable to establish a relationship between themselves and objects

                c. Use of long cane

                d. Difficulty walking at night, on moving walkways, escalators

                e. Difficulty with bus, subway, or crowded areas

        b. Library of Congress: Large-print materials and talking resources, including books, magazines, sheet music

        c. Large-print books and audio books: Many available from local libraries or bookstores and also book clubs that individuals can join

        d. Radio reading services: Often in conjunction with university radio stations; information is read over the air, such as local and national newspapers and advertisements, magazines

        e. Operator assistance: Available for assistance with dialing and locating a phone number; only available from some phone companies

    II. Lighting

        a. When possible, increase available room lighting.

        b. Increase task lighting; explore use of different types of lighting (incandescent, fluorescent, halogen, full spectrum, natural lighting from window).

        c. For near tasks, position lighting closest to the better eye; for fine motor tasks, place light opposite writing hand to minimize shadows.

        d. Control glare; adjust blinds and window shades; yellow sunglasses may help indoors, and yellow and amber sunglasses, hats, and visors may help control glare outdoors.

   III. Scanning training

      a. Educate client about field boundaries and perceptual completion or a CNS process in which a visual scene is completed although only part of the information is seen visually.

      b. Train use of organized search patterns (left to right, up and down, etc.); increase speed and scope and organization and accuracy; generalize patterns into everyday ADL.

      c. Functional activities include card search, word search, locating items in cupboard or on grocery shelf, wiping off counter, sorting laundry, scanning courses.

   IV. Safety adaptations

      a. Educate client and caregiver about safety hazards in the home and how to maximize safe completion of ADL.

      b. Provide both physical and verbal cues.

c. Contrast sensitivity deficits

(Radomski & Latham, 2008, p. 235)
(Zoltan, 2007, pp. 60–61)

   i. Purpose

      I. Contrast sensitivity: Ability to detect grayness from a background and detect an object that is on a similar color background

      II. High-contrast activities: White on black, black on white

        a. Black coffee in a white mug

        b. Mashed potatoes on a dark plate

        c. Black felt-tipped pen on white paper

      III. Low-contrast activities

        a. Faces: Facial features used to recognize and identify someone are usually similar in color (high cheekbones blend in with nose shape)

        b. Newspaper: Grayish paper with slightly darker ink

        c. Curbs, steps

   ii. Assessment

      I. Standardized testing

        a. Vistech contrast sensitivity chart (not portable)

        b. Lea charts (portable, inexpensive)

          i. Lea numbers low contrast screener (part of biVABA)

          ii. Lea symbols low contrast screener

      II. Clinical tasks

        a. Clinical observation list in biVABA

        b. Example: Have client pour water into a clear glass; have client pour cold coffee into a white mug. Compare the client's ability to complete both tasks. Is glass underfilled or overfilled? Does client use fingers with glass?

   iii. Clinical observations and affect on ADL

      I. Clinical observations

        a. Difficulty recognizing faces, trimming fingernails, distinguishing similar colors

        b. Hesitates with a subtle change in support surface; difficulty with stairs and curbs

        c. Difficulty cutting foods or eating when the food and plate are similar color

        d. Reports an increased number of falls, trips, stumbles

      II. Effect on activities

        a. Activities involving reading, writing, fine motor tasks: Difficulty reading low contrast or colored print; difficulty reading or writing with pencil, blue, or black pens; difficulty with disorganized space, clutter, or patterned backgrounds; difficulty with sewing, pouring, trimming fingernails, putting on makeup evenly; difficulty cleaning up spills

    b. Activities involving mobility: Difficulty with curbs, stairs, steps; difficulty detecting subtle changes in surfaces

    c. Socialization and communication with others: Difficulty recognizing others, distinguishing faces; difficulty cutting foods or seeing foods on a similar color plate

    d. Safety during ADL: Reaching into oven; steps, stairs, curbs; cuts and infection when trimming nails; trips over pets that are same color as floor

iv. OT intervention

  I. Change color to increase contrast.

    a. Change background color. Have a light- and dark-colored plate, cutting board, and cups available for use. Men can use a blue tablet in the commode water. Hang a contrasting-colored towel in bathroom to see hair in mirror. When sewing, place a solid-colored towel on lap or table; it should contrast with material being sewn.

    b. Add high-contrast colors if possible. Add high-contrast marks on appliances, letters on keyboard, and numbers on telephone. Use a black felt-tipped pen and bold-lined paper for writing.

  II. Decrease patterns.

    a. Use solid color on background and support surfaces.

    b. Examples of contrast-reducing patterns: Pencil on a flowered tablecloth, fork or spoon on a plaid placemat, or coins on patterned carpet.

  III. Reduce clutter. Clutter creates a pattern and makes items more difficult to locate.

    a. Organize spaces. Clean off counters. In kitchen, organize spice rack and cupboards. Organize medications and grooming tools.

    b. Throw out unused items. Recycle or throw out junk mail and old newspaper. Clean out clothes closet with this rule in mind: "If you have not worn it in 1 year, you probably won't wear it again." This rule can be adapted throughout house.

    c. Return items to their storage place after using them.

  IV. Environmental adaptations for safety.

    a. Add a contrasting stripe to edges of steps.

    b. Use black electrical tape to stripe a white pull cord.

    c. Use liquid level indicators for pouring hot liquids.

    d. Pull oven rack out when placing items in or removing them from the oven.

d. Deficits in oculomotor function

(Pendleton & Schultz-Krohn, 2006, pp. 564–568)
(Radomski & Latham, 2008; pp. 236–237, 240–242)
(Zoltan, 2007, pp. 61–64, 70–86)

  i. Purpose/definitions

    I. Foveation: Creates and sustains a clear, precise image

      a. Fixation: The process of locating and focusing on an object on the fovea; foundation of oculomotor control

      b. Saccades: Quick, small movements of the eye (oscillations); used when scanning; moves us from word to word (reading) or object to object (locating object or driving)

      c. Smooth pursuits/tracking: Ability to follow a moving object with the fovea

    II. Sensory fusion: The ability to merge two images into one for binocular vision; CNS function

      a. Vergence

        i. Convergence: Focusing on an object and maintaining the image as it is moving toward the face; eyes move medially toward the nose

        ii. Divergence: Focusing on an object and maintaining the image as it is moving away from the face; eyes move laterally away from the nose

      b. Accommodation: Ability to quickly change focus from near to far; uses both saccades and vergence skills

      c. Extraocular range of motion: Motor process of moving the eyes in a symmetrical manner throughout all nine cardinal directions; strabismus (also called tropia) is the misalignment of the eyes.

      d. Diplopia: Double vision occurs when the fovea of both eyes are not aligned on the same target, so the brain is not able to fuse the image. Diplopia can be horizontal or vertical, a double image, or a blur or shadow; it can be present at near, intermediate, or far distances.

ii. Clinical observations and affect on ADL

  I. Foveation

    a. Fixation deficit

      i. Clinical observations: Difficulty attaining, changing, or sustaining gaze, especially at varying locations in visual field

      ii. Effect: Decreased acuity and binocular vision problems

      iii. Assessment: biVABA

    b. Deficits in saccadic eye movements

      i. Clinical observations: Undershooting or overshooting eye movements; difficulty shifting gaze; inability to isolate head and eye movements; difficulty reading (missing words, repeating or skipping a line of text)

      ii. Effect: Problems reading, writing, scanning, searching, locating objects, driving

      iii. Assessment

        1. biVABA

        2. VSRT

        3. Hold two different targets 16 inches from the face and approximately 8 inches apart. Ask the client to look from one to the other when verbally cued. Repeat for a total of 10 fixations (five complete cycles). Observe the ability to complete all cycles, accuracy of eye movements (overshoot/undershoot), and movement of head or body.

    c. Smooth pursuits/tracking deficits

      i. Clinical observations: Unable or impaired ability to track across visual field or coordinate both eyes to move in the same direction symmetrically

      ii. Effect: Difficulty playing and watching sports; problems staying on line when reading and writing; difficulty driving

      iii. Assessment

        1. biVABA

        2. Hold a target 16 inches from the client's face. Tell the client to focus on the target and follow it without taking his or her eyes off it. Move target in a clockwise direction; repeat twice. Move target in a counterclockwise direction; repeat twice. Record the number of rotations completed and how many times the client refixates. Record any head or body movement (see Radomski & Latham, 2008, p. 242).

  II. Sensory fusion

    a. Vergence deficits (convergence and divergence)

      i. Clinical observations: Diplopia (double vision) occurs at distances greater than 4 inches from eye; client complains of intermittent diplopia, blurred vision, headache, eye strain, or fatigue when reading; eyes stinging or burning, squints or closes one eye.

      ii. Effect: Difficulty performing near tasks (sewing, cutting, reading, writing), skips lines when reading, inability to sustain focus at specific distance (results in road fatigue, computer fatigue)

      iii. Assessment: Slowly move target toward client's bridge of nose. Client indicates when two targets are seen (diplopia occurs). Measure distance. Move target in approximately 1 inch farther, and then slowly move target away from client's nose. Client reports the distance at which one image is seen. Measure distance.

  b. Accommodation: Requires convergence, lens thickening, and pupil constriction

      i. Clinical observations: Blinks excessively, light sensitivity, blurring when changing the focal distance, swirling or moving print, blurred vision, headaches, eye strain or fatigue

      ii. Effect: Difficulty with near tasks (sewing, cutting, reading), dialing phone from a written number (phone directory), buttoning, shaving, copying from a chalkboard

      iii. Assessment: Same test as for convergence. Hold pen at near point of convergence (the point at which fixation is broken and usually one eye moves outward). Ask client to look at your face, then look at the pen and focus on it. Record the amount of time before the client loses fixation or looks away.

  c. Extraocular range of motion

      i. Clinical observations: Slowness or unequal eye movements, overshoots or undershoots, clumsiness, difficulty focusing, frequently closes one eye, diplopia; client may complain of nausea, motion sickness, vertigo

      ii. Effect: Difficulty with eye–hand or foot coordination tasks, difficulty with depth perception, misidentification

      iii. Assessment: biVABA

  d. Diplopia

      i. Clinical observations:

        1. Clients with tropias will complain of constant diplopia when viewing objects and often must close one eye to complete tasks.

        2. Clients with phorias will complain of diplopia that comes and goes and is most noticeable with fatigue.

      ii. Effect: Spatial judgment, disorientation, eye–hand coordination deficits, mobility problems, reading difficulties; specifically, difficulty with stairs, pouring, measuring, weeding, golf, getting in and out of bathtub, hammering, threading a needle, cutting, writing

      iii. Assessment

        1. Question client:

          a. When? Near, far, constant, or intermittent?

          b. Where? Straight ahead, right, left, up, or down?

          c. How? Vertical, horizontal, shadows, or ghosting?

        2. Cover/uncover test for when a tropia is suspected: Ask client to fixate on target held at eye level. Cover one eye while observing the movement of the other eye. Record if there is movement. The uncovered eye will move to obtain fixation.

          a. Esotropia: Inward deviation of the eye when the other is focusing on an object.

          b. Exotropia: Outward turning of the eye when the other is focusing on an object.

          c. Hypertropia: Upward turning of the eye when the other is focusing on an object.

          d. Hypotropia: Downward turning of the eye when the other is focusing on an object.

        3. Alternate cover test when a phoria is suspected: Ask client to fixate on target held at eye level. Occlude one eye then the other every 2 seconds. Record the direction of movement. The covered eye will move to obtain fixation when it is uncovered.

       a. Esophoria: Tendency for eyes to turn inward when both eyes are fixating on an object; controlled by fusion.

       b. Exophoria: Tendency for eyes to turn outward when both eyes are fixating on an object; controlled by fusion.

       c. Hyperphoria: Tendency for eyes to turn upward when both eyes are fixating on an object; controlled by fusion.

       d. Hypophoria: Tendency for eyes to turn downward when both eyes are fixating on an object; controlled by fusion.

    iii. OT intervention

      I. Refer to ophthalmologist or optometrist. Provide your clinical observations and affect on ADL performance, if possible. Monitor visual fatigue, stress, and endurance during activities.

      II. Eye movement activities and visual–motor coordination tasks, such as tracing exercises on paper or chalkboard, bird watching or tracking children running and playing, playing video games, crossword puzzles, laser pointer tag, reading a map, sweeping, balloon activities, beanbag throw, finding car in parking lot, coloring, or painting

      III. Scanning tasks

      IV. Increase endurance during tasks

e. Perception deficits: Perception is the way by which the brain interprets information received by the body's sensory systems

    i. Basic OT approaches

      I. Restorative or remedial approach

(Pendleton & Schultz-Krohn, 2006, p. 576)
(Zoltan, 2007, p. 4)

       a. Goal is to develop increased organization in the brain by enhancing brain recovery; change client and client's abilities during completion of ADL.

       b. Activities are chosen that meet the client's current level of function, and more difficult tasks are slowly introduced to improve independence.

       c. Repetition of exercises working on a particular component skill

      II. Adaptive approach

(Pendleton & Schultz-Krohn, 2006, p. 576)
(Zoltan, 2007, pp. 4–5)

       a. Encourages adaptation to the environment for ADL completion.

       b. Compensatory techniques based on activity analysis: Modify the environment or activity to change client performance.

       c. Adaptations practiced in a variety of settings so they become automatic.

    ii. Attention (unilateral neglect)

(Pendleton & Schultz-Krohn, 2006, pp. 540, 557–564)
(Radomski & Latham, 2008, pp. 242–245, 734–744)
(Zoltan, 2007, pp. 87–96, 107–129)

      I. General information

       a. Results in impaired scanning

       b. Attention is required for the CNS to use the information for an adaptive response

      II. Purpose and types

       a. Sensory neglect (input or attentional)

         i. Called visual inattention, visual attention deficit, hemi-inattention

         ii. Lack of or impaired awareness of information to one side of the body or in the space to one side of the body

         iii. Goals of visual attention

        1. Careful observation of objects

        2. Obtain information about specific features, relationships of self to environment

        3. Shift focus from object to object

    iv. Assessment of deficits

        1. Cancellation tests

        2. biVABA

        3. Figure and shape copying tests, line bisection test

    v. Clinical observations and ADL effects

        1. Difficulty scanning into personal and extrapersonal space

        2. Disorganized, asymmetrical, quick scanning during task

        3. Sidetracked by motion on right

        4. Impulsive behavior; does not rescan or recheck work

        5. Breakdown of scanning to left

        6. Loses items

        7. Difficulty with grooming and dressing

        8. Difficulty finding way in familiar environments

  vi. OT intervention

        1. Emphasize scanning to left using organized search patterns; correction of errors by careful inspection; slowly increase cognitive demands during activity

        2. Scanning needs to be automatic and spontaneous and integrated into all aspects of ADL

        3. Use of anchoring techniques, or cuing to redirect client's attention back to the impaired side

        4. Occlusion: Carried out under the direction of the eye care physician

            a. Total or partial occlusion, although total is usually avoided

            b. As control of muscles increases, occluded area is decreased

        5. Prisms

            a. Prescribed by an eye care physician

            b. A lens used to bend light and move an image to a specific area of the fovea; lens is thicker on one side than the other

            c. Fresnel prism: Temporary, inexpensive, plastic sheet stuck to a client's glasses; may cause some distortion

b. Motor neglect (output or intentional): Breakdown of the ability to begin or perform a movement

  i. Definitions

(Radomski & Latham, 2008, p. 245)

        1. Praxis: The ability to perform a movement

        2. Limb akinesia: Absence of ability to move limb

        3. Hypokinesia: Delayed movement of limb

        4. Hypometria: Decreased amplitude of movement

        5. Impersistence: Difficulty sustaining movement or posture

        6. Motor perseveration: Difficulty ending movement

        7. Extinction: Lack of awareness of one object when objects are presented in both sides of the body at a time, even though they are recognized when presented individually

  ii. Apraxia: Inability to carry out a movement even though the sensory system, muscles, and coordination are intact

        1. Limb apraxia

        2. Ideational apraxia: Difficulty with sequencing steps within a task

            a. Ideomotor apraxia: Production error; can use tools but appears awkward or clumsy

      b. Conceptual apraxia: Difficulty with use of tools

      c. Constructional apraxia: Difficulty copying, drawing, constructing designs

    3. Dressing apraxia: Inability to complete dressing tasks

III. Assessment

(Radomski & Latham, 2008, pp. 250, 252–253)

    a. Florida Apraxia Screening Test-Revised

    b. Screening for apraxia

    c. Assessment of apraxia

    d. Assessment of disabilities in clients with stroke and apraxia

IV. OT intervention

    a. Provide and combine tactile, kinesthetic, and proprioceptive feedback during tasks.

    b. Use hand-over-hand guidance during tasks.

    c. Use specific, simple verbal directions.

    d. Use chaining techniques during tasks. Chaining is a method of breaking the task into smaller steps. The client then relearns the task by completing steps and sequencing the steps together. Backward chaining, or allowing the client to first complete the last step and then the second-to-the-last step, can be used.

    e. Establish a routine for activities and perform training during appropriate time.

    f. Use cue cards for daily tasks with step-by-step instructions.

    g. Maximize safety and ease of completion by modifying the environment.

iii. Agnosia: Impairment in the ability to recognize and identify objects using only visual means; caused by lesions to the right occipital lobe.

(Pendleton & Schultz-Krohn, 2006, pp. 577–578)
(Zoltan, 2007, p. 171–180)

I. Color agnosia: Inability to recognize or remember specific colors for common object; client should be able to state if two colors are the same or different.

    a. Assessment: Present client with two common items that are correctly colored and two that are incorrectly colored. Ask client to pick out the two inaccurately colored items. An incorrect answer indicates color agnosia.

    b. OT intervention: Ask client to recognize, identify, and name various colors of objects within the environment during functional tasks or ADL training.

II. Color anomia: Inability to name the specific color of the objects

    a. Assessment: Ask client to name the color of various objects in the environment. Inability to correctly identify indicates a color anomia. OT can provide clients with aphasia color choices and answer "yes" or "no."

    b. OT intervention: Ask client to recognize, identify, and name various colors of objects within the environment during functional tasks or ADL training.

III. Object agnosia and metamorphopsia

    a. Object agnosia: Inability to recognize objects using only vision.

    b. Metamorphopsia: Visual distortion of objects although they might be recognizable to the client.

    c. Assessment: Place several common objects (comb, key, glass, ball) on table in front of client. Ask client to identify object and demonstrate its use. Present client with various objects of different weight, size, or color (drinking glasses filled with water, balls, and puzzle pieces). Ask client to put each object in order using only observation.

    d. OT intervention: Provide items in their natural environments, allowing client to use other senses to identify. Provide auditory description of the object and allow the client to feel it. Progress from simple to complex objects. Provide real objects before line drawings or objects in their functional environments versus at clinic table. Identify the object itself before the larger group to which it belongs (e.g., fork versus utensil).

    e. Prosopagnosia (facial agnosia): Inability to recognize or identify a known face or individual

    f. Assessment

        i. Standardized test of facial recognition: Multiple choice matching of faces

        ii. Informal tests: Using family photographs, have client identify the people pictured. Using photographs from magazines, ask client to identify the famous people pictured. Examples of famous people may include a political or religious person who has recently been in the news, a famous talk show host, or a movie actor. Family may confirm if client should recognize the famous person. Deficit is indicated if client cannot visually identify family members or famous people.

    g. OT intervention: Provide pictures of family members, friends, and famous people; assist client in identifying unique physical characteristics or mannerisms. Provide face-matching exercises. Teach client to make a mental list of features when they are introduced.

IV. Simultanagnosia: Inability to recognize and interpret an entire visual array (more than one thing) at a time; usually due to damage to the right hemisphere of the brain.

    a. Assessment: Present client with a photograph that includes a detailed visual array (picture with several people, animals, and details). Ask client to describe what is seen. Deficit is indicated when client can identify one particular object, person, or detail at a time but cannot describe the meaning of the entire scene.

    b. OT intervention: Assist client in learning to see the whole picture by offering verbal feedback and by questioning client about the details and how they relate to the entire picture; start simple then move to more complex situations (home or work then community outings).

iv. Visual spatial perception deficits (also called visual discrimination deficits)

    I. General information

        a. Definition: The ability to distinguish the space around one's body, objects in relation to the body and environment, and the relationship between objects in the environment.

(Pendleton & Schultz-Krohn, 2006, pp. 578–581)
(Zoltan, 2007, pp. 151–166)

        b. Processes are controlled by right hemisphere in an instant; deficits may be absent response or a slowed response, although the response may be correct. Slowed responses can still affect ADL function, such as driving.

    II. Figure ground: Ability to recognize the foreground from the background based on differences in color, luminance, depth, texture, or motion.

(Pendleton & Schultz-Krohn, 2006, p. 579)
(Radomski & Latham, 2008, p. 237)
(Zoltan, 2007, pp. 156, 158, 165–166)

        a. Assessment

            i. Functional: Locate white washcloth on white sink; locate cooking or eating utensil in cluttered drawer

            ii. Standardized

                1. Ayres' Figure-Ground Visual Perception Test (subset of Southern California Sensory Integration Test)

        2. Overlapping Figures Subtest of the Lowenstein Occupational Therapy Cognitive Assessment (LOTCA)

        3. Developmental Test of Visual Perception-Adolescent and Adult

        4. Motor-Free Visual Perception Test, Third Edition (MVPT)

  b. OT intervention

    i. Remedial approach: Place a number of objects in front of the client. Ask client to pick out particular objects (of similar color to the background), increasing the number of objects on the table as the client improves.

    ii. Adaptive approach: Modify the environment. Organize items, removing objects that are not necessary for the task. Label or mark commonly used items so they are easily identified.

    iii. Multicultural approach (Toglia): Assist client in increasing recognition of compensatory strategies, such as scanning and organization. Assist client in learning to integrate general skill to other ADL situations.

  c. Affect on ADL: Dressing and self-care activities; locating objects in cluttered environments

III. Form constancy or discrimination: The ability to distinguish a form, shape, or object despite its location, position, color, or size.

  a. Assessment

    i. Functional: Ask client to locate and identify different objects of similar forms, such as eating utensils in a kitchen or a cup on its side. A deficit is indicated if the client cannot identify an object in a different position/color/location than normal (see Pendleton & Schultz-Krohn, 2006, p. 579).

    ii. Standardized (see Zoltan, 2007, pp. 152, 165–166)

        1. Developmental Test of Visual Perception-Adolescent and Adult

        2. Motor-Free Visual Perception Test, Third Edition (MVPT)

        3. Form board test

  b. OT intervention

(Pendleton & Schultz-Krohn, 2006, p. 579)

(Zoltan, 2007, p. 153)

    i. Remedial approach: Have client practice sorting commonly used items in different forms. Encourage client to identify differences and similarities using tactile cues.

    ii. Adaptive approach: Necessary objects should be placed in upright positions and should be labeled so they are easily identified. Organization strategies should be implemented.

  c. Affect on ADL: Inability to recognize common objects needed to complete ADL; safety affected

IV. Spatial relations (position in space): The ability to perceive the position of one's self in relation to objects in the environment.

  a. Assessment

(Pendleton & Schultz-Krohn, 2006, p. 580)

(Radomski & Latham, 2008, p. 237)

    i. Functional: Ask client to place an object in a certain position. Use terms such as up/down, above/below, on/off, top/bottom, over/under. Deficits are indicated if the client is unable to complete the task.

    ii. Standardized (see Zoltan, 2007, pp. 161, 166)

        1. Cross Test

        2. Ayres' Space Visualization Test (subtest of the Southern California Sensory Integration Test)

        3. MVPT

b. OT intervention

(Pendleton & Schultz-Krohn, 2006, p. 580)
(Zoltan, 2007, p. 163)

    i. Remedial approach: Present client with opportunities to follow directions during ADL. Use directional terms (up/down, on/off, etc.). Ask client to point to objects in room and describe their location in relation to self or other objects. Incorporate use of tactile and kinesthetic senses to demonstrate position or distances.

    ii. Adaptive approach: Arrange client's environment so that items needed for ADL have a designated, consistent location.

c. Affect on ADL: Unable to align zipper or buttons, difficulty determining front or back of clothing, transfers are unsafe, difficulty ambulating through crowds

V. Depth perception (the ability to judge distances and depth) and stereopsis (the ability to see things in three dimensions). Lack of stereopsis can affect depth perception and makes the environment appear flat.

  a. Basic concepts

    i. Can be impaired without any signs of diplopia

    ii. May be affected if eyes are misaligned (strabismus present)

    iii. Other visual functions may also affect depth perception, such as visual acuity and contrast sensitivity

    iv. If client has one eye patched for diplopia or does not have use of one eye, depth perception will be affected

  b. Assessment

    i. Functional

(Pendleton & Schultz-Krohn, 2006, p. 580)
(Zoltan, 2007, p. 154)

      1. Ask client to estimate distances of several objects on a table. Which is closer? Farther away? A deficit is indicated if the client cannot complete the task and demonstrates other difficulties in ADL.

      2. Place an object on a table and ask the client to pick it up. Hold the object in front of the client and ask him or her to take it from you. A deficit is indicated if the client cannot complete the tasks and demonstrates other difficulties in ADL.

    ii. Instructo Clinic Depth Perception Test (see Zoltan, 2007, p. 155)

  c. OT intervention

    i. Remedial approach: During ADL, allow client to use tactile and kinesthetic senses to increase awareness.

    ii. Adaptive approach: Modify the environment and label objects to maximize safety. Use other senses and provide verbal cues to compensate for deficit. Train client and family to maximize safety.

  d. Affect on ADL: Difficulty ambulating up or down stairs, difficulty transferring, driving, threading a needle, sewing, knitting, stabbing food with a fork, pouring, hammering, placing denture adhesive on teeth

VI. Topographical orientation: The ability to navigate from one place to the next; requires ability to determine current location, goal location, and problem solving to implement an action

(Radomski & Latham, 2008, p. 237)
(Zoltan, 2007, pp. 164–165)

  a. Assessment: After being shown a route several times, ask client to find his or her way to a specific place (clinic to room, clinic to outside door, room to clinic). This task is dependent on intact cognition, such as memory.

    b. OT intervention: Assist client in learning landmarks on route. Landmarks should be consistently available and not change from day to day. Landmarks should be easily identified (high in contrast). Verbally describe the route plan to the client prior to beginning a task.

    c. Affect on ADL: Difficulty completing a return trip; difficulty locating rooms, buildings, etc., in familiar or unfamiliar environments; gets lost easily when driving or walking

v. Deficits of tactile perception

(Pendleton & Schultz-Krohn, 2006, pp. 580–582)
(Zoltan, 2007, pp. 133–148, 180)

I. Stereognosis: Ability to identify everyday objects using their tactile properties and no vision. The inability to complete the task is called astereognosis (tactile agnosia). Requires integration of tactile information to complete.

    a. Assessment: Occlude person's vision or objects from vision. Ask client to identify common objects without looking. Record the number of trials as well as the number of errors. A correct response would include identification of the object within 5 seconds. Also record the response to the object (quickly/slowly identified, object described but name not identified, only one property of an object). Objects that could be used include pen, key, screw, safety pin, fork, dime, penny, button, playing card, small ball, banana, pair of glasses.

    b. OT intervention: Graded intervention programs can be used in which the client looks, feels, and listens to the object. The vision is then occluded and the client identifies the object. The client then locates and identifies objects in sand or rice. Lastly, the client is required to pick out a small item from a group of items.

    c. Affect on ADL: Difficult tasks in which the hand needs to guide include locating something in a drawer, pocket, or bag without using vision; knitting while watching television; stabbing food with fork while talking; locating a light switch; cooking

II. Graphesthesia: Ability to identify forms, numbers, letters written on hand; absence of ability is called agraphesthesia

    a. Assessment: Occlude client's vision and trace letters, numbers, and shapes on the palm of the client's hand using a dull pencil, pencil eraser, or the therapist's finger. The inability to identify the correct letter, number, and shape is recorded.

    b. OT intervention: Provide clients with opportunities to practice having letters, numbers, or shapes drawn on their hand. This can be done by a therapist, family member, or the client.

III. Body scheme

    a. General information

        i. Autotopagnosia

            1. Inability to identify body parts on self or someone else or the relationship between parts (see Radomski & Latham, 2008, p. 236; Zoltan, 2007, pp. 134, 185).

            2. Ask client to follow your directions. Ask client to point to or identify the body part named on his body, your body, or on a doll (e.g., show me your right foot, touch your left eye with your right hand, show me your knee).

        ii. Finger agnosia

            1. Inability to recognize which finger was touched or is being used; may have difficulty identifying fingers when asked; may display clumsiness with fingers (see Pendleton & Schultz-Krohn, 2006, p. 581; Zoltan, 2007, pp. 145–146).

2. Assessment: Occlude the client's eyes and ask him or her to tell you which finger was touched.

    iii. Anosognosia

       1. Lack of recognition or awareness of one's deficits (see Radomski & Latham, 2008, p. 236; Zoltan, 2007, pp. 142, 185)

       2. Both cognitive impairment and sensory (proprioception) impairment (see Zoltan, 2007, p. 142)

  b. OT intervention: Focus on providing reinforcements of body parts using tactile and proprioceptive awareness. The client should integrate the use of affected body parts during functional ADL tasks.

  c. Affect on ADL: Safety (burns, cuts) during ADL; need to monitor hands during ADL

IV. Right/left discrimination: Ability to identify, discriminate, and understand the concept of right and left; can be affected by short-term memory, aphasia.

  a. Assessment

    i. Ask client to identify body parts or to do something with particular body part (e.g., show me your left foot, touch your right ear, take the paper with your left hand). Client should be able to follow the direction in a reasonable amount of time.

    ii. Ayres' Right/Left Discrimination Test (subtest of Southern California Sensory Integration Test)

  b. OT intervention: Focus on providing reinforcements of body parts using tactile and proprioceptive awareness. The client should integrate use of affected body parts during functional ADL tasks.

  c. Affect on ADL: Safety (burns, cuts) during ADL; difficulty following directions

6. Cognition

  a. Definitions

    i. Cognition: Mental skills and processes.

    ii. Metacognition: The ability to choose and use specific mental skills to complete a task.

  b. General assessment information

(Pendleton & Schultz-Krohn, 2006, pp. 602–603)
(Radomski & Latham, 2008, pp. 267–268)

    i. Evaluate the client's history (intellectual capacity, substance abuse history, age), prior ADL status, goals, and future plans.

    ii. Establish current level of functioning (baselines).

    iii. Complete appropriate assessments.

       I. Static assessments: Standardized testing

       II. Dynamic assessments: Focus on client performance; allows for manipulation of environment

    iv. Formulate interventions and discharge plan.

    v. Refer for neuropsychological evaluations when appropriate (includes a battery of tests to evaluate cognitive function).

  c. Skills of cognition

    i. Orientation: Attentiveness to self, others, environments, and time

(Pendleton & Schultz-Krohn, 2006, p. 599)
(Radomski & Latham, 2008, p. 262)
(Zoltan, 2007, pp. 189–190)

       I. Deficit can frequently lead to increased confusion and anxiety.

       II. Deficits may be transitory or last longer.

       III. Dimension of time seems to be weakest; time is also multidimensional.

IV. May be connected with memory deficits

V. Multiple areas of brain control function

ii. Attention

(Pendleton & Schultz-Krohn, 2006, pp. 591–593, 849)

(Radomski & Latham, 2008, p. 262)

(Zoltan, 2007, pp. 193–201)

I. Types
  a. Sustained: Maintain over time
  b. Selective: Maintain attention on one item while ignoring competing stimuli (ignoring fighting children when driving).
  c. Divided: Ability to attend to several stimuli at once (listening to radio while driving)
  d. Alternating: The ability to maintain attention on multiple tasks (reading directions while driving)

II. Assessment
  a. Lesion site: Mainly frontal and parietal in the right hemisphere, but multiple areas affect attention
  b. Clinical observation (see Zoltan, 2007, p. 199)
    i. Observe the client participating in ADL tasks in a variety of locations and at various times of day.
    ii. Considerations: When can they attend and for how long? With what types of tasks does attention break down?
    iii. Outside impacts: Memory deficits, problem-solving deficits, processing limitations
  c. Test of Everyday Attention (TEA) (see Radomski & Latham, 2008, p. 270)
  d. Cognitive Assessment of Minnesota (see Radomski & Latham, 2008, p. 275)
  e. Cognistat (Neurobehavioral Cognitive Status Examination) (see Radomski & Latham, 2008, p. 275)
  f. Mini-Mental State Examination (MMSE) (see Radomski & Latham, 2008, p. 274)

III. Treatment: Engage clients in activities of interest. Assist client in improving organization skills and listening skills. Client can vocalize steps aloud. Adapt environment to grade tasks (e.g., reduce noise).

iii. Memory

(Pendleton & Schultz-Krohn, 2006, pp. 594–598, 849)

(Radomski & Latham, 2008, pp. 261–263)

(Zoltan, 2007, pp. 207–227)

I. Types
  a. Short-term memory (STM): Temporary storage
    i. Primary memory: Simple storage information in STM; little processing occurs here
    ii. Working memory
      1. Interim storage and manipulation of information
      2. Conscious or controlled recovery of information
  b. Long-term memory: Permanent storage
    i. Implicit memory related to the steps of doing something (also called nondeclarative memory or procedural memory)
      1. Becomes automatic and effortless (automatic process, habitual)
      2. Most extensive and permanent memory
      3. Aids motor or mental functions
    ii. Explicit: Learned or experienced; also called declarative
      1. Episodic: Personal knowledge of an event; linked to a person, place, time

       2. Semantic: General wisdom of factual information
          a. Not dependent on episodic memory
          b. Uses visual perception and visual spatial information
       3. Procedural memory: Most complex form of memory used to complete a task; combination of skills from many of the body's systems

II. Cognitive Information Processing Model: Information is altered, saved, expanded, and retrieved to be used during cognitive tasks.

III. Assessments
    a. Lesion site: Several areas of brain, including frontal lobe, parietal lobe, thalamus
    b. Galveston Orientation and Amnesia Test (GOAT) (see Radomski & Latham, 2008, p. 270)
    c. Rivermead Behavioral Memory Test (RBMT) (see Pendleton & Schultz-Krohn, 2006, p. 603; Radomski & Latham, 2008, p. 270)
    d. Contextual Memory Test (see Radomski & Latham, 2008, p. 270)
    e. Cognitive Assessment of Minnesota (CAM) (see Pendleton & Schultz-Krohn, 2006, p. 603; Radomski & Latham, 2008, p. 275)
    f. Cognistat (Neurobehavioral Cognitive Status Examination) (see Pendleton & Schultz-Krohn, 2006, p. 603; Radomski & Latham, 2008, p. 275)

iv. Executive function

(Pendleton & Schultz-Krohn, 2006, pp. 589–605, 849–850)
(Radomski & Latham, 2008, pp. 261–278)
(Zoltan, 2007, pp. 231–284)

    I. Definition: Higher level cognition, higher order thinking abilities
       a. Involves decision making, planning, sequencing, executing
       b. Generalization occurs with intact executive function and short-term memory. Generalization is the ability to apply learned compensatory strategies to new environments or situations.
       c. Self-correction component
    II. Categories
       a. Self-awareness
          i. Judgment of individual traits
          ii. Problem recognition
          iii. Anticipatory knowledge
       b. Initiation and termination: Start and end tasks; needed for independent living
       c. Planning: Ability to sequence events prior to and during a task
       d. Problem solving, decision making, reasoning
          i. Definitions
             1. Problem solving: The active process of making a decision
             2. Reasoning: The ability to use information to arrive at a conclusion
          ii. Occurs during everyday tasks when one is unsure of what to do next
          iii. Complex process involving problem identification, solution development, and a choice of solution
          iv. Key terms
             1. Abstract thinking: Ability to differentiate between pertinent and nonpertinent information as well as recognize the relationships within the situation (events, people, objects, thoughts); thinking symbolically
            2. Concrete thinking: Tangible, specific
            3. Convergent thinking: Central idea
            4. Divergent thinking: Conflicting or alternative ideas
            5. Deductive reasoning: Reach conclusions

        6. Inductive reasoning: Use generalizations to reach a specific result.

        7. Dyscalculia: Inability to solve a simple problem; includes dyslexia and dysgraphia

   v. Impacts: Inability to recognize consequences; limitations in judgment and safety awareness

e. Assessments

   i. Multiple areas are impacted but mainly a frontal lobe function

   ii. Dynamic investigative approach: Using an ADL as a method to evaluate cognition using questioning, cuing and grading (see Pendleton & Schultz-Krohn, 2006, p. 591; Radomski & Latham, 2008, p. 269)

   iii. Toglia's Category Assessment (TCA) (see Radomski & Latham, 2008, p. 269, 272)

   iv. Toglia's Deductive Reasoning Test (see Radomski & Latham, 2008, p. 272)

   v. Tinkertoy Test (see Radomski & Latham, 2008, p. 273)

   vi. Client Competency Rating Scale (PCRS) (see Radomski & Latham, 2008, p. 273)

   vii. Self-Awareness of Deficits Interview (SADI) (see Radomski & Latham, 2008, p. 274)

   viii. Cognitive Assessment of Minnesota (CAM) (see Pendleton & Schultz-Krohn, 2006, p. 603; Radomski & Latham, 2008, p. 275)

   ix. Cognistat (Neurobehavioral Cognitive Status Examination) (see Pendleton & Schultz-Krohn, 2006, p. 603; Radomski & Latham, 2008, p. 275)

   x. Lowenstein Occupational Therapy Cognitive Assessment (LOTCA) (see Pendleton & Schultz-Krohn, 2006, p. 603; Radomski & Latham, 2008, p. 275)

   xi. Executive Function Route-Finding Task (EFRT) (see Radomski & Latham, 2008, p. 277)

   xii. Observed Tasks of Daily Living-Revised (OTDL-R) (see Radomski & Latham, 2008, p. 278)

d. Influences on cognition

   i. Neurobiological: Alterations or declines (see Radomski & Latham, 2008, p. 266)

   ii. Affective: Emotional factors (anxieties, pain, depression, fatigue, adjustment issues) (see Pendleton & Schultz-Krohn, 2006, pp. 851–852; Radomski & Latham, 2008, p. 266)

   iii. Social, cultural, and experiential (see Radomski & Latham, 2008, p. 266)

   iv. Environmental and task components (see Radomski & Latham, 2008, p. 267)

e. General intervention strategies for cognitive deficits

   i. Definitions

(Radomski & Latham, 2008, pp. 749–750)

   I. Cognitive rehabilitation

   II. Cognitive retraining

   ii. Approaches

      I. Remediate deficits

(Pendleton & Schultz-Krohn, 2006, p. 604)
(Radomski & Latham, 2008, pp. 750, 753–755, 758)

      a. Restoration of cognitive abilities

      b. Use practice exercises (usually computer based, pen and paper) to increase abilities.

      c. Complexity and demands of task (grading) controlled by therapist

      d. One deficit area can be treated independent of others.

II. Adaptive therapy: Changes in context, habits, routines, strategies

(Radomski & Latham, 2008, pp. 755–767)

a. Context
   i. Lower cognitive demands
   ii. Effective with dementia
   iii. Physical context
      1. Modify physical properties to aid client
      2. Decrease tools, items in environment, distractions
      3. Increase physical cues
   iv. Social context: Train family and caregivers to maximize success using prompts and cues
b. Habits and routines
   i. Automatic behaviors that are completed with little to no cognitive effort
   ii. Achieved through practice and repetition
   iii. In conjunction with family, caregivers, and client, develop new habits and routines that can be accomplished successfully by client.
   iv. Especially effective for ADL
c. Learn compensatory strategies
   i. New strategies to be used in ADL to offset deficits and aid client in successful completion
   ii. Multicontext approach: Uses self-awareness, acquisition of new information, processing strategies, activity analysis, integration of strategy, opportunities for practice
   iii. Cognitive compensatory strategy: Improve self-awareness through anticipation, acquisition, application, adaptation

REFERENCES

Jose, R. T. (1983). *Understanding low vision.* New York: American Foundation for the Blind.

Pendleton, H. M., & Schultz-Krohn, W. (Eds.). (2006). *Pedretti's occupational therapy: Practice skills for physical dysfunction* (6th ed.). St. Louis, MO: Mosby.

Radomski, M. V., & Latham, C. A. T. (Eds.). (2008). *Occupational therapy for physical dysfunction* (6th ed.). Philadelphia: Lippincott Williams & Wilkins.

Warren, M. (1998). *Brain injury visual assessment battery for adults.* Lenexa, KS: visAbilities Rehab Services.

Warren, M. (2008). *Low vision: Occupational therapy evaluation and intervention with older adults, revised edition* (2nd ed.). Bethesda, MD: American Occupational Therapy Association.

Watson, G., Whittaker, S., & Steciw, M. (1995). *Pepper visual skills for reading test* (2nd ed.). Lilburn, GA: Bear Consultants.

Zoltan, B. (2007). *Vision, perception, and cognition: A manual for the evaluation and treatment of the adult with acquired brain injury* (4th ed.). Thorofare, NJ: SLACK.

Exhibit 1-1 Stress Vulnerability Scale

In modern society, most of us can't avoid stress. But we can learn to behave in ways that lessen its effects. Researchers have identified a number of factors that affect one's vulnerability to stress—among them are eating and sleeping habits, caffeine and alcohol intake, and how we express our emotions. The following questionnaire is designed to help you discover your vulnerability quotient and to pinpoint trouble spots. Rate each item from 1 (always) to 5 (never), according to how much of the time the statement is true of you. Be sure to mark each item, even if it does not apply to you—for example, if you don't smoke, circle 1 next to item six.

		Always	Sometimes		Never
1. I eat at least one hot, balanced meal a day.	1	(2)	3	4	5
2. I get 7–8 hours of sleep at least four nights a week.	(1)	2	3	4	5
3. I give and receive affection regularly.	(1)	2	3	4	5
4. I have at least one relative within 50 miles on whom I can rely.	1	2	3	4	(5)
5. I exercise to the point of perspiration at least twice a week.	1	2	3	(4)	5
6. I limit myself to less than half a pack of cigarettes a day.	(1)	2	3	4	5
7. I take fewer than five alcohol drinks a week.	1	2	(3)	4	5
8. I am the appropriate weight for my height.	1	(2)	3	4	5
9. I have an income adequate to meet basic expenses.	(1)	2	3	4	5
10. I get strength from my religious beliefs.	1	(2)	3	4	5
11. I regularly attend club or social activities.	(1)	2	3	4	5
12. I have a network of friends and acquaintances.	(1)	2	3	4	5
13. I have one or more friends to confide in about personal matters.	(1)	2	3	4	5
14. I am in good health (including eyesight, hearing, and teeth).	1	(2)	3	4	5
15. I am able to speak openly about my feelings when angry or worried.	1	(2)	3	4	5
16. I have regular conversations with the people I live with about domestic problems—for example, chores and money.	(1)	2	3	4	5
17. I do something for fun at least once a week.	(1)	2	3	4	5
18. I am able to organize my time effectively.	(1)	2	3	4	5
19. I drink fewer than three cups of coffee (or other caffeine-rich drinks) a day.	(1)	2	3	4	5
20. I take some quiet time for myself during the day.	(1)	2	3	4	5

Exhibit 1-1 Stress Vulnerability Scale *(continued)*

Scoring Instructions: To calculate your score, add up the figures and subtract 20.

(14)

Score Interpretation:
A score below 10 indicates excellent resistance to stress.
A score over 30 indicates some vulnerability to stress.
A score over 50 indicates serious vulnerability to stress.

Self-Care Plan: Notice that nearly all the items describe situations and behaviors over which you have a great deal of control. Review the items on which you scored three or higher. List those items in your self-care plan. Concentrate first on those that are easiest to change—for example, eating a hot, balanced meal daily and having fun at least once a week—before tackling those that seem difficult.

Source: Exhibit courtesy Copyright 2009 Stress Directions, Inc., Lyle H. Miller and Alma Dell Smith, Boston, MA
www.stressdirections.com

Exhibit 5-1 Reflection Question Journal

1. What? (What have I accomplished? What have I learned?)

2. So what? (What difference did it make? Why should I do it? How is it important? How do I feel about it?)

3. Now what? (What's next? Where do we go from here?)

Source: Exhibit courtesy of Live Wire Media.

Exhibit 5-2 Screening for Visual Impairment Using Clinical Observations

PATIENT NAME: _____ DX.: _____ DATE: _____

VISUAL ACUITY DEFICITS (Near)

_____ Complains of needing more light or brighter light

_____ Complains of print being too faint or too small

_____ Complains of blurred or fuzzy print

_____ Moves the reading material to one side of midline (horizontal or vertical)

_____ Moves the reading material toward the eyes, then away as if trying to bring print into focus

_____ Changes head position often trying to locate a clear area of vision (head–fishing)

_____ Uses a flashlight to complete ADL in areas with low light (thermostat, appliance dials, reading menus and price tags)

_____ Unable to take accurate phone messages

_____ Complains of difficulty reading small print (expiration dates, price tags, nutrition labels, medicine labels, own handwriting)

_____ Unable to stay on the line when writing or loses pen-tip when writing

VISUAL ACUITY DEFICITS (Intermediate/Distance)

_____ Complains of difficulty reading signs (room numbers, store signs, directional signs, restroom signs, etc.)

_____ Complains of difficulty seeing the television

_____ Complains of difficulty reading the computer monitor, sheet music, playing cards or bingo cards

_____ Has difficulty navigating or driving

_____ Has difficulty seeing bowling pins or following a ball on the golf course

CONTRAST SENSITIVITY DEFICIT

** Ask patient to fill a clear glass with water. Next ask the patient to fill a black cup with milk. Compare the 2 performances.

_____ Has difficulty recognizing faces

_____ Reports an increased number of falls and/or stumbles, especially when transitioning between support surfaces of similar colors (sidewalk to ramp to street)

_____ Hesitates when there is a subtle change in the support surface

_____ Has difficulty with stairs and curbs (misses curbs, does not see drop-off until directly on top of it)

_____ Difficulty trimming fingernails

_____ Complains of difficulty cutting foods or eating when the food & plate are similar color

_____ Difficulty distinguishing similar colors (dark blue, black, purple, brown or white, beige, tan)

VISUAL FIELD DEFICIT

_____ Has absent or poor eye contact

_____ Watches feet when walking

_____ Complains of seeing only one-half an image or that objects are darker on one side

(continues)

Exhibit 5-2 Screening for Visual Impairment Using Clinical Observations *(continued)*

PATIENT NAME: _____ DX.: _____ DATE: _____

_____ Has poor navigational skills and/or gets lost easily

_____ Has difficulty judging distances

_____ Avoids obstacles in familiar areas but collides or comes close to obstacles in an unfamiliar areas

_____ Stays close to one side of the wall when ambulating down a hallway

_____ Uses fingers to "trail" wall to tactually guide self

_____ Refuses to take the lead when ambulating; prefers to follow others

_____ Increased hesitancy or unable to navigate in crowded environments

_____ Stops walking when approaching or passing by another moving person or object

_____ Reluctant to change head position or holds head to one side

_____ Omits letters or words

_____ Consistently loses place on one side of page or when finding next line

_____ Uses finger to maintain place on page

_____ Displaces writing to one side when completing a form (e.g., check) or drifts off the line

_____ Has become very particular that items be returned to a specific location and becomes upset with others who leave items out or return them to a different place

OCULOMOTOR CONTROL DEFICIT (including Binocular Vision Deficits)

_____ Complains of double vision, blurring vision, shadow vision (horizontal or vertical) when viewing objects or completing tasks

_____ Has difficulty with depth perception; often overshoots or undershoots during a reaching task

_____ Deliberately positions head abnormally and is resistant to changing head position

_____ Shows difficulty focusing up close for reading and writing tasks

_____ Attempts to change the focusing distance at which the task is presented

_____ Complains of nausea or eye pain with movement of eyes

_____ Complains of blurred vision when changing the focus from a near object to a distant object

_____ Transition between 2 focal distances is slow (decreased speed or increased time is noted)

_____ Shows a sensitivity to light changes

_____ Frequently repositions self or task

_____ Complains of losing place when reading or writing

_____ Skips words or lines when reading

_____ Is unable to fixate on an object and sustain it (e.g., walk/don't walk sign)

_____ Squints when viewing objects or shuts one eye (or turns head to view from one eye) to view an object

_____ Complains that print begins to swirl or move on the page

_____ Complains of headache, fatigue, or difficulty concentrating on tasks requiring sustained focus at a near distance

Exhibit 5-2 Screening for Visual Impairment Using Clinical Observations *(continued)*

PATIENT NAME: _____ DX.: _____ DATE: _____

<u>VISUAL ATTENTION DEFICIT (Also called Visual Inattention)</u>

_____ Has decreased attention to both intrapersonal and extrapersonal space

_____ Skews body position

_____ Makes observations about objects or details to one side of a visual scene

_____ Distracted easily by motion occurring on the right side

_____ Demonstrates reduced effort on tasks which require visual discrimination

_____ Displays impulsive behavior and rushes through a task

_____ Fails to rescan or recheck work when completing a complex task

_____ Fails to initiate and scan in an organized search patterns to the left

_____ Has difficulty shifting eyes across midline toward left

_____ Has difficulty maintaining fixation on an object placed to the left of midline

_____ Grooms or dresses only one side of body (usually right) and fails to correct the mistake

_____ Reads only one side of the food menu

_____ Shows increased bumps, collisions, and near collisions on left side

_____ Avoids left turns during when walking or is reluctant to turn left

_____ Only corrects errors in performance with physical cuing (after auditory & visual cuing have been given first); often requires repeated physical cuing

Source: O'Donnell, C. and Riddering, A. T., 2005. Henry Ford Health System's Visual Rehabilitation and Research Center of Michigan, Livonia, MI

Assessment of Roles and Context: Personal, Social, and Cultural

Catherine Lysack and Rosanne DiZazzo-Miller

OBJECTIVES

1. Understand the importance of context in occupational performance assessment.
2. Describe the components of personal, social, physical, and cultural context that influence occupational therapy assessment and guide treatment planning.
3. Identify major theories and models that guide occupational therapists' use of assessments of context.
4. Identify appropriate assessments of context.
5. Demonstrate how assessment knowledge is applied to clinical situations.

INTRODUCTION

Welcome to Day 6 of your study guide. This chapter will provide you with a review of why it is important to assess the context for an individual's occupational performance and how best to do this. Occupational therapy treatment interventions work far better when therapists understand the background of their patients and clients and their real-life situations and environments. This chapter will review key concepts and assessment tools that therapists use to assess personal context and the broader social, physical, and cultural environment.

Table 6.1 Key Terms

Radomski & Latham, 2008, pp. 66, 284, 311	*Pendleton & Schultz-Krohn, 2006, p. 79*
Context	Independent living movement
Cultural context	Life roles
Culture	Medical model
Personal context	Person-first language
Physical environment	Social model of disability
Social context	Stage process of adjustment

OUTLINE

1. Overview: The importance of assessing context

(Pendleton & Schultz-Krohn, 2006, pp. 79–80)
(Radomski & Latham, 2008, pp. 285–288, 311–312)

a. Basic principles
  i. Therapists must assess the social self or person, not only the physical corporeal body. Thus, occupational therapy assessment must go beyond the physical body and impairments to include personal attributes of individuals and the life roles they assume at various points across the lifespan.
  ii. Assessing a person's occupational performance context is multidimensional. Assessment of context must include unique personal attributes (e.g., gender, age, etc.) and personal life roles (e.g., worker, mother, spouse, etc.) and also the various physical, social, and cultural contexts in which people live and interact with one another (e.g., one's home and neighborhood, one's society, etc.).
  iii. There are models and frameworks to help therapists organize how they understand and assess context.
  iv. There are well-accepted criteria, including reliability and validity, that help therapists identify useful assessments of context.
  v. Occupational therapists live and work in a personal, social, physical, and cultural context, too. What forces shape occupational therapists' perceptions of their patients and clients? Are occupational therapists aware of that context in shaping their practice?
b. Personal, social, physical, and cultural context

(Pendleton & Schultz-Krohn, 2006, pp. 79–100)
(Radomski & Latham, 2008, pp. 285–337)

  i. Personal context: Personal context refers to a person's internal unseen environment that is derived from, among other things, age, gender, personal beliefs and values, cultural background and identity, and psychological state of mind. Some of the factors in the personal context are fixed, like age, but others are very dynamic and changeable, such as one's emotional state, which is often altered in response to positive and negative conditions.
  ii. Social context: Social context refers to factors in the human environment that influence people but are external to the person her- or himself. Social context refers to a person's social roles and social networks and also to the socioeconomic resources a person has and the social position one holds in the social groups to which the person belongs.
  iii. Physical context: Physical context refers to the natural and human-made or -built environment we live in. People's homes and the objects within them, as well as neighborhoods and buildings, are examples of the physical context. Physical contexts can facilitate occupational engagement and participation, but the environment can also pose barriers.
  iv. Cultural context: Cultural context is broader than personal and social contexts and refers to the influence of norms, beliefs and values, and standards of behavior that are expected and accepted in a particular person's community or society. The effect of cultural context is often very subtle and not easy to measure because we are so much a part of our society's rules and practices and beliefs that we hardly have the ability to stand back and realize how it could be different.
c. Models and theories that guide assessment of context: Models and theories help us organize how we understand and measure things. The following models and theories used in occupational therapy all include context in some way. These theories and models stress that the whole situation or context is relevant to understanding occupational performance.

(Radomski & Latham, 2008, p. 286)

     i. Ecology of Human Performance Model (Dunn, Brown, & McGuigan, 1994): In this model, the interaction between the person and the environment affects his or her behavior and performance, and human performance can only be understood through context, which operates externally of the person. In this model, the interrelationship between person and context determines which tasks fall within the individual's expected performance range.

     ii. Person-Environment Occupational Model of Occupational Performance (Law, M., Cooper, B., Strong, S., Stewart, D., Rigby, P., et al., 1996): In this model, occupational performance is defined as a transactive relationship among people, their occupations and roles, and the environments in which they live, work, and play. This model emphasizes the interdependence of persons and their environments and the changing nature of occupational roles over time.

     iii. The World Health Organization's (WHO) International Classification of Functioning, Disability and Health (ICF) Model (WHO, 2001): The ICF model views a person's functioning and disability as a dynamic interaction between health conditions and contextual factors. In this model, contextual factors are divided into personal and environmental factors. Personal factors are internal influences on functioning like age, gender, etc. Environmental factors are external influences on functioning that include features of the physical, social, and attitudinal world.

2. **Occupational Therapy Practice Framework** (American Occupational Therapy Association, 2008): The Practice Framework states that the goal of occupational therapy is to facilitate clients' engagement in occupation to support participation in the unique context of their life situations. In this model, context is included in the domain of occupational therapy.

(Crepeau, Cohn, & Schell, 2009, p. 653)
(Pendleton & Schultz-Krohn, 2006, pp. 81–85)
(Radomski & Latham, 2008, pp. 289–295)

    a. Fixed personal attributes
      i. Age
        I. Life roles differ at various developmental ages and stages
        II. Life roles differ for generational cohorts
      ii. Gender
        I. Traditional gender roles
        II. Gender is social; sex is biologically determined.
      iii. Sexual orientation
      iv. Personality
        I. Extraversion
        II. Self-efficacy
    b. Dynamic personal attributes
      i. Educational background
      ii. Marital status
      iii. Employment status
      iv. Life roles
        I. Role Checklist: Assesses productive roles in adulthood, including motivation to assume roles and perceptions of role shifting
        II. Interest Checklist: Assesses interest patterns and characteristics (adolescence to adulthood), including ADL, sports, social, educational, and recreational activities
        III. Occupational Performance History Interview-II (OPHI): Assesses occupational adaptation over time (adolescence to adulthood), with a focus on critical life events, daily routines, and occupational behavior roles and settings
        IV. Canadian Occupational Performance Measure (COPM): A client-centered tool for persons aged 7 years and older that evaluates clients' perceptions of their occupational performance over time
        V. Worker Role Interview: Gathers data on adults' evaluation of the psychosocial and environmental factors that affect work and the workplace

v. Perceived health and functioning (e.g., independence)

   I. Self-rated health: A single-item question that asks, "In general, would you say your health is . . ." with response options of 1 = excellent, 2 = very good, 3 = good, 4 = fair, and 5 = poor

   II. Disability and function

   a. Functional Independence Measure (FIM): A very well-known 18-item measure of disability consisting of 13 motor items and five cognitive/communication items

   b. Barthel Index: One of many assessments of inpatients' ADL status

vi. Stress, coping, and adjustment to disability

   I. Stage process of adjustment

   II. Depression

   a. Beck Depression Inventory: Assesses the intensity of depression in persons aged 13 to 80 years

   III. Life satisfaction and quality of life

   a. Diener Satisfaction with Life Scale (SWLS): Very well-known five-item scale to assess overall life satisfaction

   IV. Spirituality

   a. Religiosity

   b. Fatalism

   V. Stress

   a. Perceived stress scale: 10-item scale to assess current stress

   b. Family violence screening and response scale

   c. CAGE screening for alcoholism: Four questions that screen for alcohol abuse

   VI. Fatigue

   a. Fatigue severity scale: A brief scale, developed in the context of multiple sclerosis, to measure fatigue severity

   VII. Pain

   a. McGill Pain Questionnaire: A 5-minute test that measures intensity and quality of pain

   b. Visual Analogue Scale: A 2-minute test in which individuals indicate their current pain intensity on a 10 cm line

3. Social context

(Crepeau, et al., 2009, pp. 69–53, 94–97)
(Pendleton & Schultz-Krohn, 2006, pp. 85–88)
(Radomski & Latham, 2008, pp. 295–298)

a. Socioeconomic status (SES) and social class: Socioeconomic resources are not distributed evenly in society. When certain groups systematically have less, their health is much worse. Visible minorities, women, and children are vulnerable groups who have less. Over many years, the disadvantages associated with having fewer economic resources accumulate and lead to higher rates of disability.

   i. SES and poverty

   ii. Health inequalities and disparities

   iii. Occupational deprivation

b. Social network and social support: Research shows all people need access to tangible hands-on help and emotional support if they wish to have good health throughout their lives. Caring for the caregivers is also critical because caregiving itself can put a stress on one's health.

   i. Multidimensional Scale of Perceived Social Support

   ii. Norbeck Social Support Questionnaire: A nine-item tool that measures individuals within their social networks and their contributions regarding affect, affirmation, and tangible aid

   iii. Caregiver Reaction Assessment: A 24-item tool that measures caregivers' reactions to caregiving for aged persons with physical and mental health conditions

   c. Therapist-client interactions

(Pendleton & Schultz-Krohn, 2006, pp. 81, 95–96)

      i. Independent living movement
      ii. Client-centered practice
      iii. Person-first language
      iv. Social model of disability

4. Physical context

(Pendleton & Schultz-Krohn, 2006, pp. 85–90)
(Radomski & Latham, 2008, pp. 315–337)

   a. Barrier-free design and universal design
   b. Home accessibility
      i. Safety Assessment of Function and the Environment for Rehabilitation (SAFER) and SAFER Home: Evaluates home safety for older adults
      ii. Westmead Home Safety Assessment: Evaluates potential fall hazards in the home
   c. Access to the workplace
      i. Workplace Environment Impact Scale: Semistructured interview to evaluate a person's perceptions of his or her work environment
   d. Access to the community

(Radomski & Latham, 2008, pp. 326–327)

      i. Physical and environmental barriers
         I. Craig Handicap Inventory of Environmental Factors (CHIEF): A brief assessment of perceived environmental barriers
         II. Measure of the Quality of the Environment: Developed in the context of spinal cord injury but used to measure facilitators and obstacles to social participation for all persons with disabilities
         III. Accessibility Checklist: An assessment that identifies problems in community access, including compliance to ADA policies and regulations
      ii. Community integration and participation
         I. Community Integration Measure (CIM): A 10-item assessment focused on feelings of belonging and independence in one's community
         II. Community Integration Questionnaire (CIQ): A 15-item survey relevant to home integration, social integration, and productive activities
         III. Reintegration to Normal Living Index (RNL): Assesses how well a person reintegrates into normal living after severe disability

5. Cultural context

(Pendleton & Schultz-Krohn, 2006, pp. 85–94)
(Radomski & Latham, 2008, pp. 298–299)

   a. Societal context
      i. Western (dominant) culture: Ideas of full adult personhood, self-sufficiency (independence), and individualism that may be very difficult to fulfill if a person is living with a chronic illness or disability
      ii. Culture of disability
         I. Social status and disability: Idea of disability as deficit and deficiency, not full adult persons
         II. Disability as a collective experience

WORK SHEETS

Work Sheet 6-1

Please match each assessment with its *most* appropriate category. Assessments will be used more than once (Radomski & Latham, 2008, pp. 70–79).

Table 6-2 Asessment Worksheet

_A_ Occupational Performance History Interview-II (OPHI)	A.	Occupational performance
_D_ Safety Assessment of Function and the Environment for Rehabilitation (SAFER)	B.	Roles and community integration
_B_ Community Independence Measure (CIM)		
_F_ Interest Checklist	C.	ADL
_A D_ Kitchen Task Analysis (KTA)	D.	IADL
_B_ Craig Handicap Assessment and Reporting Technique (CHART)	E.	Work
_C_ Barthel Index	F.	Leisure
_D_ The Assessment of Motor and Process Skills (AMPS)		
_C_ Katz Index of Independence in Activities of Daily Living		
_E_ Worker Role Interview		
_C_ Klein-Bell Activities of Daily Living Scale		
_C D_ The Kohlman Evaluation of Living Skills (KELS)		
_B_ Role Checklist		
_B_ Reintegration to Normal Living Index (RNL)		
_A D_ Rabideau Kitchen Evaluation Revised		
_E_ VALPAR Component Work Samples		
_C_ Functional Independence Measure (FIM)		
_A_ Canadian Occupational Performance Measure (COPM)		

REFERENCES

American Occupational Therapy Association. (2008). Occupational therapy practice framework: Domain and process (2nd ed.). *American Journal of Occupational Therapy, 62,* 625–683.

Crepeau, E. B., Cohn, E. S., & Schell, B. A. B. (Eds.). (2009). *Willard & Spackman's occupational therapy* (11th ed.). Philadelphia: Lippincott Williams & Wilkins.

Dunn, W., Brown, C., & McGuigan, A. (1994). The ecology of human performance: A framework for considering the effect of context. T*he American Journal of Occupational Therapy, 48,* 595–607.

Pendleton, H. M., & Schultz-Krohn, W. (Eds.). (2006). *Pedretti's occupational therapy: Practice skills for physical dysfunction* (6th ed.). St. Louis, MO: Mosby.

Radomski, M. V., & Latham, C. A. T. (Eds.). (2008). *Occupational therapy for physical dysfunction.* (6th ed.). Philadelphia: Lippincott Williams & Wilkins.

WORK SHEET ANSWERS

Work Sheet 6-1

Table 6-3 Asessment Work Sheet Answers

__A__ Occupational Performance History Interview-II (OPHI)	A. Occupational performance
__D__ Safety Assessment of Function and the Environment for Rehabilitation (SAFER)	B. Roles and community integration
__B__ Community Independence Measure (CIM)	C. ADL
__F__ Interest Checklist	D. IADL
__D__ Kitchen Task Analysis (KTA)	E. Work
__B__ Craig Handicap Assessment and Reporting Technique (CHART)	F. Leisure
__C__ Barthel Index	
__D__ The Assessment of Motor and Process Skills (AMPS)	
__C__ Katz Index of Independence in Activities of Daily Living	
__E__ Worker Role Interview	
__C__ Klein-Bell Activities of Daily Living Scale	
__D__ The Kohlman Evaluation of Living Skills (KELS)	
__B__ Role Checklist	
__B__ Reintegration to Normal Living Index (RNL)	
__D__ Rabideau Kitchen Evaluation Revised	
__E__ VALPAR Component Work Samples	
__C__ Functional Independence Measure (FIM)	
__A__ Canadian Occupational Performance Measure (COPM)	

Exhibit 6-1 Perceived Stress Scale (PSS-14)

INSTRUCTIONS

The questions in this scale ask you about your feelings and thoughts during *the last month*. In each case, you will be asked to indicate your response by placing an X over the circle that represents *how often* you felt or thought a certain way. Although some of the questions are similar, there are differences among them, and you should treat each one as a separate question. The best approach is to answer fairly quickly. That is, don't try to count up the number of times you felt a particular way, but rather indicate the alternative that seems like a reasonable estimate.

	Never	Almost Never	Sometimes	Fairly Often	Very Often
	1	2	3	4	5
1. In the last month, how often have you been upset because of something that happened unexpectedly?	○	○	○	○	○
2. In the last month, how often have you felt that you were unable to control the important things in your life?	○	○	○	○	○
3. In the last month, how often have you felt nervous and stressed?	○	○	○	○	○
4. In the last month, how often have you dealt successfully with day-to-day problems and annoyances?	○	○	○	○	○
5. In the last month, how often have you felt that you were effectively coping with important changes that were occurring in your life?	○	○	○	○	○
6. In the last month, how often have you felt confident about your ability to handle your personal problems?	○	○	○	○	○
7. In the last month, how often have you felt that things were going your way?	○	○	○	○	○
8. In the last month, how often have you found that you could not cope with all the things that you had to do?	○	○	○	○	○
9. In the last month, how often have you been able to control irritations in your life?	○	○	○	○	○
10. In the last month, how often have you felt that you were on top of things?	○	○	○	○	○
11. In the last month, how often have you been angered because of things that happened that were outside of your control?	○	○	○	○	○
12. In the last month, how often have you found yourself thinking about things that you have to accomplish?	○	○	○	○	○
13. In the last month, how often have you been able to control the way you spend your time?	○	○	○	○	○
14. In the last month, how often have you felt difficulties were piling up so high that you could not overcome them?	○	○	○	○	○

PSS-14 SCORING

PSS-14 scores are obtained by reversing the scores on the seven positive items (i.e., 0 = 4, 1 = 3, 2 = 2, etc.) and then summing across all 14 items. Items 4, 5, 6, 7, 9, 10, and 13 are the positively stated items.

The PSS-14 was designed for use with community samples whose members have at least a junior high school education. The items are easy to understand, and the response alternatives are simple to grasp. Moreover, as previously noted, the questions are quite general in nature and hence relatively free of content specific to any subpopulation group.

Source: Exhibit courtesy of Dr. Sheldon Cohen, Carnegie Mellon University, Pittsburgh, PA, USA.

Exhibit 6-2 Interest Checklist

Activity	What has been your level of interest						Do you currently participate in this activity?		Would you like to pursue this in the future?	
	In the past 10 years			In the past year						
	Strong	Some	No	Strong	Some	No	Yes	No	Yes	No
Gardening/yard work										
Sewing/ needle work										
Playing cards										
Foreign languages										
Church activities										
Radio										
Walking										
Car repair										
Writing										
Dancing										
Golf										
Football										
Listening to popular music										
Puzzles										
Holiday activities										
Pets/livestock										
Movies										
Listening to classical music										
Speeches/lectures										
Swimming										
Bowling										
Visiting										
Mending										
Checkers/chess										
Barbecues										
Reading										
Traveling										
Parties										
Wrestling										
Housecleaning										
Model building										
Television										
Concerts										
Pottery										

Source: Exhibit courtesy of MOHO Clearinghouse, University of Illinois at Chicago, USA

(continues)

Exhibit 6-2 Interest Checklist *(continued)*

Activity	What has been your level of interest						Do you currently participate in this activity?		Would you like to pursue this in the future?	
	In the past 10 years			In the past year						
	Strong	Some	No	Strong	Some	No	Yes	No	Yes	No
Camping										
Laundry/ironing										
Politics										
Table games										
Home decorating										
Clubs/lodge										
Singing										
Scouting										
Clothes										
Handicrafts										
Hairstyling										
Cycling										
Attending plays										
Bird watching										
Dating										
Auto racing										
Home repairs										
Exercise										
Hunting										
Woodworking										
Pool										
Driving										
Child care										
Tennis										
Cooking/baking										
Basketball										
History										
Collecting										
Fishing										
Science										
Leatherwork										
Shopping										
Photography										
Painting/drawing										

Source: Exhibit courtesy of MOHO Clearinghouse, University of Illinois at Chicago, USA

Exhibit 6-3 Safety Assessment of Function and the Environment for Rehabilitation Report

COTA

Community Occupational Therapists and Associates
3101 Bathurst St., Suite 200
Toronto, Ontario M6A 2A6
Telephone: (416) 785-8797 Fax: 785-9358

S	Safety
A	Assessment of
F	Function and the
E	Environment for
R	Rehabilitation

CLIENT'S NAME: _____John Doe_____ DATE: ___M/D/Y___ TIME: ____1:30pm____

THERAPIST: _____ CLIENT'S AGE: ___80___

TYPE OF HOUSING: House/Apartment/Other

ADDRESSED   - A
NOT APPLICABLE   - N/A
PROBLEM   - P

		A	N/A	P	COMMENTS
	LIVING SITUATION				
1.	Access/entrance/security	✓			
2.	Lives alone/with others	✓			– lives with wife, very supportive
3.	Support – family/friends	✓			
4.	Stairs/ramps – condition	✓			
5.	Railings	✓		✓	– railing on one side only – both sides preferable
6.	Elevator	✓	✓		
7.	Environment cluttered	✓			
8.	Scatter rugs/flooring	✓			
9.	Wires/cords	✓			
	MOBILITY				
10.	Positioning	✓			
11.	Transfers	✓			
12.	Walking/devices	✓		✓	– uses walker but height seems inappropriate – too low
13.	Wheelchair/scooter	✓	✓		
14.	Venturing outside	✓			
15.	Public/disabled transport	✓			
16.	Car/driving	✓			– wife drives, this is acceptable to client

Source: Exhibit courtesy of COTA Health, Toronto, Canada

Exhibit 6-4 Craig Hospital Inventory of Environmental Factors Short Form

Being an active, productive member of society includes participating in such things as working, going to school, taking care of your home, and being involved with family and friends in social, recreational and civic activities in the community. Many factors can help or improve a person's participation in these activities, but other factors can act as barriers and limit participation.

First, please tell me how often each of the following has been a barrier to your own participation in the activities that matter to you. Think about the past year, and tell me whether each item on the list below has been a problem **daily, weekly, monthly, less than monthly, or never.** If the item occurs, then answer the question as to how big a problem the item is with regard to your participation in the activities that matter to you.

(Note: If a question asks specifically about **school or work** and you neither work nor attend school, check not applicable.)

	Daily	Weekly	Monthly	Less than monthly	Never	Not applicable	Big problem	Little problem
1. In the past 12 months, how often has the availability of transportation been a problem for you?	○	○	○	○	○			
When this problem occurs has it been a big problem or a little problem?							○	○
2. In the past 12 months, how often has the natural environment – temperature, terrain, climate—made it difficult to do what you want or need to do?	○	○	○	○	○			
When this problem occurs has it been a big problem or a little problem?							○	○
3. In the past 12 months, how often have other aspects of your surroundings – lighting, noise, crowds, etc.— made it difficult to do what you want or need to do?	○	○	○	○	○			
When this problem occurs has it been a big problem or a little problem?							○	○
4. In the past 12 months, how often has the information you wanted or needed not been available in a format you can use or understand?	○	○	○	○	○			
When this problem occurs has it been a big problem or a little problem?							○	○
5. In the past 12 months, how often has the availability of healthcare services and medical care been a problem for you?	○	○	○	○	○			
When this problem occurs has it been a big problem or a little problem?							○	○
6. In the past 12 months, how often did you need someone else's help in your home and could not get it easily?	○	○	○	○	○			
When this problem occurs has it been a big problem or a little problem?							○	○
7. In the past 12 months, how often did you need someone else's help at school or work and could not get it easily?	○	○	○	○	○	○		
When this problem occurs has it been a big problem or a little problem?							○	○

Exhibit 6-4 Craig Hospital Inventory of Environmental Factors Short Form *(continued)*

	Daily	Weekly	Monthly	Less than monthly	Never	Not applicable	Big problem	Little problem
8. In the past 12 months, how often have other people's attitudes toward you been a problem at home?	○	○	○	○	○			
When this problem occurs has it been a big problem or a little problem?							○	○
9. In the past 12 months, how often have other people's attitudes toward you been a problem at school or work?	○	○	○	○	○	○		
When this problem occurs has it been a big problem or a little problem?							○	○
10. In the past 12 months, how often did you experience prejudice or discrimination?	○	○	○	○	○			
When this problem occurs has it been a big problem or a little problem?							○	○
11. In the past 12 months, how often did the policies and rules of businesses and organizations make problems for you?	○	○	○	○	○			
When this problem occurs has it been a big problem or a little problem?							○	○
12. In the past 12 months, how often did government programs and policies make it difficult to do what you want or need to do?	○	○	○	○	○			
When this problem occurs has it been a big problem or a little problem?							○	○

Source: Exhibit courtesy of Craig Hospital, Englewood, Colorado, USA (for information contact charrison-felix@craighospital.org or dmellick@craighospital.org)

Exhibit 6-5 Community Integration Measure (CIM)

For this first questionnaire, I want you to think about the community you live in, and for each of the following statements, please indicate whether you agree or disagree:

☐ 1. I feel like part of this community, like I belong here.

__ always agree __ sometimes agree __ neutral __ sometimes disagree __ always disagree

☐ 2. I know my way around this community.

__ always agree __ sometimes agree __ neutral __ sometimes disagree __ always disagree

☐ 3. I know the rules in this community and I can fit in with them.

__ always agree __ sometimes agree __ neutral __ sometimes disagree __ always disagree

☐ 4. I know that I am accepted in this community.

__ always agree __ sometimes agree __ neutral __ sometimes disagree __ always disagree

☐ 5. I can be independent in this community.

__ always agree __ sometimes agree __ neutral __ sometimes disagree __ always disagree

☐ 6. I like where I'm living now.

__ always agree __ sometimes agree __ neutral __ sometimes disagree __ always disagree

☐ 7. There are people I feel close to in this community.

__ always agree __ sometimes agree __ neutral __ sometimes disagree __ always disagree

☐ 8. I know a number of people in this community well enough to say hello and have them say hello back.

__ always agree __ sometimes agree __ neutral __ sometimes disagree __ always disagree

☐ 9. There are things that I can do in this community for fun in my free time.

__ always agree __ sometimes agree __ neutral __ sometimes disagree __ always disagree

☐ 10. I have something to do in this community during that main part of my day that is useful and productive.

__ always agree __ sometimes agree __ neutral __ sometimes disagree __ always disagree

Coding:

5, always agree; 4, sometimes agree; 3, neutral; 2, sometimes disagree; 1, always disagree

Source: Exhibit courtesy of Dr. Mary Ann McColl, PhD, Queen's University, Kingston, Ontario, Canada.

Therapeutic Interventions: Physical Disabilities (Days 7–15)

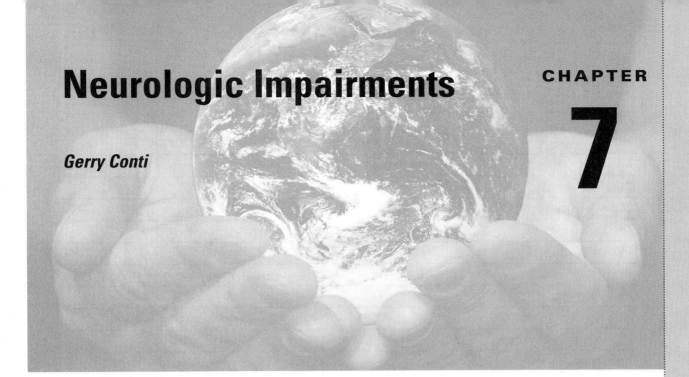

Neurologic Impairments

Gerry Conti

CHAPTER

7

OBJECTIVES

1. Describe briefly the etiology and pathology of each condition.
2. Describe the common signs and symptoms associated with each condition.
3. Cite the precautions and contraindications for each condition that a therapist must be aware of prior to intervention.
4. Apply the knowledge of conditions to intervention strategies.

INTRODUCTION

Welcome to Days 7 and 8 of your study guide. In this chapter you will review medical conditions that affect adults. Work through the outline to review each set of conditions, then complete the work sheets without referring back to the outline. If you can identify the major aspects of each condition, go on to the next set of conditions. Knowing this foundation information will provide a sound basis for assessment and intervention questions. You will have a quick understanding of the common problems seen with a particular impairment and will be able to identify types of interventions that may be needed. This will save time while you take the certification examination so that you can spend more time thinking about the appropriate intervention for the specific question.

OUTLINE

1. **Common adult physical conditions**
2. **Stroke**

(Atchison & Dirette, 2007, pp. 167–194)
(Pendleton & Schultz-Krohn, 2006, pp. 802–808)
(Radomski & Latham, 2008, pp. 1002–1011)

Table 7-1 Key Terms 7a

Radomski & Latham, 2008, p. 1010	Pendleton & Schultz-Krohn, 2006, pp. 802, 838	Atchison & Dirette, 2007, p. 167
Aphasia	Dysarthria	Agnosia
Apraxia	Ischemia	Aneurysm
Cognitive deficits	Stroke	Apraxia
Depression	Transient ischemic attack	Arteriovenous
Dysarthria	Traumatic brain injury	Atheroma
Dysphagia		Atherosclerosis
Hemianopsia		Brain attack
Hemiplegia/hemiparesis		Cerebrovascular accident
Incontinence		Stroke
Somatosensory deficits		
Stroke		

i. Etiology and pathology

(Atchison & Dirette, 2007, pp. 168, 170–173)
(Pendleton & Schultz-Krohn, 2006, pp. 803–808)
(Radomski & Latham, 2008, pp. 1002, 1008)

    I.   Syndromes leading to stroke

ii. Signs and symptoms

(Atchison & Dirette, 2007, pp. 179–180)
(Pendleton & Schultz-Krohn, 2006, pp. 803–808)
(Radomski & Latham, 2008, pp. 1009–1010)

    I.   *Note:* Damage to the middle cerebral artery (MCA) is most common cause of stroke. Therefore, you should know the common impairments resulting from MCA damage (see especially Pendleton & Schultz-Krohn, 2006, pp. 805–806).

    II.   Contralateral hemiplegia, hemiparesis

    III.   Contralateral somatosensory deficits

    IV.   Aphasia

        a. Types: Broca, Wernicke, global, anomic (see especially Pendleton & Schultz-Krohn, 2006, p. 822)

        b. *Note:* Persons with right hemiplegia (left lesion) tend to have aphasia.

    V.   Dysarthria

    VI.   Dysphagia (see Radomski & Latham, 2008, p. 1325)

    VII.   Visual deficits, including homonymous hemianopsia

    VIII.   Perceptual deficits, including visual inattention (unilateral neglect, hemi-inattention, spatial–body neglect), apraxia (motor, ideational), figure–ground

        a. *Note:* Persons with left hemiplegia (right lesion) tend to have perceptual deficits.

    IX.   Cognitive deficits, including attention, organization and sequencing, initiation and perseverance, and executive function, including problem solving

    X.   Neurobehavioral deficits, including perseveration, lability, poor judgment, apathy, and depression

    XI.   Incontinence

iii. Precautions and contraindications

(Atchison & Dirette, 2007, p. 181)
(Pendleton & Schultz-Krohn, 2006, pp. 815–831)
(Radomski & Latham, 2008, pp. 1022–1023)

    I. Deep venous thrombosis, respiratory infections, cardiac disease, and bowel and bladder dysfunction (see also Pendleton & Schultz-Krohn, 2006, p. 809)
    II. Subluxation
    III. Pressure ulcers (see also Atchison & Dirette, 2007, pp. 326–327; Pendleton & Schultz-Krohn, 2006, p. 908)
    IV. Falls (see only Radomski & Latham, 2008, p. 1023)
    V. Dysphagia (see also Pendleton & Schultz-Krohn, 2006, p. 625; Radomski & Latham, 2008, p. 1325)
    VI. Visual inattention (see also Pendleton & Schultz-Krohn, 2006, p. 557; Radomski & Latham, 2008, p. 734)
    VII. Seizures (see only Pendleton & Schultz-Krohn, 2006, pp. 821–822)
iv. Impact on occupational performance and performance skills
    I. Impairment of activities of daily living (ADL) and instrumental activities of daily living (IADL) occupational performance. Impairment depends on severity of stroke. If severe, all areas of ADL and IADL will be affected.
    II. Impairment of sensorimotor performance skills. The major motor impairment is hemiplegia contralateral to the lesion site. ***Note:*** Read the exam question carefully to determine whether it refers to the lesion site or the side of the body with hemiplegia.
    III. Impairment of perceptual and cognitive performance skills. Persons with left cerebral impairment (right hemiplegia) typically have difficulty expressing and/or understanding communication. Persons with right cerebral impairment (left hemiplegia) typically have difficulty with perceptual and behavioral impairments. Homonymous hemianopsia is the most common visual impairment in stroke.
    IV. Impairment of psychosocial adjustment
b. Traumatic brain injury (TBI)

(Atchison & Dirette, 2007, pp. 231–246)
(Pendleton & Schultz-Krohn, 2006, pp. 838–872)
(Radomski & Latham, 2008, pp. 1042–1078)

Table 7-2 Key Terms 7b

Radomski & Latham, 2008, p. 1043	Pendleton & Schultz-Krohn, 2006, p. 838	Atchison & Dirette, 2007, p. 231
Agitation	Decerebrate rigidity	Anterograde amnesia
Anterograde amnesia	Decorticate rigidity	Aspiration
Diffuse axonal injury	Diffuse axonal injury	Coma
Hematoma	Posttraumatic amnesia	Decerebrate rigidity
Mild brain injury		Decorticate rigidity
Posttraumatic amnesia		Hydrocephalus
		Mild traumatic brain injury
		Moderate traumatic brain injury
		Severe traumatic brain injury

i. Etiology and pathology

(Atchison & Dirette, 2007, pp. 232–233)
(Pendleton & Schultz-Krohn, 2006, pp. 840–842)
(Radomski & Latham, 2008, pp. 1043–1045)

I. Etiology: The three leading causes of TBI are moving vehicle accidents, violence, and falls.

II. Level of disability: Mild, moderate, severe (Glasgow Coma Scale, RLAH Levels of Cognitive Functioning). ***Note:*** The level of disability determines the severity of signs and symptoms. At all levels there are cognitive and/or neurobehavioral symptoms.

III. Primary brain damage may be focal or diffuse.

    a. Focal: Contusion, laceration, intracranial hematoma (epidural, subdural)

    b. Diffuse axonal injury: Damaged brainstem, cerebellar pathways

IV. Secondary brain damage results from hypoxia.

    a. Coma

    b. Hydrocephalus or increased intracranial pressure

    c. Brain ischemia or hemorrhage

    d. Hypothermia

    e. Electrolyte imbalances

    f. Hyperventilation

    g. Abnormal responses of autonomic nervous system

V. Common associated pathology

    a. Posttraumatic seizures (see especially Pendleton & Schultz-Krohn, 2006, pp. 841–842)

    b. Increased intracranial pressure and cerebral edema

    c. Fractures

    d. Cardiovascular complications

    e. Respiratory dysfunction

    f. Cranial nerve damage, for example, olfactory (I) and visual nerves (II, III, IV, VI)

ii. Signs and symptoms

(Atchison & Dirette, 2007, pp. 234–239)
(Pendleton & Schultz-Krohn, 2006, pp. 842–853)
(Radomski & Latham, 2008, p. 1047)

I. Coma/level of consciousness

II. Decorticate rigidity, decerebrate rigidity, and motor rigidity (see especially Pendleton & Schultz-Krohn, 2006, pp. 845–846)

III. Cranial nerve dysfunction (see especially Atchison & Dirette, 2007, pp. 236–237)

IV. Abnormal muscle tone

V. Primitive reflexes

VI. Muscle weakness

VII. Ataxia

VIII. Tremor (see especially Pendleton & Schultz-Krohn, 2006, p. 847)

IX. Decreased sensation

X. Dysphagia (see also Pendleton & Schultz-Krohn, 2006, p. 625; Radomski & Latham, 2008, p. 1325)

XI. Postural deficits

XII. Joint motion limitations

XIII. Decreased functional endurance

XIV. Poor integration of total body movements

iii. Precautions and contraindications

(Pendleton & Schultz-Krohn, 2006, pp. 842–851)
(Radomski & Latham, 2008, p. 1051)

    I. Posttraumatic seizures
    II. Increased intracranial pressure and cerebral edema
    III. Fractures
    IV. Cardiovascular complications
    V. Respiratory dysfunction
    VI. Cranial nerve damage
    VII. Pressure ulcers
    VIII. Aspiration pneumonia (see especially Pendleton & Schultz-Krohn, 2006, pp. 615–616)

iv. Impact on occupational performance and performance skills
    I. Impairment of ADL and IADL occupations. All are affected, irrespective of severity of TBI.
    II. Impairment of sensorimotor performance skills. All are affected.
    III. Impairment of visual, perceptual, cognitive, and neurobehavioral performance skills. All are affected, although perceptual deficits may be less affected than visual deficits.
    IV. Impairment of psychosocial adjustment.

c. Spinal cord injury (SCI)

(Atchison & Dirette, 2007, pp. 311–340)
(Pendleton & Schultz-Krohn, 2006, pp. 903–930)
(Radomski & Latham, 2008, pp. 1171–1213)

Table 7-3 Key Terms 7c

Radomski & Latham, 2008, p. 1172	Pendleton & Schultz-Krohn, 2006, p. 903	Atchison & Dirette, 2007, p. 311
Complete injury	Autonomic dysreflexia	Autonomic dysreflexia (hyperreflexia)
Dermatome	Heterotopic ossification	Cauda equina
Incomplete injury	Paraplegia	Heterotopic ossification
Paraplegia	Pressure ulcer	Pressure ulcer
Tenodesis grasp	Spasticity	Scoliosis
Tetraplegia	Tetraplegia/quadriplegia	Spinal shock

i. Etiology and pathology

(Atchison & Dirette, 2007, pp. 314, 317–318)
(Pendleton & Schultz-Krohn, 2006, p. 904)
(Radomski & Latham, 2008, p. 1172)

    I. Male young adults most common
    II. Motor vehicle accidents most common

ii. Signs and symptoms

(Atchison & Dirette, 2007, pp. 319–322)
(Pendleton & Schultz-Krohn, 2006, pp. 905–906)
(Radomski & Latham, 2008, pp. 1173–1174)

    I. Neurological classification
        a. Upper motor neuron
        b. American Spinal Injury Association (ASIA) classification system

        i. Sensory and motor systems are rated as complete, incomplete, or normal

    c. Syndromes: Anterior cord, Brown-Séquard, central (cervical) cord

    d. Cauda equina injury

    e. *Note:* C5, C6, and T10 are the most common levels of injury. Know the available function especially for these injury levels.

   II. Paralysis and loss of all or some sensation below the neurological level

iii. Precautions and contraindications

(Atchison & Dirette, 2007, pp. 322–327)
(Pendleton & Schultz-Krohn, 2006, pp. 908–909)
(Radomski & Latham, 2008, pp. 1175–1180)

    I. Decreased vital capacity
    II. Autonomic dysreflexia (hyperreflexia)
    III. Orthostatic hypotension (postural hypotension)
    IV. Pressure ulcers
    V. Bowel and bladder dysfunction
    VI. Thermal dysregulation
    VII. Pain
    VIII. Fatigue
    IX. Deep vein thrombosis
    X. Spasticity and spasms
    XI. Heterotopic ossification (ectopic bone)
    XII. Osteoporosis
    XIII. Decreased motor skill for sexual intimacy

iv. Impact on occupational performance and performance skills

(Atchison & Dirette, 2007, pp. 330–332)
(Pendleton & Schultz-Krohn, 2006, pp. 917–925)
(Radomski & Latham, 2008, pp. 1199–1210)

    I. Impairment of ADL and IADL occupations based on neurological level.

        a. *Note:* Know the possible functional outcomes, equipment requirements, and assistance requirements for C5, C6, and T10.

        b. *Note:* Also know at what level respiration is present, hand musculature is fully innervated, and at what level trunk balance, independent wheelchair mobility, and ambulation become feasible.

    II. Impairment of all sensorimotor performance skills below the neurological level

    III. Impairment of visual, perceptual, cognitive, and neurobehavioral performance skills. Not typically affected, unless there is a combination of brain and spinal injury.

    IV. Impairment of psychosocial adjustment

d. Neurodegenerative diseases

(Atchison & Dirette, 2007, pp. 261–274)
(Pendleton & Schultz-Krohn, 2006, pp. 873–902)
(Radomski & Latham, 2008, pp. 1079–1105)

Table 7-4 Stroke, TBI, and SCI Work Sheet

Condition	Etiology & Pathology	Signs & Symptoms	Precautions & Contraindications	Application to Practice Framework
Stroke (CVA)				
Traumatic brain injury (TBI)				
Spinal cord injury (SCI)				

Table 7-5 Key Terms 7d

Radomski & Latham, 2008, p. 1080	Pendleton & Schultz-Krohn, 2006, p. 873	Atchison & Dirette, 2007, p. 261
Akinesia	Chorea	Agnosia
Axonal transaction	Exacerbation	Cogwheel rigidity
Bradykinesia	Fasciculation	Demyelination
Cogwheel rigidity	Remission	Dysarthria
Fasciculation	Rigidity	Dysesthesia
Festinating gait		Myelin
Myelin		Nystagmus
Rigidity		Optic neuritis

Discussions of neurogenerative diseases are presented in the following outline sections. ***Note:*** Remember that myasthenia gravis and muscular dystrophy are also neurodegenerative diseases (Atchison & Dirette, 2007, multiple sclerosis, Parkinson disease, amyotrophic lateral sclerosis; Pendleton & Schultz-Krohn, 2006, multiple sclerosis, Parkinson disease, amyotrophic lateral sclerosis, Guillain-Barré syndrome; Radomski & Latham, 2008, multiple sclerosis, Parkinson disease, amyotrophic lateral sclerosis, Alzheimer disease, Huntington disease, pp. 1083–1096)

   i.   Multiple sclerosis
   I.   Etiology and pathology

(Atchison & Dirette, 2007, p. 262)
(Pendleton & Schultz-Krohn, 2006, p. 889)
(Radomski & Latham, 2008, p. 1083)

   a. Cause unknown
   II.   Signs and symptoms

(Atchison & Dirette, 2007, pp. 265–266)
(Pendleton & Schultz-Krohn, 2006, pp. 889–890)
(Radomski & Latham, 2008, pp. 1084–1086)

   a. Symptoms, intensity, and effect on function are highly individual and variable
   b. Characterized by periods of exacerbation and remission
   c. The most common deficit is fatigue.
   d. Diagnostic criteria include:
      i. Weakness
      ii. Visual deficits: Diplopia, nystagmus, loss of vision in one eye, blurred vision
      iii. Dysmetria
      iv. Sensory deficits: Vibration, position sense
   e. Additional motor symptoms may include:
      i. Tremor and ataxia
      ii. Dysphagia
      iii. Dysarthria
      iv. Neurogenic bladder
   f. Additional sensory disturbances may include pain.
   g. Cognitive disturbances may include:
      i. Memory loss
      ii. Decreased attention span
   h. Psychological disturbances may include:
      i. Depression or euphoria
      ii. Impulsivity
      iii. Lability
   III.   Precautions and contraindications for each condition are embedded within the information on signs and symptoms.
   IV.   Impact on occupational performance and performance skills
   a. Refer to texts on neurodegenerative diseases. Information on occupational performance is embedded within the text.
   b. ***Note:*** The ability to perform routine and preferred occupations deteriorates.
   c. All ADL and IADL deteriorate.
   d. There is increasing impairment of sensorimotor performance.
   e. There is increasing impairment of visual, perceptual, cognitive, and neurobehavioral performance skills.
   f. There is difficulty with psychosocial adjustment.

ii. Parkinson disease

    I. Etiology and pathology

(Atchison & Dirette, 2007, p. 265)
(Pendleton & Schultz-Krohn, 2006, p. 893)
(Radomski & Latham, 2008, p. 1090)

        a. Typically after age 55 years
        b. Slowly progressive and degenerative
        c. Hereditary and/or environmental cause
        d. Damage to basal ganglia

    II. Signs and symptoms

(Atchison & Dirette, 2007, pp. 265–266)
(Pendleton & Schultz-Krohn, 2006, pp. 893–897)
(Radomski & Latham, 2008, pp. 1090–1092)

        a. Hoen and Yahr scale for identification of stages
            i. Stage I: Signs are unilateral
            ii. Stage II: Signs are bilateral
            iii. Stage III: Signs are bilateral, balance is impaired
            iv. Stage IV: Disabling signs
            v. Stage V: Confined to bed or wheelchair
        b. Diagnostic criteria include:
            i. Resting tremor (pill-rolling)
            ii. Cogwheel rigidity
             iii. Voluntary movement deficits
                 1. Akinesia (freezing, that is, difficulty initiating movement)
                 2. Bradykinesia and akinesia
        c. Additional motor deficits may include:
            i. Gait disturbances (festinating gait, shuffle)
            ii. Masked facial expression
            iii. Dysphagia – *swallowing*
            iv. Dysarthria – *no articulation*
            v. Oculomotor deficits (blink, fixation, scanning)
            vi. Bowel and bladder dysfunction
        d. Sensory disturbances may include:
            i. Numbness, tingling, burning
            ii. Fatigue
        e. Visual/perceptual disturbances may include visuospatial impairment.
        f. Cognitive disturbances may include:
            i. Difficulty with:
                 1. Abstract reasoning
                 2. Processing information provided simultaneously
            ii. Decreased attention span
            iii. Potential for dementia in late stages
        g. Psychological disturbances may include depression

    III. Precautions and contraindications for each condition are embedded within the information on signs and symptoms.

    IV. Impact on occupational performance and performance skills
        a. Refer to texts on neurodegenerative diseases. Information on occupational performance is embedded within the text.
        b. *Note:* ADL and IADL deteriorate.
        c. There is increasing impairment of sensorimotor performance.
        d. There is increasing impairment of visual, perceptual, cognitive, and neurobehavioral performance skills.
        e. There is difficulty with psychosocial adjustment.

   iii. Amyotrophic lateral sclerosis (Lou Gehrig disease)
      I. Etiology and pathology

(Atchison & Dirette, 2007, p. 268)
(Pendleton & Schultz-Krohn, 2006, pp. 875–876)
(Radomski & Latham, 2008, p. 1092)

        a. Fatal
        b. Most common motor neuron disease in adults
        c. More common in males than females
      II. Signs and symptoms

(Atchison & Dirette, 2007, pp. 268–269)
(Pendleton & Schultz-Krohn, 2006, pp. 876–877)
(Radomski & Latham, 2008, pp. 1092–1094)

        a. Fatal; survival after diagnosis is 1–5 years, with a mean of 3 years.
        b. Diagnostic criteria are variable and may include:
          i. Focal weakness: Arm, leg, or bulbar
          ii. Fatigue
          iii. Emotional lability
        c. Later signs may include:
          i. Muscle atrophy
          ii. Muscle cramping and fasciculations (twitching)
          iii. Spasticity
          iv. Dysphagia
          v. Dysarthria
          vi. Difficulty in respiration
        d. Sensory is not affected at any stage.
        e. Vision is not affected at any stage.
        f. Cognition is not affected at any stage.
        g. Psychological disturbances may include depression.
     III. Precautions and contraindications for each condition are embedded within the information on signs and symptoms.
     IV. Impact on occupational performance and performance skills
        a. Refer to texts on neurodegenerative diseases. Information on occupational performance is embedded within the text.
        b. *Note:* ADL and IADL deteriorate.
        c. There is increasing impairment of sensorimotor performance.
        d. There is difficulty with psychosocial adjustment.
  iv. Guillain-Barré syndrome
      I. Etiology and pathology

(Radomski & Latham, 2008, p. 1096)

        a. Inflammatory disease resulting in demyelinization of peripheral nerves
        b. Rapidly progressive, ascending paralysis from feet
        c. Etiology unknown
      II. Signs and symptoms

(Radomski & Latham, 2008, pp. 1096–1097)

        a. Motor deficits include weakness or paralysis.
          i. Phase 1: Distal to proximal paralysis
          ii. Phase 2: Plateau
          iii. Phase 3: Partial or full recovery proximal to distal
        b. Sensory disturbances may include:
          i. Paresthesias

          ii. Fatigue

          iii. Vision is not affected at any stage.

          iv. Cognition is not affected at any stage.

          v. Psychological disturbances may include depression.

III. Precautions and contraindications for each condition are embedded within the information on signs and symptoms.

IV. Impact on occupational performance and performance skills

    a. Refer to texts on neurodegenerative diseases. Information on occupational performance is embedded within the text.

    b. *Note:* ADL and IADL deteriorate then partially or fully recover.

    c. There is increasing impairment of sensorimotor performance.

    d. There is difficulty with psychosocial adjustment.

v. Alzheimer disease

I. Etiology and pathology

(Pendleton & Schultz-Krohn, 2006, pp. 880–881)

    a. Age and family history are primary risk factors

II. Signs and symptoms

(Pendleton & Schultz-Krohn, 2006, pp. 881–886)

    a. Life expectancy 8–10 years following diagnosis

    b. Diagnostic criteria include:

        i. Impairment in recent memory

        ii. Apraxia, aphasia, agnosia, or impaired executive function

    c. Cognitive disturbances

        i. Increasing impairment in memory

        ii. Aphasia, apraxia, agnosia, or impaired executive function

    d. Visuospatial dysfunction

    e. Behavioral disturbances may include:

        i. Irritability in early stages

        ii. Agitation in later stages

    f. Sensory and motor changes may occur in mid- to late stages

III. Precautions and contraindications for each condition are embedded within the information on signs and symptoms.

IV. Impact on occupational performance and performance skills

    a. Refer to texts on neurodegenerative diseases. Information on occupational performance is embedded within the text.

    b. *Note:* ADL and IADL deteriorate.

    c. There is increasing impairment of sensorimotor performance.

    d. Visual, perceptual, cognitive, and neurobehavioral performance deteriorate in later stages.

    e. There is difficulty with psychosocial adjustment.

vi. Huntington disease

I. Etiology and pathology

(Pendleton & Schultz-Krohn, 2006, pp. 886–887)

    a. Hereditary; neurogenetic basis

    b. Fatal

    c. Damage to basal ganglia

II. Signs and symptoms

(Pendleton & Schultz-Krohn, 2006, pp. 887–889)

    a. Fatal

    b. Motor, cognitive, and behavioral signs

    c. Initial symptoms vary but most commonly include:
- **i.** Changes in behavior
- **ii.** Changes in cognition
- **iii.** Choreiform movements (rapid, involuntary, irregular movements)

    d. Additional motor changes include:
- **i.** Staggering gait with disease progression
- **ii.** Dysphagia in later stages
- **iii.** Dysarthria

    e. Visual changes may include:
- **i.** Nystagmus
- **ii.** Difficulty with ocular pursuit, saccades

    f. Cognitive changes include decreased:
- **i.** Executive function
- **ii.** Memory

    g. Behavioral changes include:
- **i.** Irritability
- **ii.** Depression
- **iii.** Behavioral outbursts

III. Precautions and contraindications for each condition are embedded within the information on signs and symptoms.

IV. Impact on occupational performance and performance skills
    a. Refer to texts on neurodegenerative diseases. Information on occupational performance is embedded within the text.
    b. *Note:* ADL and IADL deteriorate.
    c. There is increasing impairment of sensorimotor performance.
    d. There is increasing impairment of visual, perceptual, cognitive, and neurobehavioral performance skills.
    e. There is difficulty with psychosocial adjustment.

Table 7-6 Neurodegenerative Diseases Work Sheet

Condition	Etiology & Pathology	Signs & Symptoms	Precautions	Application to Practice Framework
Multiple sclerosis				
Parkinson disease				
Amyotrophic lateral sclerosis				
Guillain-Barré syndrome				
Alzheimer disease				
Huntington disease				

REFERENCES

Atchison, B., & Dirette, D. (Eds.). (2007). *Conditions in occupational therapy: Effect on occupational performance.* Philadelphia: Lippincott Williams & Wilkins.

Pendleton, H. M., & Schultz-Krohn, W. (Eds.). (2006). *Pedretti's occupational therapy: Practice skills for physical dysfunction* (6th ed.). St. Louis, MO: Mosby.

Radomski, M. V., & Latham, C. A. T. (Eds.). (2008). *Occupational therapy for physical dysfunction* (6th ed.). Philadelphia: Lippincott Williams & Wilkins.

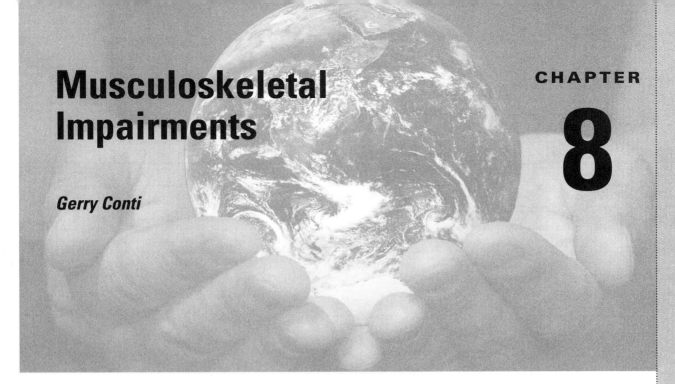

Musculoskeletal Impairments

CHAPTER

8

Gerry Conti

OBJECTIVES

1. Describe briefly the etiology and pathology of each condition.
2. Describe the common signs and symptoms associated with each condition.
3. Cite the precautions and contraindications for each condition that a therapist must be aware of prior to intervention.
4. Apply the knowledge of conditions to intervention strategies.

INTRODUCTION

Welcome to Days 9 and 10 of your study guide. In this chapter you will review medical conditions that affect adults. Work through the outline to review each set of conditions, then complete the work sheets without referring back to the outline. If you can identify the major aspects of each condition, go on to the next set of conditions. Knowing this foundation information will provide a sound basis for assessment and intervention questions. You will have a quick understanding of the common problems seen with a particular impairment and will be able to identify types of interventions that may be needed. This will save time while you take the certification examination so that you can spend more time thinking about the appropriate intervention for the specific question.

OUTLINE

1. **Common orthopedic conditions**
   a. Hip fractures and hip replacements

   (Pendleton & Schultz-Krohn, 2006, pp. 1020–1024)
   (Radomski & Latham, 2008, pp. 1117–1121)

      i. ***Note:*** These are very common conditions seen by occupational therapists (OTs). Know these conditions and their corresponding assessments and interventions.

Table 8-1 Key Terms 8a

Radomski & Latham, 2008, p. 1107	Pendleton & Schultz-Krohn, 2006, pp. 1022–1024
Clinical union	Arthroplasty
	Avascular necrosis
	Minimally invasive technique
	Open reduction and internal fixation
	Osteoporosis

ii. Etiology and pathology

(Pendleton & Schultz-Krohn, 2006, p. 1117)
(Radomski & Latham, 2008, p. 1022)

    I. Trauma
    II. Osteoporosis, in aging, is often a contributing factor
    III. More common in women

iii. Signs and symptoms

(Pendleton & Schultz-Krohn, 2006, p. 1117)
(Radomski & Latham, 2008, p. 1022)

    I. Pain
    II. Reduced trunk and lower extremity mobility following surgery

iv. Precautions and contraindications

(Pendleton & Schultz-Krohn, 2006, p. 1117)
(Radomski & Latham, 2008, p. 1022)

    I. Weight-bearing restrictions (***Note:*** Know these.)
    II. Movement restrictions (***Note:*** Know these.)
    III. Common comorbid conditions
        a. Osteoporosis
        b. Diabetes mellitus
        c. Hypertension

v. Impact on occupational performance and performance skills

(Pendleton & Schultz-Krohn, 2006, p. 1117–1118)
(Radomski & Latham, 2008, p. 1028)

    I. Impairment of activities of daily living (ADL) and instrumental activities of daily living (IADL) on occupational performance during the healing process
    II. Altered sensation and/or pain at incision site
    III. Fear of movement or falling again may be present.

b. Back impairment: Low back pain

(Pendleton & Schultz-Krohn, 2006, pp. 1036–1056)
(Radomski & Latham, 2008, pp. 1121–1124)

Table 8-2 Key Terms 8b

Radomski & Latham, 2008	Pendleton & Schultz-Krohn, 2006, p. 1044
None	Neutral spine

i. Etiology and pathology

(Pendleton & Schultz-Krohn, 2006, p. 1037)
(Radomski & Latham, 2008, p. 1122)

    I.   Low back pain is found in 80% of the adult population of the world; less than 1% is due to serious spinal disease.

    II.   Types of low back pain

(Pendleton & Schultz-Krohn, 2006, p. 1039)

        a. Acute
            i.   90% resolves within the first 6 weeks.
            ii.   An additional 5% resolves within 12 weeks.
        b. Chronic: Pain occurs beyond 3 months following surgery

ii. Etiology

(Pendleton & Schultz-Krohn, 2006, p. 1039)
(Radomski & Latham, 2008, p. 1122)

    I.   Cumulative postural stress is the primary factor

    II.   Other contributing factors
        a. Poor physical fitness
        b. Obesity
        c. Reduced muscle strength and endurance

iii. Pathology may include:

(Pendleton & Schultz-Krohn, 2006, p. 1039)

    I.   Scoliosis
    II.   Kyphosis
    III.   Sciatica
    IV.   Spinal stenosis
    V.   Facet joint pain
    VI.   Spondylolysis
    VII.   Spondylolisthesis
    VIII. Herniated nucleus pulposus

iv. Signs and symptoms

(Radomski & Latham, 2008, p. 1122)

    I.   Acute symptoms (present less than 3 months)
        a. Pain
        b. Spasms
        c. Muscle guarding
        d. Limited postural flexibility
        e. Anxiety
    II.   Chronic symptoms (present beyond 3 months postinjury)
        a. Pain
        b. Illness behavior
        c. Impaired sleep

v. Precautions and contraindications
    I.   Exacerbation of pathology
    II.   Comorbid conditions
    III.   Muscle fatigue

vi. Impact on occupational performance and performance skills
    I.   Impairment of ADL and IADL occupational performance
    II.   Altered sensation and/or pain at incision site

Table 8-3 KeyTerms 8c

Radomski & Latham, 2008, pp. 1264–1270, 1132	Pendleton & Schultz-Krohn, 2006, pp. 1095–1130
Above-knee amputation	Acquired amputation
Below-knee amputation	Transfemoral amputation
Neuroma	Transhumoral amputation
Phantom limb	Transradial amputation
Phantom sensations	Transtibial amputation
Residual limb	Syme amputation

     III.   Fear of lifting or movement may be present

c. Amputations

(Pendleton & Schultz-Krohn, 2006, pp. 1095–1130)
(Radomski & Latham, 2008, pp. 1264–1294)

   i.   Etiology and pathology

(Pendleton & Schultz-Krohn, 2006, p. 1096)
(Radomski & Latham, 2008, p. 1265)

     I.   The ratio of upper : lower limb loss is 1:3
     II.   In adults, frequently work related
     III.   Lower extremity (LE) amputation
         a. Primary cause: Peripheral vascular disease (PVD) associated with smoking and diabetes
         b. Trauma
     IV.   Upper extremity (UE) amputation
         a. Primary cause is trauma
     V.   Other causes of amputation
         a. Peripheral vasospastic diseases
         b. Chronic infection (diabetes mellitus as comorbid condition)
         c. Chemical, thermal, or electrical injuries
         d. Malignant tumor
     VI.   Classification system

(Radomski & Latham, 2008, p. 1265)

         a. Transhumeral (past terminology: short above-elbow amputation)
         b. Transhumeral (past terminology: above-elbow amputation)
         c. Transfemoral amputation (past terminology: above-knee amputation)
         d. Transtibial amputation (past terminology: below-knee amputation)
         e. Syme amputation (ankle disarticulation)

  ii. Signs and symptoms

(Pendleton & Schultz-Krohn, 2006, pp. 1098–1100)

     I.   Potential development of bone spurs
     II.   Sensory deficits
         a. Residual limb hyperesthesia
         b. Neuroma
         c. Phantom limb sensation
         d. Phantom limb pain

III. Psychological
   a. Initial responses may include:
      i. Shock, disbelief, rage, suicidal impulses
      ii. Grieving
   b. Later responses may include:
      i. Grieving, hopelessness, depression, bitterness, anger
iii. Precautions and contraindications

(Pendleton & Schultz-Krohn, 2006, pp. 1107–1110)
(Radomski & Latham, 2008, pp. 1267–1268)

I. Joint complications
   a. Potential decreased range of motion
II. Skin complications
   a. Preprosthetic phase
      i. Delayed healing
      ii. Extensive skin grafts
      iii. Reduction of edema
   b. Prosthetic phase
      i. Decubitus ulcers (i.e., pressure sores or ulcers)
      ii. Infected sebaceous cysts
      iii. Allergic reactions
   c. Postprosthetic phase
      i. Skin breakdown
      ii. Scar adhesions
III. Sensory complications
   a. Pain
   b. Altered body scheme or image
IV. Psychological complications
   a. Severe depression
   b. Suicidal impulses
iv. Affect on occupational performance and performance skills
      I. Impairment of ADL and IADL occupational performance
2. Altered sensation and/or pain

Table 8-4 Common Orthopedic Conditions Work Sheet

Condition	Etiology & Pathology	Signs & Symptoms	Precautions & Contraindications	Application to Practice Framework
Hip fracture or hip replacement				
Back injury or low back pain				
Amputation				

a. Arthritis conditions

    i. Osteoarthritis (degenerative joint disease)

(Pendleton & Schultz-Krohn, 2006, pp. 950–982)
(Radomski & Latham, 2008, pp. 1214–1243)

    I. Key term

        a. Crepitus (audible or palpable crunching or popping in joints)

    II. Etiology and pathology

        a. Common after age 65 years

            i. Under age 50 years, males are more affected.

            ii. Over age 50 years, females are more affected.

        b. Develops over years

        c. Risk factors include age, gender, heredity, obesity, anatomical joint abnormalities, injury, and occupational overuse of joints

        d. Affected by local, systemic, genetic, environmental, and mechanical factors

    III. Signs and symptoms

        a. Diagnostic criteria

            i. According to Altman et al., (1990) hand pain, aching, or stiffness of three or four of the following are required for a classification of osteoarthritis of the hand (p. 1601):

                1. Hard tissue enlargement of 2 or more of 10 selected joints

                2. Hard tissue enlargement of two or more distal interphalangeal joints

                3. Fewer than three swollen metacarpal joints

                4. Deformity of at least 1 of 10 selected joints

            ii. History and physical examination

            iii. Radiographic information

                1. Presence of osteophytes

                2. Asymmetrical joint space narrowing

                3. Subchondral bone sclerosis

        b. Classified as primary or secondary

            i. Primary

                1. Localized: Involvement of one or two joints

                2. Generalized: Three or more joints

            ii. Secondary

                1. Related to an identifiable cause, such as trauma, infection, aseptic necrosis

        c. Comparison to rheumatoid arthritis

            i. Affects individual joints; is *not* systemic

            ii. Noninflammatory (secondary inflammation caused by joint damage is possible)

        d. Commonly affected joints

            i. Distal/proximal interphalangeal joints

                1. *Note:* Know these deformities and implications for intervention

                2. Swan neck deformity

                3. Boutonnière deformity

            ii. Thumb carpometacarpal joints

            iii. Neck

            iv. Spine

            v. Hips

            vi. Knees

            vii. Metatarsophalangeal joints

        e. Joint pain

        f. Stiffness

            i. Morning stiffness that lasts less than 30 minutes

            ii. After periods of inactivity (gelling)

     iii. Tenderness

     iv. Limited movement

     v. Variable degree of local inflammation

  g. Crepitus

  h. Precautions and contraindications

(Pendleton & Schultz-Krohn, 2006, p. 967)

(Radomski & Latham, 2008, p. 1218)

     i. Osteophytes, erosions, joint narrowing, other skeletal problems

     ii. Pain

     iii. Fatigue

     iv. Inflamed or unstable joints

     v. Performs resistive activity or exercise with caution

     vi. Possible sensory impairments

     vii. Fragile skin due to disease or pharmaceutical side effects

IV. Effect on occupational performance and performance skills

  a. Impairment of ADL and IADL occupational performance. Impairment depends on severity of condition; if severe, all areas of ADL and IADL will be affected;

  b. Impairment of motor performance skills

  c. There is typically no impairment of perceptual and cognitive performance skills

  d. Impairment of psychosocial adjustment

ii. Rheumatoid arthritis

(Atchison & Dirette, 2007, pp. 275–310)

(Pendleton & Schultz-Krohn, 2006, pp. 950–982)

(Radomski & Latham, 2008, pp. 1214–1243)

Table 8-5 Key Terms 8d

Radomski & Latham, 2008, p. 1215	Pendleton & Schultz-Krohn, 2006, pp. 950–982	Atchison & Dirette, 2007, pp. 275–310
Crepitus	Crepitus	Anemia
Hyperalgesia	Flare	Ankylosis
Morning stiffness	Gelling	Antibodies
Rheumatoid nodules	Joint laxity	Apophyseal
	Nodes	Boutonnière deformity
	Nodules	Diarthroses
	Subluxation	Inflammation
	Synovitis	Pannus
	Systemic	Rheumatoid factor
	Tenosynovitis	Sjögren syndrome
		Swan neck deformities
		Synovial
		Tenosynovitis

I. Etiology and pathology

(Atchison & Dirette, 2007, pp. 275–279)
(Pendleton & Schultz-Krohn, 2006, pp. 951, 954–955)
(Radomski & Latham, 2008, p. 1215)

    a. Peak incidence between age 40 and 60 years; predominantly in females
    b. Insidious onset (develops within weeks or months)
    c. Multifactorial etiology: Genetic history, environment

II. Signs and symptoms

(Atchison & Dirette, 2007, pp. 295–297, see especially Table 15-3)
(Pendleton & Schultz-Krohn, 2006, pp. 955–956)
(Radomski & Latham, 2008, p. 1215)

    a. Systemic disease; the entire body is affected
    b. Characterized by inflammation of the synovial membrane (synovitis)
        i. *Note:* Know the cardinal signs of inflammation: swelling, heat, and redness. The cardinal signs of inflammation are present in many health conditions.
    c. Variable for different people and variable over the course of the disease
    d. Characterized by periods of exacerbation (flare) and remission of the disease
    e. Stages of the inflammatory process
        i. Stages may overlap, with forward and backward movement among stages
        ii. Common systemic signs and symptoms at all stages
            1. Symmetrical polyarticular pain and swelling.
            2. Morning stiffness typically 1–2 hours or more
            3. Malaise
            4. Fatigue
            5. Low-grade fever
            6. Chronic pain from joint damage
        iii. Acute signs and symptoms
            1. Rheumatoid nodules may develop.
            2. Limited movement in affected joints
            3. Pain and tenderness at rest; increases with movement
            4. Overall stiffness, weakness, tingling, or numbness
            5. Hot, red joints
            6. Low endurance
        iv. Subacute signs and symptoms
            1. Limited movement in affected joints
            2. Tingling
            3. Decreased pain and tenderness
            4. Morning, not all-day, stiffness
            5. Joints pink and warm
            6. Low endurance
        v. Chronic–active signs and symptoms
            1. Increased activity tolerance
            2. No signs of inflammation
            3. Less tingling, pain, and tenderness
            4. Endurance remains low.
    f. Characteristic joint deformities
        i. Wrist radial deviation
        ii. Metacarpophalangeal ulnar deviation
        iii. Swan neck deformity
        iv. Boutonnière deformity
        v. Thumb deformity: Nalebuff Types I, II, III

g. Other joints commonly affected

    i. Upper extremity: elbows, shoulders

    ii. Lower extremity: ankles, metatarsal joints, hips, knees

    iii. Temporomandibular joints

    iv. Cervical spine

    v. Heberden nodes (***Note:*** Know what these are.)

    vi. Subluxation, especially at the metacarpophalangeal joints

h. Precautions and contraindications

(Atchison & Dirette, 2007, pp. 291–294)
(Pendleton & Schultz-Krohn, 2006, pp. 966–969)
(Radomski & Latham, 2008, pp. 1221–1227)

    i. Fatigue is present with the systemic disease of rheumatoid arthritis.

    ii. Potential intolerance of thermal modalities

    iii. See precautions previously noted for osteoarthritis.

i. Effect on occupational performance and performance skills

    i. Impairment of ADL and IADL occupational performance. Impairment depends on severity of condition. If severe, all areas of ADL and IADL will be affected.

    ii. Impairment of motor performance skills

    iii. There is typically no impairment of perceptual and cognitive performance skills.

    iv. Impairment of psychosocial adjustment (e.g., depression)

iii. Fibromyalgia

(Radomski & Latham, 2008, pp. 1235–1237)

I. Key terms:

    a. Allodynia: Pain in response to a stimulus that is normally not painful

    b. Hyperalgesia: Increased pain in response to a stimulus that is normally painful

II. Etiology and pathology

    a. More common in women

    b. May occur in children or adults

    c. Onset is typically gradual over months or years.

III. Signs and symptoms

    a. Characterized by spontaneous exacerbations and remissions

    b. Widespread soft tissue pain, especially in neck and lower back

    c. Fatigue

    d. Nonrestorative sleep is found in 90% of people with fibromyalgia

    e. Cognitive disorders may include decreased memory, decreased organized thought processing (thinking clearly)

    f. Depression or anxiety may occur in 20–40% of persons with fibromyalgia

    g. Symptoms may be exacerbated by "moderate physical exercise, inactivity, poor sleep, emotional stress, and humid weather" (Radomski & Latham, 2008, p. 1235).

    h. Commonly associated conditions include:

        i. Chronic fatigue syndrome

        ii. Bowel disorders, such as irritable bowel syndrome

        iii. Headache

        iv. Temporomandibular joint dysfunction

IV. Precautions and contraindications

    a. Fatigue

    b. Pain

    c. Stress

  V. Effect on occupational performance and performance skills
  - **a.** Impairment of ADL and IADL occupational performance depends on severity of condition; if severe, all areas of ADL and IADL will be affected.
  - **b.** Impairment of motor performance skills
  - **c.** Impairment of perceptual and cognitive performance skills
  - **d.** Depression or anxiety may be present, in addition to impairment of psychosocial adjustment.
- **b.** Cardiopulmonary conditions
  - **i.** Coronary artery disease

(Atchison & Dirette, 2007, pp. 195–218)
(Pendleton & Schultz-Krohn, 2006, pp. 1139–1147)
(Radomski & Latham, 2008, pp. 1295–1307)

Table 8-6 Arthritis Conditions Work Sheet

Condition	Etiology & Pathology	Signs & Symptoms	Precautions & Contraindications	Application to Practice Framework
Osteoarthritis				
Rheumatoid arthritis				
Fibromyalgia				

Table 8-7 Key Terms 8e

Radomski & Latham, 2008, p. 1296	Pendleton & Schultz-Krohn, 2006, pp. 1139–1147	Atchison & Dirette, 2007, pp. 195–218
Acute coronary syndrome	Blood pressure	Congestive heart failure
Angina	Heart rate	Diastolic
Atherogenic	Ischemic heart disease	Dyspnea
Atrial fibrillation	Myocardial infarction	Ecchymosis

(continues)

Table 8-7 Key Terms 8e *(continued)*

Radomski & Latham, 2008, p. 1296	Pendleton & Schultz-Krohn, 2006, pp. 1139–1147	Atchison & Dirette, 2007, pp. 195–218
Cardioversion	Rate pressure product	Hypertension
Congestive heart failure		Myocardial infarction
Diaphoresis		Pneumonia
Sternotomy		Sphygmomanometer
Tachypnea		Systolic

I.   Etiology

(Atchison & Dirette, 2007, pp. 210, 212)
(Pendleton & Schultz-Krohn, 2006, pp. 1142–1144)
(Radomski & Latham, 2008, pp. 1296–1297)

  a. Heart disease is leading cause of death in United States.
  b. More common in males than females
  c. Risk factors
   i.   Risk factors that can't be controlled
      1. Age
      2. Family history
      3. Gender
   ii. Risk factors that can be controlled
      1. Cigarette smoking
      2. Hyperlipidemia
      3. Hypertension
      4. Sedentary lifestyle
   iii. Factors that contribute to heart disease and may be controlled
      1. Diabetes
      2. Obesity
      3. Stress

II.   Pathology
  a. Myocardial infarction (MI): Atherosclerosis or thrombic or embolic occlusion
  b. Congestive heart failure: Primarily due to coronary artery disease. Other causes include a history of MI, hypertension, abnormal heart valves, heart muscle disease (cardiomyopathy), congenital heart defects, severe lung disease, and diabetes.

III.   Signs and symptoms

(Atchison & Dirette, 2007, pp. 210–214)
(Pendleton & Schultz-Krohn, 2006, p. 1146, Table 44-3)
(Radomski & Latham, 2008, p. 1299, Safety Note 47-1)

  a. Stage two hypertension: Systolic pressure of 160 or more, diastolic pressure of 100 or more; no symptoms are associated with this pressure
  b. Myocardial infarction
   i.   Angina: Substernal chest pain or pressure; may radiate to jaw, teeth, ear, arm, or midback
   ii. Diaphoresis
   iii. Shortness of breath
   iv. Nausea and/or vomiting
   v.   Fatigue
   vi. *Note:* Not everyone will have these symptoms.

    c. Congestive heart failure
        i. Increased weight of 2–5 pounds over several days
        ii. Inability to sleep
        iii. Persistent dry, hacking cough
        iv. Shortness of breath with normal activities
        v. Swelling in ankles or feet
        vi. Fatigue
  IV. Precautions and contraindications

(Atchison & Dirette, 2007, p. 211, Table 10-3)
(Pendleton & Schultz-Krohn, 2006, p. 1146, Table 44-3)
(Radomski & Latham, 2008, p. 1299, Safety Note 47-1)

    a. Angina or chest pain
    b. Excessive fatigue
    c. Shortness of breath
    d. Lightheadedness or dizziness
    e. Nausea or vomiting
    f. Unusual weight gain over several days
  V. Affect on occupational performance and performance skills
    a. Impairment of ADL and IADL occupational performance, decreasing depending on extent of recovery and rehabilitation
    b. Impairment of motor performance skills
    c. No impairment of perceptual and cognitive performance skills anticipated.
    d. Impairment of psychosocial adjustment; depression or anxiety may be present.
 ii. Respiratory diseases

(Atchison & Dirette, 2007, pp. 195–218)
(Pendleton & Schultz-Krohn, 2006, pp. 1147–1156)
(Radomski & Latham, 2008, pp. 1307–1320)

  I. Etiology and pathology

(Atchison & Dirette, 2007, p. 210)
(Pendleton & Schultz-Krohn, 2006, pp. 1149–1150)
(Radomski & Latham, 2008, p. 1307)

    a. Respiratory disease is fourth greatest cause of death in United States
    b. Risk factors
        i. Smoking and exposure to second-hand smoke
        ii. Air pollution
        iii. Industrial chemical exposures
        iv. Frequent childhood respiratory infections

Table 8-8 Key Terms 8f

Radomski & Latham, 2008, p. 1296	Pendleton & Schultz-Krohn, 2006, p. 1149	Atchison & Dirette, 2007, pp. 195–218
Oxygen saturation	Chronic obstructive pulmonary disease	Chronic obstructive pulmonary disease
		Dyspnea
		Oxygen transport
		Pneumonia
		Spirometry

II. Signs and symptoms

(Atchison & Dirette, 2007, p. 199)
(Pendleton & Schultz-Krohn, 2006, p. 1150)
(Radomski & Latham, 2008, pp. 1307–1308)

    a. Chronic obstructive pulmonary disease
       i. Dyspnea; breathlessness is a key symptom
       ii. Fatigue
       iii. Chronic cough
       iv. Sputum production
       v. Chest tightness

III. Precautions and contraindications

(Atchison & Dirette, 2007, p. 202)
(Pendleton & Schultz-Krohn, 2006, pp. 1149–1150)
(Radomski & Latham, 2008, p. 1307)

    a. Oxygen saturation below 90 percent
    b. Altered breathing patterns
    c. Shortness of breath
    d. Perspiration
    e. Anxiety
    f. Cough
    g. Cyanosis

IV. Affect on occupational performance and performance skills
    a. Increasing impairment of all ADL and IADL occupational performance
       i. Difficulty maintaining adequate nutrition
       ii. Difficulty sleeping
       iii. Difficulty with social and family activities
    b. Impairment of motor performance skills, including normal physical exertions
    c. No impairment of perceptual and cognitive performance skills is anticipated.
    d. Impairment of psychosocial adjustment; depression and anxiety are common.

Table 8-9 Cardiopulmonary Conditions Work Sheet

Condition	Etiology & Pathology	Signs & Symptoms	Precautions & Contraindications	Application to Practice Framework
Myocardial infarction				
Congestive heart failure				
Chronic obstructive pulmonary disease				

Table 8-10 Key Terms 8g

Radomski & Latham, 2008, p. 1359	Pendleton & Schultz-Krohn, 2006, p. 1157
Carcinoma	Cancer
Hematopoiesis	Edema
Leukemia	Lymphedema
Lymphoma	Metastasis
Lytic	
Sarcoma	

c. Oncology conditions

(Pendleton & Schultz-Krohn, 2006, pp. 1157–1168)
(Radomski & Latham, 2008, pp. 1358–1375)

    i. Etiology and pathology
        I. Factors affecting development of cancer
            a. Environmental
                i. Diet
                ii. Obesity
                iii. Level of physical activity
                iv. Smoking
                v. Exposure to chemicals, radiation, or infectious processes
            b. Cellular
                i. Genetic predisposition
        II. Risk factors by gender
            a. Males are at risk for cancers that include the following:
                i. Prostate
                ii. Lung
                iii. Colon and rectum
            b. Females are at risk for cancers that include the following:
                i. Breast
                ii. Lung
                iii. Colon and rectum
    ii. Signs and symptoms
        I. *Note:* These vary by type and location of cancer.
        II. Lung cancer
            a. Weight loss
            b. Fatigue
            c. Osteoarthropathy
            d. Weakness
            e. Shortness of breath
            f. Dyspnea
        III. Hematological cancers (cancers of the blood system; e.g., leukemia)
            a. Anemia
            b. Low endurance
            c. Bone and joint pain
            d. Susceptibility to bruising
            e. Susceptibility to infection
        IV. Sarcomas (soft tissue and bone tumors)

a. General
   i. Loss of motion
   ii. Weakened body structures
   iii. Edema
   iv. Muscle, bone, and joint pain
   v. Impaired mobility
b. Colon; changes in pattern of bowel movements
c. Prostate
   i. Urinary incontinence
   ii. Sexual dysfunction
d. Brain
   i. Motor dysfunction
   ii. Sensory dysfunction
   iii. Cognitive dysfunction
   iv. Visual dysfunction
   v. Behavioral dysfunction
iii. Precautions and contraindications
   I. Increased blood pressure
   II. Increased edema
   III. Pathological bone fractures
iv. Effect on occupational performance and performance skills
   I. *Note:* This varies based on type, stage, and location of cancer
   II. Impairment of all ADL and IADL occupational performance
   III. Impairment of motor performance skills
   IV. Impairment of visual perceptual and cognitive performance skills may be anticipated with primary brain tumor or metastasis to the brain.
   V. Impairment of psychosocial adjustment; depression is common following diagnosis.

3. Burn Injuries

(Atchison & Dirette, 2007, pp. 247–260)
(Pendleton & Schultz-Krohn, 2006, pp. 1056–1094)
(Radomski & Latham, 2008, pp. 1244–1263)

Table 8-11 Key Terms 8h

Radomski & Latham, 2008, p. 1245	Pendleton & Schultz-Krohn, 2006, pp. 1056–1094	Atchison & Dirette, 2007, pp. 247–260
Deep partial-thickness burn	Allograft	Allograft
Dermis	Autograft	Autograft
Epidermis	Compartment syndrome	Burn scar contracture
Eschar	Deep partial-thickness burn	Collagen
Full-thickness burn	Dermis	Eschar
Superficial burn	Epidermis	Full-thickness burn
Superficial partial-thickness burn	Eschar	Hypertrophic scar
Wound contracture	Escharotomy	Partial-thickness burn
	Full-thickness burn	Superficial burn
	Heterotopic ossification	

(continues)

Table 8-11 Key Terms 8H *(continued)*

Radomski & Latham, 2008, p. 1245	Pendleton & Schultz-Krohn, 2006, pp. 1056–1094	Atchison & Dirette, 2007, pp. 247–260
	Hypertrophic scar	
	Ischemia	
	Keloid scar	
	Scar maturation	
	Superficial burn	
	Superficial partial-thickness burn	
	Xenograft	

a. Etiology and pathology
   i. Etiology: Accident related to:
      I. Fire
      II. Scalding
      III. Radiation
      IV. Chemicals
      V. Electricity
b. Signs and symptoms
   i. Classification of burns
      I. No longer termed first, second, and third degree injury
      II. Superficial burn: Damage to epidermis
         a. Painful, red wounds
         b. Heals spontaneously in approximately 7 days
         c. No potential for scarring or contracture
      III. Superficial partial-thickness burn: Damage to epidermis and upper level of dermis
         a. Wet blisters
         b. Significant pain
         c. Heals spontaneously in 7–21 days
         d. "Minimal potential for hypertrophy or contractures if healing is not delayed by secondary infection or further trauma" (Pendleton & Schultz-Krohn, 2006, p. 1060).
      IV. Deep partial-thickness burn: Damage to epidermis and severe damage to dermis
         a. Red and white blotchy appearance
         b. Broken blisters on hairy skin, large intact blisters over glabrous skin
         c. Severe to even light touch
         d. Light touch is diminished; pressure is intact
         e. Delayed healing, 3–5 weeks
         f. High potential for scarring and contracture
            i. Joints and web spaces
            ii. Facial contours
            iii. Boutonnière deformities if distal joint involved
         g. Surgical grafting may occur
      V. Full-thickness burn: Damage to both epidermis and dermis
         a. White and waxy appearance
         b. No sensation; sensory endings destroyed
         c. Painful
         d. Surgical grafts are required
      VI. Subdermal burn: Damage to fatty layer, fascia, muscle, tendon, or bone

c. Precautions and contraindications
  i. Superficial and superficial partial-thickness burns
    I. Dry, itchy, and susceptible to excoriation when healed
  ii. Deep partial- and full-thickness burns
    I. Extremely high potential for deep scars and contracture formation
  iii. Pain
  iv. Potential complications
    I. Subcutaneous edema
    II. Sepsis
    III. Fluid loss leading to hypervolemia or burn shock
    IV. Muscle atrophy
    V. Tendon adherence
    VI. Joint stiffness
    VII. Capsular shortening
    VIII. Pruritis: Persistent itching
    IX. Microstomia: Limited mouth opening
    X. Heterotopic ossification
    XI. Heat intolerance
d. Effect on occupational performance and performance skills
  i. *Note:* Impact varies depending on extent of injury.
  ii. Disruption of all ADL and IADL occupational performance
  iii. Impairment of motor performance skills
  iv. No impairment of visual perceptual and cognitive performance skills is anticipated.
  v. Impairment of psychosocial adjustment including depression, withdrawal, grief, behavioral regression, anxiety, increased hostility, or existential crisis

Table 8-12 Cancer and Burn Injuries Work Sheet

Condition	Etiology & Pathology	Signs & Symptoms	Precautions & Contraindications	Application to Practice Framework
Cancer				
Burns				

REFERENCES

Altman, R., Alarcon, G., Appelrouth, D., Bloch, D., Borenstein, D., Brandt, K., et al. (1990). The American College of Rheumatology criteria for the classification and reporting of osteoarthritis of the hand. *Arthritis and Rheumatism, 33*(11), 1601–1610.

Atchison, B., & Dirette, D. (Eds.). (2007). *Conditions in occupational therapy: Effect on occupational performance.* Philadelphia: Lippincott Williams & Wilkins.

Pendleton, H. M., & Schultz-Krohn, W. (Eds.). (2006). *Pedretti's occupational therapy: Practice skills for physical dysfunction* (6th ed.). St. Louis, MO: Mosby.

Radomski, M. V., & Latham, C. A. T. (Eds.). (2008). *Occupational therapy for physical dysfunction* (6th ed.). Philadelphia: Lippincott Williams & Wilkins.

Exhibit 1-1 Stress Vulnerability Scale

In modern society, most of us can't avoid stress. But we can learn to behave in ways that lessen its effects. Researchers have identified a number of factors that affect one's vulnerability to stress—among them are eating and sleeping habits, caffeine and alcohol intake, and how we express our emotions. The following questionnaire is designed to help you discover your vulnerability quotient and to pinpoint trouble spots. Rate each item from 1 (always) to 5 (never), according to how much of the time the statement is true of you. Be sure to mark each item, even if it does not apply to you—for example, if you don't smoke, circle 1 next to item six.

		Always	Sometimes		Never
1.	I eat at least one hot, balanced meal a day.	1 **2** 3		4	5
2.	I get 7–8 hours of sleep at least four nights a week.	**1** 2 3		4	5
3.	I give and receive affection regularly.	**1** 2 3		4	5
4.	I have at least one relative within 50 miles on whom I can rely.	1 2 3		4	**5**
5.	I exercise to the point of perspiration at least twice a week.	1 2 **3**		4	5
6.	I limit myself to less than half a pack of cigarettes a day.	**1** 2 3		4	5
7.	I take fewer than five alcohol drinks a week.	1 **2** 3		4	5
8.	I am the appropriate weight for my height.	1 **2** 3		4	5
9.	I have an income adequate to meet basic expenses.	**1** 2 3		4	5
10.	I get strength from my religious beliefs.	1 **2** 3		4	5
11.	I regularly attend club or social activities.	**1** 2 3		4	5
12.	I have a network of friends and acquaintances.	**1** 2 3		4	5
13.	I have one or more friends to confide in about personal matters.	**1** 2 3		4	5
14.	I am in good health (including eyesight, hearing, and teeth).	1 **2** 3		4	5
15.	I am able to speak openly about my feelings when angry or worried.	1 **2** 3		4	5
16.	I have regular conversations with the people I live with about domestic problems—for example, chores and money.	**1** 2 3		4	5
17.	I do something for fun at least once a week.	**1** 2 3		4	5
18.	I am able to organize my time effectively.	**1** 2 3		4	5
19.	I drink fewer than three cups of coffee (or other caffeine-rich drinks) a day.	**1** 2 3		4	5
20.	I take some quiet time for myself during the day.	**1** 2 3		4	5

32

Exhibit 1-1 Stress Vulnerability Scale *(continued)*

Scoring Instructions: To calculate your score, add up the figures and subtract 20.

Score Interpretation:
A score below 10 indicates excellent resistance to stress.
A score over 30 indicates some vulnerability to stress.
A score over 50 indicates serious vulnerability to stress.

Self-Care Plan: Notice that nearly all the items describe situations and behaviors over which you have a great deal of control. Review the items on which you scored three or higher. List those items in your self-care plan. Concentrate first on those that are easiest to change—for example, eating a hot, balanced meal daily and having fun at least once a week—before tackling those that seem difficult.

Source: Exhibit courtesy Copyright 2009 Stress Directions, Inc., Lyle H. Miller and Alma Dell Smith, Boston, MA www.stressdirections.com

Exhibit 5-1 Reflection Question Journal

1. What? (What have I accomplished? What have I learned?)

2. So what? (What difference did it make? Why should I do it? How is it important? How do I feel about it?)

3. Now what? (What's next? Where do we go from here?)

Source: Exhibit courtesy of Live Wire Media.

Musculoskeletal Assessments and Interventions

Gerry Conti

OBJECTIVES

1. Describe basic, intermediate, and advanced levels of assessments and know when to use each level of assessment.
2. Apply knowledge of assessments appropriately to a condition, person, and environment and develop interventions.
3. Identify common intervention strategies appropriate to the given conditions.

INTRODUCTION

Welcome to Days 11, 12, and 13 of your study guide. In this chapter you will review assessments and interventions, especially for adults. Work through the outline to review the assessments and interventions discussed; then complete the work sheet without referring back to the outline. If you can identify the major aspects of each assessment or intervention, go on to the next group of assessments or interventions. Be sure that you know basic as well as detailed assessments and the information provided so that you can quickly decide, based on a given condition, whether the assessment is necessary and the level of information that is required. For example, someone with a spinal cord injury may require a manual muscle test, but a young adult with a mild traumatic brain injury may require just a screening of muscle strength.

To develop an appropriate set of assessments and interventions, you will need to put together your knowledge of the person, the condition, and the environment. ***Note:*** For the purposes of the certification exam, the introduction to the question will give you all the information you need to answer the question. Although you may be able to think of other issues that could be considered, based on your fieldwork experience, remember that the introduction to the question will provide all the information you need. Don't get sidetracked by the many other concerns that come to mind based on your experience.

OUTLINE

1. **To put together an appropriate assessment and intervention sequence, you must combine your knowledge of the person, the condition and common deficits, and the environment.**
   a. Personal information provided by the person (i.e., client)
   b. Condition: See Chapters 7 and 8
      i. Categories of deficits

        I. Sensorimotor

        II. Visual–cognitive–perceptual–behavioral (VCPB)

        III. Psychosocial–emotional

        IV. Activities of daily living (ADL): Basic and instrumental

    ii. Not all conditions have deficits in all areas. VCPB deficits typically are not present in orthopedic conditions, for example.

  c. Environmental considerations for assessment and intervention planning

    i. The environment in which the person is seen by the occupational therapist (OT)

    ii. The person's home environment: physical, spiritual, social

        I. Past, present, future

2. Sensorimotor assessments and interventions; order of testing

  a. Sensation

    i. If sensation is impaired or absent, all other tests will require vision and/or be impaired because of the confounding problem of decreased sensation

  b. Range of motion

    i. Range of motion precedes muscle testing. If full range of motion is present against gravity (upper extremity muscles from the scapula to the wrist), then the muscle grade is at least 3 (fair). This can eliminate unnecessary testing.

  c. Strength testing

  d. Coordination

    i. Coordination tests require sensation, range of motion, and strength for completion and are therefore completed last during sensorimotor testing.

3. Sensory assessment

(Pendleton & Schultz-Krohn, 2006, pp. 513–531)

(Radomski & Latham, 2008, pp. 212–233)

  a. Purposes of sensory testing

(Radomski & Latham, 2008, p. 214)

    i. Assess sensory loss

    ii. Evaluate sensory recovery

    iii. Aid in diagnosis

    iv. Determine function and limitations

    v. Provide direction for intervention

Table 9-1 Key Terms 9a

Radomski & Latham, 2008, p. 213	Pendleton & Schultz-Krohn, 2006, pp. 513–531
Aesthesiometer	Chemoreceptor
Hypersensitivity/hyperesthesia	Desensitization
Kinesthesia	Habituation
Monofilament	Mechanoreceptors
Paresthesia	Neuropathy
Proprioception	Nociceptor
Stereognosis	Proprioception
Vibrometer	Sensory threshold
	Stereognosis
	Thermoreceptors

b. Principles of sensory testing in persons with neurologic injury (e.g., CVA, TBI, CP, MS)

(Radomski & Latham, 2008, p. 216)

    i. Quickly screen areas of the body expected to be intact; test more thoroughly those areas where a deficit may be expected (e.g., side of hemiplegia).

    ii. Pain and temperature are mediated at a lower level of the brain, and fine touch and proprioception are mediated at higher levels. Therefore, the two sets of sensations are correlated.

        I. If fine touch and proprioception are present, do not assess pain and temperature. These more basic sensations will be intact.

        II. If pain and temperature are absent, do not assess fine touch and proprioception because they will also be absent.

        III. In persons with severe cortical impairment, test pain and temperature first.

        IV. In sensory recovery, pain and temperature precede light touch and proprioception.

        V. Testing in neurologic conditions should occur along the distribution of dermatomes.

            a. Testing one location in a dermatome (e.g., C5) is sufficient to identify whether the sensation is present in the whole dermatome.

c. Principles of sensory testing in persons with spinal cord injury (a special case of neurologic injury)

(Pendleton & Schultz-Krohn, 2006, p. 911)
(Radomski & Latham, 2008, p. 216)

    i. In a complete spinal cord injury, there will be a total absence of sensation below the level of a complete lesion. Therefore, sensory testing is not needed below the level of a complete injury.

    ii. Sensory testing below the level of an *incomplete* spinal cord injury may provide important information about the potential for motor recovery at the level of the dermatome.

    iii. There are patterns of sensory deficit due to the configuration of ascending sensory fibers in the spinal cord.

        I. Anterior spinal cord lesion: Pain, temperature, and touch are lost below the level of the lesion, but proprioception and vibration are intact.

        II. Posterior spinal cord lesion: Touch, proprioception, and vibration are lost below the level of the lesion, but pain, temperature, and touch are intact.

        III. Brown-Séquard syndrome: Loss of ipsilateral proprioception (on the side of the lesion); loss of pain, temperature, and touch on the contralateral side

        IV. Central cord syndrome: Bilateral loss of pain and temperature below the level of the lesion

            a. This syndrome may be seen in older adults with arthritic changes to the neck.

d. Principles of sensory testing in persons with peripheral nerve injuries

(Pendleton & Schultz-Krohn, 2006, pp. 519–520)
(Radomski & Latham, 2008, pp. 217–218)

    i. Testing is recorded in peripheral nerve distribution patterns (e.g., median nerve rather than C7 dermatome).

    ii. Sensory mapping of the hand is frequently indicated.

        I. Demonstration on the unaffected side occurs prior to testing on the affected side.

e. General procedures for all sensory tests

(Radomski & Latham, 2008, p. 219, Box 7-1)

    i. Test in a quiet environment.

  ii. Ensure that the person is relaxed and comfortable.

  iii. Verify if the person can understand and speak English. If not, modify your testing procedure to ensure reliable communication.

   I. Example: Person with limited English comprehension

   II. Example: Person with aphasia

  iv. Stabilize the body part being tested and ensure that vision is occluded.

   I. This is important to avoid providing inadvertent sensory cues to the person.

   II. Occluded vision can be accomplished by having the person close his or her eyes, using a blindfold, placing a folder between the eyes and the body part being tested, or placing the body part behind a barrier.

  v. Demonstrate the test on an area of skin with intact sensation while the person observes the process.

  vi. State instructions clearly, and verify the person's understanding of them.

  vii. Apply stimuli irregularly or provide catch trials to ensure accuracy of response.

  viii. Observe the person's response to testing (e.g., hypersensitivity, delay, confidence in responding).

  ix. Tests and retests should be done by the same therapist to avoid differences of test administration and/or test interpretation.

   I. *Note:* This means you may need to test your client either before or after a vacation, but don't ask the person who is covering to do it for you!

  x. Decision-making tips

   I. Decide first how in-depth your sensory tests need to be.

    a. You do not want to waste evaluation time with unnecessary sensory testing.

    b. Be aware of what tests have already been performed by other team members, and do not duplicate these results.

   II. Determine what sensory information is needed.

    a. If the client has normal cognition and reports no problem with sensation, either do not test (and document the client's statement) or test quickly with a high-level test, such as stereognosis.

    b. Listen to the client. If a certain sensory loss can be inferred, test for that sensation specifically.

    c. If you know typical sensory losses for the condition, test for them first.

   III. Neurologic conditions: Tests of proprioception pain and temperature (protective sensation) are important for treatment planning.

   IV. Spinal cord injury: Tests of proprioception, pain, temperature, and touch by dermatome level are important for treatment planning.

   V. Peripheral nerve injuries: Sophisticated sensory testing with monofilaments is frequently indicated.

   VI. General medical conditions: Sensory screening may be adequate.

f. Screening tests of sensation

(Pendleton & Schultz-Krohn, 2006, pp. 519–520)

  i. Client description of sensory problems, location, and effect

  ii. Observations

   I. Skin temperature, color, cold intolerance

   II. Sweating; lack of sweating correlates with lack of discriminative (touch) sensation.

   III. Pilomotor change (lack of goose bumps)

   IV. Trophic changes (atrophy of nails or finger pulps, slower healing, hair changes)

   V. Absence of wear marks

   VI. Atrophy of soft tissue

  iii. Functional sensory test

   I. Useful when the goal is to confirm that sensation appears to be intact

   II. Stereognosis (person must be able to understand and communicate and have sufficient cognition)

    III. Test of median nerve function (injury suspected)
        a. Test thumb tip, index tip, index proximal phalanx
    IV. Test of ulnar nerve function (injury suspected)
        a. Test distal and proximal little finger, proximal ulnar palm
    V. Test of radial nerve function (injury suspected)
        a. Test thumb web space

g. Proprioception

(Pendleton & Schultz-Krohn, 2006, p. 520)
(Radomski & Latham 2008, p. 224)

    i. Measures awareness of the static position of the body part
        I. Equipment: None
        II. Nonstandardized
        III. See text for specific test procedure.

h. Kinesthesia

(Radomski & Latham, 2008, p. 224)

    i. Measures awareness of the position of the moving body part
        I. Equipment: None
        II. Nonstandardized
        III. See text for specific test procedure.

i. Vibration

(Radomski & Latham, 2008, p. 222)

    i. Measures awareness of vibration
    ii. Equipment: Specialized vibration tools
        I. Standardized for each specific tool
        II. See text for specific test procedure.
        III. Comment: Less often performed

j. Pain (pinprick)

(Pendleton & Schultz-Krohn, 2006, pp. 521–522)
(Radomski & Latham, 2008, p. 223)

    i. Measures protective sensation
    ii. Equipment: Pin
    iii. Nonstandardized
    iv. See text for specific test procedure.

k. Temperature

(Pendleton & Schultz-Krohn, 2006, pp. 522–523)
(Radomski & Latham, 2008, p. 223)

    i. Measures protective sensation
    ii. Equipment: Test tubes filled with hot and cold water
    iii. Nonstandardized
    iv. See text for specific test procedure.

l. Touch awareness

(Radomski & Latham, 2008, p. 223)

    i. Measures general awareness of touch sensation
    ii. Equipment: Cotton swab, fingertip, or pencil eraser
    iii. Nonstandardized
    iv. See text for specific test procedure.
    v. *Note:* Often a higher-level touch test will provide more information, such as the ability to localize or distinguish between one or two points.

m. Touch localization

(Pendleton & Schultz-Krohn, 2006, p. 523)
(Radomski & Latham, 2008, p. 223)

    i. Measures ability to identify spatial location of touch sensation
    ii. Equipment: Semmes-Weinstein monofilament (smallest size the client can feel), pen, or pencil eraser
    iii. Standardized
    iv. See text for specific test procedure.

n. Light touch: Touch–pressure

(Pendleton & Schultz-Krohn, 2006, pp. 523–524)
(Radomski & Latham, 2008, p. 221)

    i. Measures
        I. Light touch, important for discriminatory hand use
        II. Pressure, important as a protective sensation
    ii. Equipment: Semmes-Weinstein pressure aesthesiometer (monofilaments) or WEST monofilaments
    iii. Standardized
    iv. See text for specific test procedure.
    v. Considered to be the gold standard for testing nerve entrapments, such as carpal tunnel syndrome

o. Two-point discrimination

(Pendleton & Schultz-Krohn, 2006, pp. 524–525)
(Radomski & Latham, 2008, pp. 221–222)

    i. Measures discriminatory sensation
    ii. Equipment: Disk-Criminator or aesthesiometer
    iii. Standardized
    iv. See text for specific test procedure.
    v. Comments
        I. Moving two-point discrimination returns before static two-point discrimination
        II. To avoid error due to pressure, press only to point of blanching the skin

p. Stereognosis

(Pendleton & Schultz-Krohn, 2006, pp. 520–521)
(Radomski & Latham, 2008, p. 223)

    i. Composite measure of touch, proprioception, cognition, speech, and coordination
    ii. Equipment: Small common objects that are known to the client
    iii. Nonstandardized
    iv. See text for specific test procedure.
    v. Comments
        I. Touch, proprioception, cognition, speech, coordination, and the ability to manipulate objects must all be present to complete this test successfully.
        II. Frequently used as a high-level screening tool to assess overall sensory function of the hand

q. Functional tests of sensation
    i. Moberg Pick-Up Test

(Pendleton & Schultz-Krohn, 2006, p. 525)
(Radomski & Latham, 2008, p. 223)

        I. Nonstandardized
        II. See text for specific test procedure

      ii.   Modified Pick-Up Test (Dellon)

(Pendleton & Schultz-Krohn, 2006, p. 525)
(Radomski & Latham, 2008, p. 222)

            I.   Standardized
            II.   See text for specific test procedure.
           III. *Note:* When possible, a standardized test is preferred to a nonstandardized test. For a functional sensory test, the Modified Pick-Up Test is preferred to the Moberg Pick-Up Test.

4. Sensory intervention
   a.   Sensory reeducation

(Pendleton & Schultz-Krohn, 2006, pp. 527–530)
(Radomski & Latham, 2008, pp. 719–724)

      i.   Purposes
            I.   Protect from sharp objects or temperature extremes
            II.   Decrease force used in gripping
      ii.   Techniques following peripheral nerve injury
            I.   Minimal requirements to initiate program
                a.   Perception of vibration (30 cps) and moving touch in area
                b.   Motivation to follow through with program
            II.   Components of intervention
                a.   Localization of moving touch with added visual stimulation
                b.   Graded sensory discrimination
           III. Stages of sensory reeducation program
                a.   Object recognition using feature detection strategies
                b.   Refined grasp and pinch of objects
                c.   Control of force while holding objects
                d.   Maintenance of force while transporting objects
                e.   Object manipulation
    iii. Techniques following cerebrovascular accident
            I.   Minimal requirements to initiate program
                a.   Perception of vibration (100 cps)
                b.   Motivation to follow through with program
            II.   Components of program
                a.   Vibration with and without vision
                b.   Incorporation of normal hand function into daily activities with enhanced sensory stimulation
                c.   Sensory treatment activities (see especially Radomski & Latham, 2008, p. 722)
                d.   Studies of effectiveness following stroke are limited.

5. Range of motion assessments

(Pendleton & Schultz-Krohn, 2006, pp. 437–468)
(Radomski & Latham, 2008, pp. 91–125)

Table 9-2 Key Terms 9b

Radomski & Latham, 2008, p. 92	Pendleton & Schultz-Krohn, 2006, pp. 437–468
Active range of motion	Active range of motion
Anatomical position	End-feel
Calibrate	Functional range of motion
Contracture	Goniometer
Limits of motion	Joint measurement
Passive range of motion	Palpation
Tenodesis	Passive range of motion
	Range of motion

    a. Definitions

(Pendleton & Schultz-Krohn, 2006, p. 438)
(Radomski & Latham, 2008, p. 93)

        i.   Passive range of motion
        ii.   Active range of motion
        iii. Active assistive range of motion
    b. *Note:* Levels of range of motion assessments
        i.   Gross: Based on observation during active movement
        ii.   Functional: Assessment of selected joints with visual identification of approximate range of motion during active movement (see especially Radomski & Latham, 2008, p. 93, Box 5-1)
        iii. Goniometric: Formal assessment of all or selected joints with goniometric measurement
    c. Precautions and contraindications for goniometric range of motion

(Pendleton & Schultz-Krohn, 2006, p. 440)

        i.   *Note:* Gross assessment through observation is still feasible.
        ii.   Inflammation or infection
        iii. Medications include pain medication or muscle relaxants
        iv. Osteoporosis; hypermobility; subluxation
        v.   Hemophilia
        vi. Hematoma
        vii. Recent soft tissue injury
        viii. Newly united fracture
        ix. Prolonged immobilization
        x.   Bony ankylosis is suspected
        xi. Bone carcinoma or any fragile bone condition
    d. Principles of goniometric range of motion assessments

(Pendleton & Schultz-Krohn, 2006, pp. 445–468)
(Radomski & Latham, 2008, pp. 97–124)

        i.   Visual observation of limb and joint
        ii.   Palpation of joint
        iii. Passive movement of limb to determine end-feel
    e. Positioning of therapist and support of limb
        i.   Positions for testing of specific joints are provided
        ii.   Be aware of possible substitutions.

Table 9-3 Key Terms 9c

Radomski & Latham, 2008, p. 92	Pendleton & Schultz-Krohn, 2006, pp. 469–512
Maximum voluntary contraction	Against gravity
Mechanical advantage	Gravity-minimized
	Manual muscle test
	Muscle endurance
	Muscle grades
	Resistance
	Screening tests
	Substitutions

6. **Range of motion interventions**

(Pendleton & Schultz-Krohn, 2006, pp. 670–671, 967–969)
(Radomski & Latham, 2008, pp. 581–582)

    a. Passive stretching to several degrees beyond the point of discomfort, with stretch maintained for 15–30 seconds (see especially Radomski & Latham, 2008, pp. 581–582)
    b. Active stretching
    c. Passive stretching
    d. *Note:* Understand the concept of tenodesis action—what is it, why it might be used, and at what level of spinal cord injury it might be used.

7. **Strength assessments**

(Pendleton & Schultz-Krohn, 2006, pp. 469–512)
(Radomski & Latham, 2008, pp. 125–185)

    a. Muscle testing grading system (see especially Pendleton & Schultz-Krohn, 2006, p. 475, Table 21-1; Radomski & Latham, 2008, p. 127, Table 5-1)
        i. *Note:* Know this so that you can interpret information given in questions.
    b. Levels of strength testing
        i. Observation of ability to use key muscles against gravity so that a grade of at least 3 (fair) can be recorded
        ii. Functional muscle testing: Selected testing of key muscles and muscle groups (e.g., shoulder flexors, elbow flexors)
        iii. Manual muscle testing: Specific strength testing of selected muscles
    c. Precautions and contraindications

(Pendleton & Schultz-Krohn, 2006, p. 474)

        i. True effort from the client is required.
        ii. Inflammation or pain to the region
        iii. Unhealed fracture or dislocation
        iv. Recent surgery, especially of the musculoskeletal system
        v. Myositis ossificans
        vi. Bone carcinoma or fragile bone condition
        vii. Osteoporosis, hypermobility, and joint subluxation
        viii. Hemophilia or cardiovascular risk or disease
        ix. Abdominal surgery or hernia
        x. Fatigue that exacerbates the client's condition
    d. Principles of muscle testing

(Pendleton & Schultz-Krohn, 2006, pp. 476–477)
(Radomski & Latham, 2008, p. 127, Box 5-3)

8. Strengthening intervention

(Pendleton & Schultz-Krohn, 2006, pp. 670–674, 1011–1012)
(Radomski & Latham, 2008, pp. 582–590)

- **a.** Contraindications
  - **i.** Poor general health
  - **ii.** Inflamed joints
  - **iii.** Recent surgery (unless prescribed by physician)
  - **iv.** In presence of severe contractures
  - **v.** In presence of dyskinetic contractures
  - **vi.** Spasticity
    - **I.** *Note:* Strengthening is warranted, but special care is needed.
- **b.** Types of strengthening
  - **i.** Isometric
    - **I.** Appropriate for any grade muscle
    - **II.** Contraindicated in the presence of cardiac disease
    - **III.** May be used with or without resistance
    - **IV.** In rheumatoid arthritis, may be used to improve muscle tone, static endurance, and strength, and to prepare joints for more vigorous activity
  - **ii.** Active-assistive
    - **I.** Concentric or eccentric contraction through maximum range of motion the person can achieve; device or person assists with completion of motion
    - **II.** Appropriate for grade 2 or 3 muscles
    - **III.** The underlying concept behind use of mobile arm supports
  - **iii.** Active
    - **I.** Typically concentric contraction through part of full range of motion, in gravity-minimized plane or with gravity plane
    - **II.** Appropriate for grade 2 or 3 muscles
    - **III.** Many activities and occupations can be developed for this type of strengthening.
  - **iv.** Resistive
    - **I.** Contraction through full range of motion against gravity and with device- or person-aided resistance
    - **II.** Appropriate for grade 3+ to 4+ muscles
    - **III.** Use of weights, springs, bands, special devices
    - **IV.** Some activities and occupations can be developed for this type of strengthening.

9. Coordination assessments
- **a.** Coordination is not separately addressed in the two major texts.
- **b.** Effective coordination requires functional sensation, range of motion, strength, and endurance. Cognition and the ability to understand and use communication are also required.
- **c.** Types of coordination
  - **i.** Gross: Partial or full upper limb movement with grasp and manipulation of larger objects.
  - **ii.** Fine: Limited upper limb movement with grasp of manipulation of small objects.
- **d.** Examples of coordination tests
  - **i.** Gross coordination tests
    - **I.** Box and Block
    - **II.** Minnesota Manual Dexterity Test
  - **ii.** Fine coordination tests
    - **I.** Purdue Pegboard
    - **II.** 9-Hole Peg test

          III. Crawford Small Parts Dexterity Test
- **e.** Composite coordination tests
  - **i.** Carroll Quantitative Test of Upper Extremity Function
  - **ii.** Jebsen Test of Hand Function
  - **iii.** Bennett Hand-Tool Dexterity Test

10. Coordination intervention

(Pendleton & Schultz-Krohn, 2006, p. 675)
(Radomski & Latham, 2008, p. 361)

- **a.** *Note:* Participation in graded activity is excellent to improve coordination.
- **b.** Principles for activity grading
  - **i.** Slow to fast movement
  - **ii.** Simple to complex movement
  - **iii.** Few to more joints
  - **iv.** Gross to precise movement
  - **v.** Voluntary to involuntary control

WORK SHEET

Work Sheet 9-1. Summary Assessment and Intervention

Complete this work sheet beginning with your basic working assumptions about a person with the identified condition and stage. Recognize that these working assumptions may need to be altered based on variations in the condition and the individual. The first table is provided as a partial example. A: Assessment. P: Plan of intervention.

Pendleton & Schultz-Krohn, 2006, pp. 802–837; Radomski & Latham, 2008, pp. 1001–1041	ADL IADL Environment	Sensorimotor	Vision (V) Perception (P) Cognition (C)	
CVA Acute	**A** 1. Self-care ADL 2. Screen for dysphagia 3. Safety with IADL 4. Recommend discharge setting **P** Educate caregivers	**A** 1. Screen ROM, sensation, motor function **P** Educate caregivers	**A** 1. Observe for neglect 2. Observe for apraxia 3. Observe for aphasia 4. Observe for other neurobehavioral signs **P** Educate caregivers	
CVA Rehabilitation	**A** Assess all ADL, IADL **P** 1. ADL: Select technique—one-handed, NDT 2. Transfers, functional use of ambulation 3. IADL 4. Environmental modification if compensation model selected	**A** Assess ROM, sensation, motor function **P** 1. Facilitation of UE, trunk motor patterns a. Select theory: Motor Control, NDT, PNF, Rood, Brunnstrom b. Select appropriate PAMs c. Select theory-appropriate application tasks	**A** Assess VCP **P** 1. Visual retraining 2. Training for neglect if present 3. Perceptual retraining when visual skills are adequate 4. Cognitive retraining a. Select functional tasks for retraining	
CVA Chronic				

Pendleton & Schultz-Krohn, 2006, pp. 838–872; Radomski & Latham, 2008, pp. 1042–1078	ADL IADL Environment	Sensorimotor	Vision (V) Perception (P) Cognition (C)
TBI Acute			
TBI Rehabilitation			
TBI Chronic			

(continues)

Pendleton & Schultz-Krohn, 2006, pp. 903–930; Radomski & Latham, 2008, pp. 1171–1213	ADL IADL Environment	Sensorimotor	Vision (V) Perception (P) Cognition (C)
SCI, C5 ASIA A Acute			
SCI, C5 ASIA A Rehabilitation			
SCI, C5 ASIA A Chronic			

	ADL IADL Environment		Sensorimotor		Vision (V) Perception (P) Cognition (C)
SCI, C6 ASIA A Acute					
SCI, C6 ASIA A Rehabilitation					
SCI, C6 ASIA A Chronic					

(continues)

	ADL IADL Environment	Sensorimotor	Vision (V) Perception (P) Cognition (C)
SCI, T4 ASIA A Acute			
SCI, T4 ASIA A Rehabilitation			
SCI, T4 ASIA A Chronic			

Pendleton & Schultz-Krohn, 2006, pp. 889–892; Radomski & Latham, 2008, pp. 1083–1090	ADL IADL Environment	Sensorimotor	Vision (V) Perception (P) Cognition (C)
MS Exacerbation			
MS Remission			

(continues)

Pendleton & Schultz-Krohn, 2006, pp. 893–897; Radomski & Latham, 2008, pp. 1090–1092	ADL IADL Environment	Sensorimotor	Vision (V) Perception (P) Cognition (C)
Parkinson disease Mild impairment			
Parkinson disease Moderate to severe impairment			

Pendleton & Schultz-Krohn, 2006, pp. 875–879; Radomski & Latham, 2008, pp. 1092–1096	ADL IADL Environment	Sensorimotor	Vision (V) Perception (P) Cognition (C)
Amyotrophic lateral sclerosis **Independent to mild impairment**			
Amyotrophic lateral sclerosis **Mild to moderate impairment**			
Amyotrophic lateral sclerosis **Moderate to severe impairment**			

(continues)

Pendleton & Schultz-Krohn, 2006, pp. 880–886	ADL IADL Environment	Sensorimotor	Vision (V) Perception (P) Cognition (C)
Alzheimer disease **Mild impairment**			
Alzheimer disease **Mild to moderate impairment**			
Alzheimer disease **Moderate to severe impairment**			

Pendleton & Schultz-Krohn, 2006, pp. 886–889	ADL IADL Environment	Sensorimotor	Vision (V) Perception (P) Cognition (C)
Huntington disease **Mild impairment**			
Huntington disease **Mild to moderate impairment**			
Huntington disease **Moderate to severe impairment**			

(continues)

Pendleton & Schultz-Krohn, 2006, pp. 934–937; Radomski & Latham, 2008, pp. 1096–1098	ADL IADL Environment	Sensorimotor	Vision (V) Perception (P) Cognition (C)
Guillain-Barré syndrome Acute			
Guillain-Barré syndrome Chronic			

Pendleton & Schultz-Krohn, 2006, pp. 1020–1035; Radomski & Latham, 2008, pp. 1117–1130	ADL IADL Environment	Sensorimotor	Vision (V) Perception (P) Cognition (C)
Hip fracture **Acute**			
Hip replacement **Acute**			

(continues)

Pendleton & Schultz-Krohn, 2006, pp. 983–1016; Radomski & Latham, 2008, pp. 1106–1117	ADL IADL Environment	Sensorimotor	Vision (V) Perception (P) Cognition (C)
Upper extremity fractures/pathology Nonsurgical			
Upper extremity fractures/pathology Postsurgical			

Pendleton & Schultz-Krohn, 2006, pp. 950–982; Radomski & Latham, 2008, pp. 1214–1243	ADL IADL Environment	Sensorimotor	Vision (V) Perception (P) Cognition (C)
Rheumatoid arthritis Exacerbation			
Rheumatoid arthritis Chronic			
Osteoarthritis			

(continues)

Pendleton & Schultz-Krohn, 2006, pp. 646–655; 1007–1008; Radomski & Latham, 2008, pp. 1121–1124, 1158, 1235–1238	ADL IADL Environment	Sensorimotor	Vision (V) Perception (P) Cognition (C)
Pain syndromes: Fibromyalgia, myofascial pain, complex regional pain syndrome			
Low back pain Acute			
Low back pain Chronic			

Pendleton & Schultz-Krohn, 2006, pp. 1139–1148; Radomski & Latham, 2008, pp. 1296–1307	ADL IADL Environment	Sensorimotor	Vision (V) Perception (P) Cognition (C)
Myocardial infarction **Acute**			
Myocardial infarction **Chronic**			
Congestive heart failure			

(continues)

Pendleton & Schultz-Krohn, 2006, pp. 1149–1155, 1160–1167; Radomski & Latham, 2008, pp. 1307–1310, 1364–1372	ADL IADL Environment	Sensorimotor	Vision (V) Perception (P) Cognition (C)
Chronic obstructive pulmonary disease Chronic			
Cancer (oncology) Postoperative			
Cancer (oncology) Palliative			

Pendleton & Schultz-Krohn, 2006, pp. 1056–1094; Radomski & Latham, 2008, pp. 1244–1236, 1301	ADL IADL Environment	Sensorimotor	Vision (V) Perception (P) Cognition (C)
Burns **Acute postoperative**			
Burns **Rehabilitation**			
Diabetes			

(continues)

Pendleton & Schultz-Krohn, 2006, pp. 1096–1129; Radomski & Latham, 2008, pp. 1265–1289	ADL IADL Environment	Sensorimotor	Vision (V) Perception (P) Cognition (C)
Upper extremity amputation Acute preprosthetic			
Upper extremity amputation Postprosthetic			

Pendleton & Schultz-Krohn, 2006, pp. 1129–1138; Radomski & Latham, 2008, pp. 1289–1293	ADL IADL Environment	Sensorimotor	Vision (V) Perception (P) Cognition (C)
Lower extremity amputation Acute preprosthetic			
Lower extremity amputation Postprosthetic			

(continues)

Pendleton & Schultz-Krohn, 2006, pp. 999–1002; Radomski & Latham, 2008, pp. 1155–1156	ADL IADL Environment	Sensorimotor	Vision (V) Perception (P) Cognition (C)
Flexor tendon repair Acute			
Flexor tendon repair Rehabilitation			

Pendleton & Schultz-Krohn, 2006, pp. 1009–1012; Radomski & Latham, 2008, pp. 1148–1149	ADL IADL Environment	Sensorimotor	Vision (V) Perception (P) Cognition (C)
Carpal tunnel syndrome Acute			
Carpal tunnel syndrome Postsurgical			
Carpal tunnel syndrome Chronic			

REFERENCES

Pendleton, H. M., & Schultz-Krohn, W. (Eds.). (2006). *Pedretti's occupational therapy: Practice skills for physical dysfunction* (6th ed.). St. Louis, MO: Mosby.

Radomski, M. V., & Latham, C. A. T. (Eds.). (2008). *Occupational therapy for physical dysfunction* (6th ed.). Philadelphia: Lippincott Williams & Wilkins.

Hand Rehabilitation and Surgical Conditions

Kurt Krueger

OBJECTIVES

1. Describe clinical presentations of common upper extremity injuries.
2. Demonstrate knowledge of the intervention strategies related to common fractures, tendon injuries, and nerve injuries.
3. Identify the phases of wound healing.
4. Describe the steps in the splint fabrication process.
5. Identify key anatomical landmarks in the splint design process.
6. Describe differences in the protocols for flexor tendon rehabilitation.
7. Review peripheral nerve function and develop intervention strategies to maximize function while healing progresses.

Table 10-1 Key Terms

Radomski & Latham, 2008, pp. 446, 1132	Pendleton & Schultz-Krohn, 2006, p. 513
Antideformity position	Axis of motion
Buddy straps	Complex regional pain syndrome (CRPS)
Carpal tunnel syndrome	Cumulative trauma disorders
Cervical screening	Dynamic splint
Claw deformity	Edema
Complex regional pain syndrome (CRPS)	Ergonomic
Contracture	Force
Counterforce strap	Friction
Cubital tunnel syndrome	Immobilization splint
de Quervain disease	Mobile arm support
Dual obliquity	Mobilization splint

(continues)

Table 10-1 Key Terms *(continued)*

Radomski & Latham, 2008, pp. 446, 1132	Pendleton & Schultz-Krohn, 2006, p. 513
Extensor lag	Orthosis
Fibroblastic phase	Peripheral nerve injury
Haldex Pinch Gauge	Provocative test
Hard end feel	Restriction splint
Inflammatory phase	Serial static splint
Maturation phase	Splinting
Neuroma	Static progressive splint
Oscillation	Static splint
Place and hold exercise	Suspension arm device
Serial static splint	Tendon injury
Soft end feel	Tenodesis
Splint	Torque
Static progressive splint	Translational force
Tenolysis	Upper quadrant

INTRODUCTION

Welcome to Days 14 and 15 of your study guide. This chapter provides an outline on hand rehabilitation and surgical conditions. After completing this chapter you will be able to understand the various conditions of the hand and be able to choose safe and appropriate intervention strategies.

OUTLINE

1. **Wound healing**
   a. Phases of wound healing

   (Pendleton & Schultz-Krohn, 2006, p. 1006)
   (Radomski & Latham, 2008, pp. 545–546, 1133–1134)

   i. Inflammation: Injury onset through at least the first 3 days
   ii. Fibroplasia: From day 4 through 6 weeks, active range of motion (ROM) may begin
   iii. Maturation/remodeling: Three months to 1 year exercise and splinting may be used to assist in the remodeling of the injured tissue.
   iv. Splinting considerations

   (Radomski & Latham, 2008, p. 469)

   b. Wound care techniques
   c. Wound evaluation

   (Radomski & Latham, 2008, pp. 546, 1136)

   i. Wound size
      I. Length
      II. Width
      III. Depth
   ii. Type of wound drainage

    iii. Presence of odor

    iv. Scar remodeling

(Radomski & Latham, 2008, p. 1142)

    v. Desensitization

    vi. Edema control techniques

2. Common fractures

a. Wrist

(Pendleton & Schultz-Krohn, 2006, pp. 994–995)
(Radomski & Latham, 2008, pp. 1152–1153)

    i. Wrist fractures can be treated in three basic ways.

        I. Closed reduction, which is followed by cast immobilization

        II. Open reduction/internal fixation (ORIF), which may require a cast or splint

        III. External fixation

    ii. Treatment is divided into two phases: immobilization and postcast/fixation removal.

        I. Immobilization

            a. Range of motion (ROM) of uninvolved joints: shoulder, elbow, and digits

            b. Edema management

(Pendleton & Schultz-Krohn, 2006, p. 1004)
(Radomski & Latham, 2008, p. 1142)

                i. Elevation

                ii. Active ROM

                iii. Compression

                iv. Retrograde massage

        c. Exercise

(Radomski & Latham, 2008, p. 1143)

            i. Differential flexor tendon gliding

            ii. Following cast removal

(Radomski & Latham, 2008, pp. 430, 1153)

                1. Continue with ROM of uninvolved joints.

                2. Edema management: Continue as previously described; addition of a compressive garment may be beneficial.

                3. Splinting: A static wrist brace may be fabricated to improve wrist ROM.

                4. Exercise

                    a. ROM of wrist and forearm may begin with physician approval.

                    b. Isolated movement of wrist extensors (extensor carpi radialis brevis, extensor carpi radialis longus, extensor carpi ulnaris)

                    c. Isolated movement of extensor digitorum communis

                    d. Restore joint mobility.

                    e. Restore fine motor control.

                    f. Add gradual strengthening.

                    g. Functional activities

b. Hand fractures

(Pendleton & Schultz-Krohn, 2006, pp. 994–999)
(Radomski & Latham, 2008, pp. 469, 1134, 1153–1155)

    i. Primary treatment of hand fractures can be classified into three groups

        I. Closed reduction/nonoperative

        II. ORIF/operative

    III. External fixation; Cast or splints may be used to maintain immobilization. If possible the hand should be placed in a safe position (metacarpal phalangeal [MP] joint flexion and interphalangeal [IP] joint extension).

  ii. Evaluation guidelines during the immobilization phase (3–5 weeks):

    I. ROM of uninvolved joints

      a. Shoulder

      b. Elbow

      c. Digits

    II. Edema control techniques: Edema management

(Pendleton & Schultz-Krohn, 2006, p. 1004)

(Radomski & Latham, 2008, p. 1142)

      a. Elevation

      b. Active ROM of noninvolved joints

      c. Compression

      d. Retrograde massage

  iii. Following the immobilization phase: Evaluate ROM and edema.

    I. Exercise

      a. Begin ROM of injured structures; may begin with physician approval.

      b. Resistive exercise, passive ROM, and functional activities can begin at 6–8 weeks with physician approval.

    II. Splinting may be used to encourage ROM and protect the area from trauma.

      a. Static splinting: Buddy straps

      b. Dynamic splinting to correct deformity may be used at 6–8 weeks with physician approval.

3. Nerve injuries

  a. Classifications

(Pendleton & Schultz-Krohn, 2006, p. 995)

    i. Neurapraxia

    ii. Axonotmesis

    iii. Neurotmesis

  b. Assessment of nerve function

(Pendleton & Schultz-Krohn, 2006, pp. 988–992)

    i. Modality tests

      I. Pain

      II. Heat/cold

      III. Touch pressure

    ii. Functional tests

      I. Two-point discrimination

      II. Moberg Pick-Up Test

    iii. Objective tests

      I. Wrinkle test

      II. Ninhydrin test

      III. Nerve-conduction studies

    iv. Provocative tests

      I. Adson maneuver

      II. Roos test

      III. Upper limb tension test

      IV. Tinel sign

      V. Phalen test/reverse Phalen test

      VI. Carpal compression test

      VII. Elbow flexion test

c. Median nerve

(Pendleton & Schultz-Krohn, 2006, p. 997)
(Radomski & Latham, 2008, p. 1151)

  i. Innervation patterns
      I. Motor
         a. Pronator teres
         b. Palmaris longus
         c. Flexor carpi radialis (FCR)
         d. Flexor digitorum profundus (FDP) to index and middle fingers
         e. Flexor digitorum superficialis
         f. Flexor pollicis longus
         g. Abductor pollicis brevis
         h. Pronator quadratus
         i. Opponens pollicis
         j. Superficial head of the flexor pollicis brevis
         k. Lumbricals to index and middle fingers
      II. Sensory
         a. Volar surface of the thumb, index finger, middle finger, and radial half of the ring finger
         b. Dorsal surface of the index finger, middle finger, and radial half of the ring finger distal to the proximal interphalangeal (PIP) joints
  ii. Clinical signs
      I. Motor tests

(Pendleton & Schultz-Krohn, 2006, p. 990)

         a. Opposition of the thumb
         b. Flexion of the fingers
      II. High nerve lesions
         a. Ulnar flexion of the wrist
         b. Loss of palmar abduction and opposition
         c. Loss of pronation
         d. Sensory loss
      III. Injury to the anterior interosseous nerve does not involve sensory loss
         a. Motor loss includes flexor pollicis longus, flexor digitorum profundus to index and middle fingers; pronator quadratus and pronator teres are not affected; pinch is affected.
      IV. Low nerve lesions
         a. Loss of thenar eminence
         b. Loss of palmar abduction
         c. Loss of opposition
         d. Sensory loss
iii. Intervention

(Radomski & Latham, 2008, pp. 449–450, 1150–1151)

      I. Prepare for tendon transfers as needed for high nerve injuries.
      II. Splinting
         a. High nerve injuries and low nerve injuries
             i. Thumb abduction splint
      III. Passive ROM to maintain (high nerve injury) splinting may be required if ROM exercises are not affected.
         a. Pronation
         b. MP flexion and IP extension
         c. Thumb abduction (low and high injuries)

      IV. Instruct in use of adaptive equipment as needed to maintain functional grip and pinch

      V. Instruct in techniques to avoid reinjury due to impaired sensation

d. Ulnar nerve

  i. Innervation patterns

(Pendleton & Schultz-Krohn, 2006, p. 998)
(Radomski & Latham, 2008, p. 1151)

      I. Motor
- **a.** Flexor digitorum profundus to ring finger and small finger
- **b.** Flexor carpi ulnaris
- **c.** Intrinsic muscles
- **d.** Palmaris brevis
- **e.** Abductor digiti minimi
- **f.** Flexor digiti minimi
- **g.** Opponens digiti minimi
- **h.** Dorsal and volar interossei
- **i.** Third and fourth lumbricals
- **j.** Medial head of flexor pollicis brevis
- **k.** Adductor pollicis

      II. Sensory
- **a.** Dorsal and volar surface of the small finger
- **b.** Dorsal and volar surface of the ulnar half of the ring finger

  ii. Low nerve lesions injury at the wrist level

      I. Muscles involved
- **a.** Abductor digiti minimi
- **b.** Flexor digiti minimi
- **c.** Opponens digiti minimi
- **d.** Intrinsic muscles
- **e.** Palmaris brevis
- **f.** Dorsal and volar interossei
- **g.** Third and fourth lumbricals

      II. Clinical signs
- **a.** Clawing of the ring and small fingers
- **b.** Loss of hypothenar muscles
- **c.** Loss of intrinsic muscles
- **d.** Greater IP flexion deformity

  iii. High nerve lesions

      I. Injury at or proximal to the elbow
- **a.** Muscles involved: Muscles previously listed along with flexor carpi ulnaris and flexor digitorum profundus

      II. Clinical signs
- **a.** Clawing of the ring and small fingers
- **b.** Wrist assumes a position of radial extension
- **c.** Slight IP joint flexion deformity
- **d.** Loss of hypothenar muscles
- **e.** Loss of intrinsic muscles
  - **i.** Motor tests

(Pendleton & Schultz-Krohn, 2006, p. 990)
(Radomski & Latham, 2008, p. 1149)

      1. Froment sign
      2. Jeanne sign
      3. Wartenberg sign

iv. Intervention

(Radomski & Latham, 2008, p. 1151)

 I. Instruct patients in techniques to avoid reinjury due to impaired sensation.

 II. Instruct patients in passive ROM exercises to maintain MP joint flexion and IP joint extension. PIP flexion contractures are common and must be avoided.

 III. Built-up handles may improve independence with activities of daily living (ADL).

 IV. Splinting

(Pendleton & Schultz-Krohn, 2006, p. 998)
(Radomski & Latham, 2008, p. 450)

  a. MP extension block that positions the MP of the ring and small fingers in slight flexion and prevents hyperextension

  b. The hand-based splint positions the hand to promote a functional grasp/release.

e. Radial nerve

(Pendleton & Schultz-Krohn, 2006, p. 997)

 i. Innervation patterns

  I. Motor

   a. Brachioradialis

   b. Extensor carpi radialis longus

   c. Extensor carpi radialis brevis (ECRB)

   d. Extensor digitorum communis

   e. Extensor digiti minimi

   f. Extensor indicis

   g. Extensor carpi ulnaris

   h. Extensor pollicis brevis (EPB)

   i. Extensor pollicis longus

   j. Supinator

   k. Abductor pollicis longus (APL)

  II. Sensory

   a. Posterior upper arm and forearm

   b. Dorsum of the thumb, index finger, middle finger, radial half of the ring finger to the PIP joints

 ii. Clinical signs

(Pendleton & Schultz-Krohn, 2006, p. 997)
(Radomski & Latham, 2008, pp. 1151–1152)

  I. High nerve lesions: Above supinator

   a. Pronation of the forearm

   b. Wrist flexion

   c. Thumb in palmar abduction

   d. Incomplete MP joint extension

   e. Loss of sensation in radial nerve distribution in forearm and hand

  II. Posterior interosseous nerve syndrome (radial nerve compression)

(Pendleton & Schultz-Krohn, 2006, p. 997)
(Radomski & Latham, 2008, p. 1150)

  a. Wrist extension is radial (extensor carpi radialis longus, extensor carpi radialis brevis remain innervated).

  b. Loss of finger and thumb extension

       c. Normal sensation

III. Low nerve lesions: Posterior interosseous palsy

(Radomski & Latham, 2008, pp. 1151–1152)

       a. Incomplete MP joint extension of the fingers and thumb
       b. Wrist extension is radial (extensor carpi radialis longus, extensor carpi radialis brevis remain innervated).
       c. Distal sensory loss

  iii. Intervention
       I. Maintain passive ROM of wrist thumb and digital extension.
       II. Splinting

(Pendleton & Schultz-Krohn, 2006, pp. 700, 702, Figures 29–18, 29–24)
(Radomski & Latham, 2008, p. 449)

       a. Dynamic extension splint: Dorsal forearm-based splint provides:
         i. Wrist extension
         ii. MP joint extension
         iii. Thumb extension
         iv. Dynamic splinting protects extensors from overstretching and allows active use of the hand with functional activities.

f. Postoperative nerve repair

(Pendleton & Schultz-Krohn, 2006, p. 998)

  i. Immobilization (2–3 weeks): A position of limited tension on the repaired nerve as prescribed by physician; most commonly flexion for the median and ulnar nerve and extension for the radial nerve.
  ii. Protective ROM (4–6 weeks)
       I. Active ROM
       II. Instruct in techniques to avoid reinjury due to impaired sensation.
  iii. Dynamic splinting
       I. Gradual reduction of contractures
       II. Assist absent or weak muscles
  iv. As sensation and motor function return:
       I. Instruct in correct patterns of motion.
       II. Asses ADL function.
       III. Revise adaptive equipment, splinting, and exercises.
       IV. Perform frequent sensory and functional testing.

4. Flexor tendon injuries
  a. Anatomy zones

(Radomski & Latham, 2008, pp. 1155–1156)

  i. Zone I: Insertion of the flexor digitorum profundus to insertion of the flexor digitorum superficialis
  ii. Zone II: Insertion of the flexor digitorum superficialis to the A1 pulley (MP joint area); this zone is also known as "no man's land"
  iii. Zone III: A1 pulley to the distal edge of the carpal tunnel
  iv. Zone IV: Carpal tunnel
  v. Zone V: Forearm

  b. Treatment protocols

(Pendleton & Schultz-Krohn, 2006, pp. 999–1000)

  i. Immobilization
       I. Use of the protocol is frequently limited to patients with multiple injuries, fracture/nerve and tendon injuries, noncompliant clients, or with children.

    II. Complete immobilization 3–4 weeks

  ii. Early controlled mobilization: These protocols require a motivated client with the ability to follow instructions closely

    I. Kleinert

      a. Dorsal blocking splint (3 weeks)

        i. Wrist 45° flexion

        ii. MPs 60° flexion

        iii. Rubber band traction from the fingertip passed through a safety pin at the palm (A pulley) then attached to a strap at the forearm level

        iv. The PIP should rest at 40° to 60° flexion.

      b. Exercise

        i. The patient is instructed to extend the digits to the limits of the splint, allowing the rubber band to flex the finger several times a day. The client must fully extend the PIP joint to prevent PIP flexion contractures.

      c. Wrist cuff with rubber band traction (week 4)

        i. May be used for 1 to 4 weeks to protect the healing tendon.

    II. Controlled passive motion/Duran

      a. Dorsal blocking splint

        i. Wrist flexed MP joint 70° flexion

      b. Exercise

        i. Instruct the patient in passive flexion and extension exercises of the digits while the wrist and MP joints remain flexed (can be performed in dorsal blocking splint).

        ii. Between exercises the hand is placed in the splint with the IP joints strapped into extension.

      c. At 4.5 weeks the dorsal blocking splint is removed and rubber band traction is attached to the wrist band.

      d. Active extension and passive flexion of the digits

  c. Postacute flexor tendon rehabilitation (following discontinuance of splint)

(Pendleton & Schultz-Krohn, 2006, pp. 1000–1001)

    i. Monitor active/passive ROM and tendon scar adhesions and modify treatment.

    ii. Tendon glides 10 repetitions two to three times a day

    iii. Blocking exercises

    iv. At 6 weeks postoperation

      I. Passive extension

      II. Splinting

        a. Serial casting

        b. Static splinting

          i. Effective with contractures greater than 25°

        c. Dynamic splinting

          i. Spring finger extension splint

          ii. Dynamic flexion if passive flexion is limited

    v. At 8 weeks resistive exercise may begin

      I. Light ADL

      II. Avoid heavy lifting

      III. Avoid sports

    vi. At 12 weeks no activity restrictions

5. **Extensor tendon injuries**

(Pendleton & Schultz-Krohn, 2006, pp. 1002–1003)

  a. Tendon zones

    i. I = Distal interphalangeal (DIP) joint

    ii. II = P2 (Middle phalanx)

   iii. III = Proximal interphalangeal (PIP) joint
   iv. IV = P1 (Proximal phalanx)
   v. V = Metacarpophalangeal (MP) joint
   vi. VI = Dorsal hand
   vii. VII = Wrist
   viii. VII = Distal forearm
  b. Common deformities

(Radomski & Latham, 2008, p. 1157)

    i. Zones I and II
      I. Ruptured terminal tendon/loss of DIP extension
      II. Immobilize DIP joint in full extension in a static extension splint for 6–8 weeks.
      III. Maintain PIP motion during immobilization.
      IV. After 6 weeks of immobilization, begin active ROM of the DIP. If DIP lags develop, resume extension splinting to maintain DIP extension.
    ii. Zones III–IV (boutonnière deformity)
      I. Splint PIP at full extension for 6 weeks DIP free, MP free.
      II. Encourage DIP flexion while in splint.
      III. After 6 weeks of immobilization, begin active ROM of the PIP. If PIP lags develop, resume extension splinting to maintain DIP extension.
    iii. Zones V and VI
      I. Immobilization
      II. Controlled early motion

6. Complex injuries of the wrist and hand

(Pendleton & Schultz-Krohn, 2006, p. 1004)

  a. Involves multiple structures of the upper extremity
  b. Skin, tendon, nerve, bone
    i. Common injuries include:
      I. Motor vehicle accidents
      II. Crush injuries
      III. Gunshot wounds
        a. Amputations, replantation, and avulsion injuries
    ii. Gather information regarding location of injuries.
    iii. Types of repairs performed
    iv. Associated injuries
    v. Sutures that were used
    vi. For structures that were injuries but not repaired, remain in frequent communication with the doctor.

7. Complex regional pain syndrome (CRPS)

(Radomski & Latham, 2008, p. 1157)

  a. Type I follows a noxious event (nonnerve injury).
    i. Pain in multiple nerve distributions
    ii. Pain that is disproportionate to the injury
    iii. Edema
    iv. Abnormal skin and sudomotor activity in the painful area
  b. Type II develops after a nerve injury
  c. Symptoms are the same as previously described
  d. Treatment Type I, II
  e. Self-immobilization increases risk factor of CRPS.
  f. Early diagnosis is key.
  g. Must learn to use the extremity in ways that are pain free and efficient

h. Normalize sensory input

8. Cumulative trauma disorders

(Radomski & Latham, 2008, pp. 1146–1150)

a. Lateral epicondylitis
  i. Involves extensor carpi radialis brevis
  ii. Pain at extensor mass and lateral epicondyle
    I. Differential diagnosis/radial tunnel
      a. Pain area
      b. Middle finger test
      c. Tinel test of radial nerve
  iii. Splint
    I. Wrist extension (0° to 30°)
    II. Counterforce strap
  iv. Exercise
    I. Proximal conditioning
    II. Scapular stabilizing
  v. ADL
    I. Built-up handles

b. Medial epicondylitis
  i. Involves flexor carpi radialis
  ii. Pain at flexor mass and medial epicondyle
  iii. Pain increases with resistive flexion and pronation
  iv. Splint
    I. Wrist neutral
    II. Counterforce strap
  v. Exercise
    I. Proximal conditioning
  vi. ADL
    I. Built-up handles

c. Trigger finger
  i. Stenosis of the flexor tendon at the A1 pulley
    I. Splint
      a. MP joint extension
      b. Tendon glides/place and hold fisting
    II. ADL
      a. Built-up handles
      b. Padded gloves
      c. Pacing

d. Carpal tunnel syndrome
  i. Median nerve compression at the carpal tunnel
    I. Symptoms
    II. Associated diagnosis
    III. Evaluation
      a. Screening neck and shoulder

      (Pendleton & Schultz Krohn, 2006, p. 986)

      b. ROM
      c. Grip
      d. Pinch
      e. Manual muscle testing (MMT)
      f. Independent excursion of flexor digitorum superficialis (FDS) and flexor digitorum profundus (FDP)
      g. Monofilament test, two-point discrimination

                  h. Tinel
                  i. Phalen

IV. Splinting
    a. Wrist neutral nighttime only

V. Exercise
    a. Tendon glides
    b. Aerobic exercise
    c. Proximal conditioning
    d. Postural training

VI. ADL
    a. Ergonomic modification
    b. Avoid extremes of forearm rotation or wrist motions.
    c. Avoid forceful grip and pinch.
    d. Padded gloves and built-up handles

VII. Postoperative carpal tunnel release (CTR)
    a. Edema control
    b. Scar management
    c. Desensitization
    d. Nerve glides tendon glides
    e. Strengthening exercises

e. de Quervain disease
  i. Involves the abductor pollicis longus and extensor pollicis brevis
  ii. Finkelstein test
  iii. Differential diagnosis
    I. Thumb carpal metacarpal (CMC) arthritis
    II. Scaphoid fracture
    III. Intersection syndrome
    IV. Flexor carpi radialis tendonitis
  iv. Splinting
    I. Forearm-based thumb spica with IP free
  v. ADL
    I. Avoid wrist deviation with pinching
    II. Built-up handles

f. Cubital tunnel
  i. Compression of the ulnar nerve between the medial epicondyle and the olecranon
  ii. Symptoms
    I. Proximal and medial forearm pain that is aching or sharp
    II. Decrease sensation in the dorsal and palmar surface of the small finger and ulnar half of the ring finger.
      a. Weakness of the flexor digitorum profundus to ring finger and small finger
      b. Flexor carpi ulnaris
      c. Dorsal and volar interossei
      d. Adductor pollicis
      e. Grip and pinch weakness
      f. Increase symptoms with repetitive elbow flexion or prolonged elbow flexion.
  iii. Evaluation
    I. Tinel
      a. Elbow flexion test with wrist neutral
      b. Wartenberg sign
      c. Froment sign
      d. Observe hand for evidence of digital clawing.
      e. Observe hand for evidence of muscle atrophy in the first web space, hypothenar, and medial forearm.
      f. Grip

        g. Pinch

        h. MMT

        i. Sensory testing

iv. Splinting

    I. Elbow pads/soft splints

    II. Anterior of posterior static elbow splints

        a. 30° of elbow flexion

        b. Use while sleeping

    III. ADL

        a. Avoid resting on elbow.

        b. Avoid prolonged flexed elbow postures.

        c. Avoid repetitive elbow activities.

        d. Splinting

        e. Ergonomic training

    IV. Exercise

        a. Ulnar nerve gliding

        b. Proximal conditioning

        c. Postural training

9. Physical agent modalities

(McPhee, Bracciano, Rose, Brayman, & Commission on Practice, 2003, pp. 650–651)
(Pendleton & Schultz-Krohn, 2006, p. 676)
(Radomski & Latham, 2008, p. 544)

  a. Thermal modalities

(Pendleton & Schultz-Krohn, 2006, pp. 676–677)
(Radomski & Latham, 2008, pp. 548–550)

  b. Superficial thermal agents

    i. Modality applied to the skin that can increase or decrease the temperature of the skin and subcutaneous tissue

        I. Thermal modalities (heat)

        II. Superficial agents can affect structures up to 1 cm in depth.

        III. To be beneficial, tissue temperature should raise between 102°F and 113°F.

        IV. Most heat modalities are applied for 20 minutes.

        V. Heat is typically used before exercise, dynamic splinting, ADL, or work simulation activities.

    ii. Types

        I. Conduction

            a. The body part comes in direct contact with the heat agent.

                i. Paraffin

                    1. Temperature of the paraffin should be checked prior to patient application (113°F to 122°F).

                    2. Frequently used with a positional stretch/finger flexion using coban or elastic wrap

                ii. Hot packs

                    1. Need six to eight towel layers

                    2. Can be placed in a positional stretch to improve extensibility

        II. Convection

            a. The body part comes in direct contact with the moving media.

                i. Whirlpool

                    1. Could be used as a cooling agent or heating agent

                    2. Can perform active ROM

                    3. Used mostly for wound care as a nonselective debridement tool

                ii. Fluidotherapy

        1. Can perform active and passive ROM

        2. Can adjust temperature

        3. Adjustable amount or particle agitation

        4. Useful for injuries that are hypersensitive

iii. Indications

    I. Increase motion

    II. Decrease joint stiffness

    III. Relieve muscle spasms

    IV. Vasodilatation

    V. Decrease pain

iv. Precautions

(Radomski & Latham, 2008, pp. 548, 1135)

    I. Diminished sensation

    II. Impaired circulation

    III. Edema

    IV. Use of anticoagulant medication

v. Contraindications

    I. Impaired sensation

    II. Tumors, cancer

    III. Cardiac disease

    IV. Acute edema

    V. Deep vein thrombophlebitis

    VI. Pregnancy

    VII. Bleeding tendencies

    VIII. Infection

    IX. Primary repair of ligament or tendon

    X. Impaired cognitive status

vi. Cryotherapy

(Pendleton & Schultz-Krohn, 2006, p. 677)

(Radomski & Latham, 2008, p. 550)

    I. Use of cold in therapy

    II. Types

        a. Ice cubes

        b. Cold packs

        c. Cold bath

        d. Controlled compression units

    III. Indications

        a. Vasoconstriction

        b. Decease edema and inflammation

        c. Decrease pain by increasing the pain threshold

        d. Decrease muscle spasms and spasticity

    IV. Contraindications

        a. Impaired circulation

        b. Cold sensitivity/Raynaud phenomenon

        c. Multiple myeloma

        d. Leukemia

        e. Cold intolerance

c. Electrical modalities

(Radomski & Latham, 2008, pp. 555–563)

    i. Transcutaneous electrical nerve stimulation (TENS)

(Pendleton & Schultz-Krohn, 2006, p. 678)

        I.   Used for pain control

  ii.   Neuromuscular electrical stimulation (NMES): Pulsating alternating current to activate a muscle through stimulation of intact peripheral nerves to cause a motor response

        I.   Indications

            a. Increase or facilitate active ROM

            b. Muscle reeducation

            c. Temporary reduction in spasticity

            d. Strengthen muscle to prevent disuse atrophy

 iii.   Functional electrical stimulation (FES): Neuromuscular electrical stimulation to target muscles for orthopedic substitution

        I.   Indications

            a. Foot drop

            b. Shoulder subluxation

  iv.   Iontophoresis: Introduction of a drug into the body by means of a direct current

(Pendleton & Schultz-Krohn, 2006, p. 678)
(Radomski & Latham, 2008, p. 564)

        I.   Indications: Inflammatory conditions

            a. Sprains and strains

            b. Trigger finger

            c. Lateral/medial epicondylitis

            d. Joint inflammation

            e. Scar adhesions

        II.   Precautions

            a. Drug interactions

d. Ultrasound

(Radomski & Latham, 2008, p. 564)

    i.   Uses sound waves

        I.   Nonthermal mode

        II.   Thermal

            a. Considered to be a deep-heating modality

            b. Most direct and effective means of heating soft tissue

10. Splinting

  a. Anatomical and biomechanical considerations

(Pendleton & Schultz-Krohn, 2006, pp. 688–694)
(Radomski & Latham, 2008, pp. 466–468)

    i.   Wrist

   ii.   Metacarpal joints

  iii. Thumb

   iv.   Interphalangeal joints

    v.   Nerve compression sites

   vi.   Arches of the hand

        I.   Distal transverse arch

        II.   Longitudinal arch

        III. Proximal transverse arch

  vii. Dual obliquity

 viii. Functional position

(Pendleton & Schultz-Krohn, 2006, pp. 711–712)
(Radomski & Latham, 2008, p. 467)

   ix.   Safe position/antideformity

(Radomski & Latham, 2008, pp. 469, 1134)

b. Forces

(Pendleton & Schultz-Krohn, 2006, pp. 698–699)

    i. Stress
    ii. Friction
    iii. Torque
    iv. Translation forces

c. Types of splints

(Pendleton & Schultz-Krohn, 2006, pp. 699–700, 708–710)
(Radomski & Latham, 2008, pp. 423, 480)

    i. Static: Static splints have no movable components. They are used to immobilize, decrease pain, or prevent contracture.
        I. Serial static splints
        II. Static progressive splints
    ii. Dynamic splints: These splints enable motion through the use of rubber bands, springs, and/or elastic cords. They are used to increase passive motion and assist with or substitute for lost motion.
        I. High-profile dynamic splints
        II. Low-profile dynamic splints

d. Splinting material characteristics

(Pendleton & Schultz-Krohn, 2006, pp. 707–708)

    i. Resistance to stretch/conformability
    ii. Memory
    iii. Rigidity
    iv. Bonding

e. Fabrication of a custom splint

(Radomski & Latham, 2008, pp. 477–481)

    i. Design
    ii. Select material
    iii. Pattern
    iv. Cut material
    v. Heat
    vi. Form splint
    vii. Finish edges
    viii. Strap padding and attachments
    ix. Evaluate splint

f. Client instruction

(Pendleton & Schultz-Krohn, 2006, pp. 703–704)
(Radomski & Latham, 2008, pp. 472–473)

    i. Precautions
    ii. Compliance
    iii. Wearing schedule

CASE STUDIES

Case Study 10-1. Chris fractured his right wrist and underwent a closed reduction 7 weeks ago; his cast was removed today. Exercise in treatment today should focus on:

A. Shoulder and elbow
B. Passive wrist flexion and extension exercise
C. Isolated extensor digitorum communis (EDC) exercises and wrist extension exercises

Case Study 10-2. The OT receives an order to splint a patient with carpal tunnel syndrome. The best splint for conservative management is:

A. Wrist cock-up splint with the wrist in neutral
B. Static MP extension splint
C. Elbow extension splint

Case Study 10-3. Which flexor tendon protocol is used with very young children or adults who are noncompliant?

A. Duran
B. Kleinert
C. Immobilization
D. Chow

WORK SHEETS

Work Sheet 10-1

Match the nerve lesion to the clinical sign.

Table 10-2 Nerve Lesion to the Clinical Sign

A. High radial nerve lesion — C Clawing of the ring and small fingers

B. Low median nerve lesion — A Incomplete MP extension

C. Low ulnar nerve lesion — B Loss of palmar abduction and opposition

D. Anterior interosseous nerve — D FDP to the index and middle fingers with no sensory loss

Work Sheet 10-2

Match the cumulative trauma disorder to the involved muscle.

Table 10-3 Cumulative Trauma Disorder to the Involved Muscle

A. Lateral epicondylitis   B Involves FCR

B. Medial epicondylitis   A Involves ECRB

C. de Quervain disease   C Involves APL and EPB

Work Sheet 10-3

Name the arches of the hand.

1. _____
2. _____
3. _____

Name the steps in splint fabrication.

1. _____
2. _____
3. _____
4. _____
5. _____
6. _____
7. _____
8. _____
9. _____

REFERENCES

McPhee, S. D., Bracciano, A. G., Rose, B. W., Brayman, S. J., & Commission on Practice. (2003). Physical agent modalities: A position paper. *American Journal of Occupational Therapy, 57*(6), 650–651.

Pendleton, H. M., & Schultz-Krohn, W. (Eds.). (2006). *Pedretti's occupational therapy: Practice skills for physical dysfunction* (6th ed.). St. Louis, MO: Mosby.

Radomski, M. V., & Latham, C. A. T. (Eds.). (2008). *Occupational therapy for physical dysfunction* (6th ed.). Philadelphia: Lippincott Williams & Wilkins.

CASE STUDY RATIONALE

Case Study 10-1.   Correct answer: C.   It is important to retrain the wrist extensors independent of the EDC. It is also important to retrain the EDC independent of the intrinsics.

Case Study 10-2.   Correct answer: A.   Static splinting of the wrist is recommended at night to minimize the pressure in the carpal tunnel.

Case Study 10-3.   Correct answer: C.   Duran uses passive flexion and extension, Kleinert uses rubber band traction, and Chow uses a combination of Kleinert and Duran. Immobilization is the only protocol that does not require client participation.

WORK SHEET ANSWERS

Work Sheet 10-1

Table 10-4 Nerve Lesion to the Clinical Sign Answers

A. High radial nerve lesion

B. Low median nerve lesion

C. Low ulnar nerve lesion

D. Anterior interosseous nerve

  C   Clawing of the ring and small fingers

  A   Incomplete MP extension

  B   Loss of palmar abduction and opposition

  D   FDP to the index and middle fingers with no sensory loss

---

Work Sheet 10-2

Table 10-5 Cumulative Trauma Disorder to the Involved Muscle Answers

A. Lateral epicondylitis

B. Medial epicondylitis

C. de Quervain disease

  B   Involves FCR

  A   Involves ECRB

  C   Involves APL and EPB

Work Sheet 10-3

Name the arches of the hand.

1. **Digital transverse arch**

2. **Longitudinal arch**

3. **Proximal arch**

Name the steps in splint fabrication.

1. **Design**

2. **Select material**

3. **Pattern**

4. **Cut material**

5. **Heat**

6. **Form splint**

7. **Finish edges**

8. **Strap padding and attachments**

9. **Evaluate splint**

Exhibit 1-1 Stress Vulnerability Scale

In modern society, most of us can't avoid stress. But we can learn to behave in ways that lessen its effects. Researchers have identified a number of factors that affect one's vulnerability to stress—among them are eating and sleeping habits, caffeine and alcohol intake, and how we express our emotions. The following questionnaire is designed to help you discover your vulnerability quotient and to pinpoint trouble spots. Rate each item from 1 (always) to 5 (never), according to how much of the time the statement is true of you. Be sure to mark each item, even if it does not apply to you—for example, if you don't smoke, circle 1 next to item six.

	Always	Sometimes			Never
1. I eat at least one hot, balanced meal a day.	1	2	3	4	5
2. I get 7–8 hours of sleep at least four nights a week.	1	2	3	4	5
3. I give and receive affection regularly.	1	2	3	4	5
4. I have at least one relative within 50 miles on whom I can rely.	1	2	3	4	5
5. I exercise to the point of perspiration at least twice a week.	1	2	3	4	5
6. I limit myself to less than half a pack of cigarettes a day.	1	2	3	4	5
7. I take fewer than five alcohol drinks a week.	1	2	3	4	5
8. I am the appropriate weight for my height.	1	2	3	4	5
9. I have an income adequate to meet basic expenses.	1	2	3	4	5
10. I get strength from my religious beliefs.	1	2	3	4	5
11. I regularly attend club or social activities.	1	2	3	4	5
12. I have a network of friends and acquaintances.	1	2	3	4	5
13. I have one or more friends to confide in about personal matters.	1	2	3	4	5
14. I am in good health (including eyesight, hearing, and teeth).	1	2	3	4	5
15. I am able to speak openly about my feelings when angry or worried.	1	2	3	4	5
16. I have regular conversations with the people I live with about domestic problems—for example, chores and money.	1	2	3	4	5
17. I do something for fun at least once a week.	1	2	3	4	5
18. I am able to organize my time effectively.	1	2	3	4	5
19. I drink fewer than three cups of coffee (or other caffeine-rich drinks) a day.	1	2	3	4	5
20. I take some quiet time for myself during the day.	1	2	3	4	5

Exhibit 1-1 Stress Vulnerability Scale *(continued)*

Scoring Instructions: To calculate your score, add up the figures and subtract 20.

Score Interpretation:
A score below 10 indicates excellent resistance to stress.
A score over 30 indicates some vulnerability to stress.
A score over 50 indicates serious vulnerability to stress.

Self-Care Plan: Notice that nearly all the items describe situations and behaviors over which you have a great deal of control. Review the items on which you scored three or higher. List those items in your self-care plan. Concentrate first on those that are easiest to change—for example, eating a hot, balanced meal daily and having fun at least once a week—before tackling those that seem difficult.

Source: Exhibit courtesy Copyright 2009 Stress Directions, Inc., Lyle H. Miller and Alma Dell Smith, Boston, MA
www.stressdirections.com

Exhibit 5-1 Reflection Question Journal

1. What? (What have I accomplished? What have I learned?)

2. So what? (What difference did it make? Why should I do it? How is it important? How do I feel about it?)

3. Now what? (What's next? Where do we go from here?)

Source: Exhibit courtesy of Live Wire Media.

Assessment of Occupational Functioning: Mental Health (Day 16)

Assessments and Evaluations of Mental Health Conditions

Regina Parnell, Doreen Head, and Sophia Kimmons

OBJECTIVES

1. Describe the core concepts and assumptions of the psychosocial frames of reference.
2. Demonstrate knowledge of psychosocial health conditions.
3. Review and reinforce best practice indications for selecting psychosocial assessments.
4. Describe the commonly used psychosocial assessments.
5. Apply knowledge of assessments into practical, clinical scenarios.

Table 11-1 Key Terms

Terms	Definitions
Affect	Sadock & Sadock, 2003, p. 280
DSM-IV	Sadock & Sadock, 2003, pp. 289–318
Dual diagnosis	Sadock & Sadock, 2003, p. 292
Negative symptoms	Sadock & Sadock, 2003, p. 490
Perceptual disturbance	Sadock & Sadock, 2003, p. 285
Positive symptoms	Sadock & Sadock, 2003, p. 490
Self-concept	Cole, 2005, p. 115
Thought disorder	Sadock & Sadock, 2003, pp. 239, 282–284

INTRODUCTION

Welcome to Day 16 of your study guide. This chapter provides a review of the content area of psychosocial assessments and evaluations. Included is a review of the major occupational therapy psychosocial frames of reference, as well as an overview of the primary mental health diagnoses. This chapter provides an in-depth review of the key assessments and evaluation tools used for the treatment of clients with mental health diagnoses. Use the outline to gather pertinent information, and complete the corresponding work sheets to reinforce your understanding of the key points and application of knowledge.

OUTLINE

1. Psychosocial theories, frames of reference, and models of practice

Occupational therapists use theory-based principles to inform and guide their treatment approaches. Theories refer to a set of statements or principles that conceptualize and interpret aspects of human occupation and behavior. Theories assist therapists with determining when, how, and why a particular human phenomenon exists.

The term "frame of reference" refers to a specific formulation of concepts, which includes four basic components: (1) the theoretical base or explanation of the concept; (2) the criteria for determining function and dysfunction as it relates to the concept; (3) statements regarding evaluation and assessment tools; and (4) statements regarding intervention methods (Bruce & Borg, 2002, pp. 9–10).

Traditional occupational therapy psychosocial frames of reference and three contemporary occupational therapy theories are reviewed.

   a. Contemporary occupational theories

(Bruce & Borg, 2002, p. 46)

     i. Person Environment Occupation
     ii. Occupational Behavior
     iii. Dynamic Interactional Model of Cognitive Rehabilitation
   b. Traditional frames of reference
     i. Behavioral (Bruce & Borg, 2002, pp. 122–155)
     ii. Cognitive–Behavioral (Bruce & Borg, 2002, pp. 162–199)
     iii. Cognitive–Disability (Bruce & Borg, 2002, pp. 244–262)
     iv. Developmental (Cole, 2005, pp. 203–213)
     v. Model of Human Occupation (MOHO) (Bruce & Borg, 2002, pp. 210–235)
     vi. Psychodynamic (Bruce & Borg, 2002, pp. 70–105)
     vii. Sensory Motor (Bruce & Borg, 2002, pp. 302–319)

2. Mental Health Conditions

(American Psychiatric Association, 2000; Bruce & Borg, 2002, pp. 29–30; Early, 2009, pp. 151–174).

Persons diagnosed with mental health conditions range in age from infancy through older adulthood. The fourth edition of the *Diagnostic and Statistical Manual of Mental Disorders* (DSM-IV) provides multiaxial guidelines for determining the range and severity of a condition based on the person's symptoms. Axis I defines the clinical disorders; mental health disorders are included here. Axis II defines the presence of any personality disorder. Axis III refers to general medical conditions. Axis IV includes information about the psychosocial and environmental problems. Axis V makes a determination about the client's global assessment of functioning (GAF).

   a. Adult disorders
     i. Psychosomatic disorders
     ii. Somatoform disorders
     iii. Anxiety disorders
     iv. Dementia
     v. Depression and mania
     vi. Suicidal behavior
     vii. Eating disorders
     viii. Personality disorders
     ix. Schizophrenic and delusional disorders
     x. Drug dependence and addiction
   b. Childhood disorders
     i. Attention-deficit/hyperactivity disorder (ADHD)
     ii. Oppositional defiant

✓**iii.** Autism and Asperger syndrome

✓**iv.** Mood disorders

3. **Selecting data-gathering assessment tool**

   a. Evidence-based practice; what is the best choice?

(Early, 2009, p. 392)

      i. Literature reviews: Higher-level result per researched topic

      ii. Expert opinion: Lower-level result per senior seasoned therapist

   b. Purpose of assessment

(Early, 2009, pp. 398–400)

      i. Identify deficits and strengths

      ii. Identify skills and habits

      iii. Identify goals and objectives

      iv. Identify functional abilities

      v. Identify values and interests

      vi. Identify contextual environments

   c. Areas of focus for data collecting

(Early, 2009, pp. 405, 413)

      i. Analysis of occupational performance (American Occupational Therapy Association [AOTA], 2008, p. 628)

      ii. Contextual

      iii. Client's goals

      iv. Impediments to engagement

   d. Concepts of assessment

      i. Standardized

      ii. Nonstandardized

4. **Psychosocial evaluations and assessments**

(Crepeau, et al., 2009, pp. 1090–1137)

    Evaluations refer to the comprehensive appraisal of a client's condition, environmental circumstance, deficits, potential for success, and recommendations for discharge setting and resources. An evaluation utilizes one or more individual assessment tools to make these determinations.

    Assessments refer to the measurement of more specific or narrow aspects of client factors, client occupational performance, and contexts. This chapter provides a review of both types of these tests and measurement tools. Some tools are appropriate for use across the lifespan while others were designed with specific ages in mind.

   a. Lifespan assessments

      i. Mini-Mental State Examiniation (MMSE)

      ii. Kohlman Evaluation of Living Skills (KELS)

      iii. Model of Human Occupation (MOHO)

      iv. Holmes-Rahe Life Change Inventory

      v. Allen Cognitive Level (ACL) Test

      vi. Role Checklist

      vii. Leisure Diagnostic Battery (LDB)

      viii. Occupational Case Analysis and Interview Rating Scales (OCAIRS)

      ix. Occupational Performance History Interview II (OPHI-II)

   b. Adolescence

      i. Adolescent Role Assessment (ARA)

      ii. Coping Inventory

   c. Adulthood

      i. Community Integration Questionnaire

      ii. Activity Card Diagnostic

WORK SHEETS

Work Sheet 11-1. Psychosocial Theories and Frames of Reference

(Bruce & Borg, 2002, pp. 70–105, 122–155, 162–199, 202–319)

(Cole, 2005, pp. 203–213)

Table 11-2 Psychosocial Theories and Frames of Reference

Theory	Author	Key Approaches
Behavioral		
Cognitive–Behavioral		
Cognitive–Disability		
Developmental		
MOHO		
Psychodynamic		
Sensorimotor		

Work Sheet 11-2. Assessments and Evaluations of Mental Health Conditions

(Early, 2009, pp. 147–177)

Table 11-3 Assessments and Evaluations of Mental Health Conditions

Mental Health Disorder	Positive Signs and Symptoms	Negative Signs and Symptoms
Attention-deficit/hyperactivity disorder		
Alzheimer disease		
Alcohol abuse		
Anxiety disorder		
Anorexia nervosa		
Bipolar II disorder		
Conduct disorder		
Depression		
Drug dependence		
Obsessive compulsive disorder		
Personality disorders		
Psychosomatic disorders		
Schizophrenic delusion		
Somatoform		

Work Sheet 11-3. Occupational Therapy Psychosocial Assessment

(Crepeau, et al., 2009, pp. 1090–1152)

Table 11-4 Occupational Therapy Psychosocial Assessment

Assessments	Population	Key Features Purpose
ACL		
MOHO		
Role Checklist		
Adolescent Role Assessment		
KELS		
MMSE		
Occupational Performance History		
Leisure Diagnostic Battery		
OCAIRS		
OPHI-II		

REFERENCES

American Occupational Therapy Association. (2008). Occupational therapy practice framework: Domain and process 2nd edition. *American Journal of Occupational Therapy, 62*(6), 625–683.

American Psychiatric Association. (2000). *Diagnostic and Statistical Manual of Mental Disorders: DSM-IV-TR.* Washington, DC: Author.

Bruce, M. A., & Borg, B. (2002). *Psychosocial frames of reference: Core for occupation-based practice* (3rd ed.). Thorofare, NJ: Slack.

Cole, M. B. (2005). *Group dynamics in occupational therapy: The theoretical basis and practice application of group intervention* (3rd ed.). Thorofare, NJ: Slack.

Crepeau, E., Cohn, E., & Schell, B. (Eds.) (2009). *Willard & Spackman's occupational therapy* (11th ed.). Philadelphia: Lippincott Williams & Wilkins.

Early, M. B. (2009). *Mental health techniques and concepts for the occupational therapy assistant* (4th ed.). Philadelphia: Lippincott Williams & Wilkins.

Sadock, B. J., & Sadock, V. A. (2003). *Kaplan & Sadock's synopsis of psychiatry: Behavioral sciences/clinical psychiatry* (9th ed.). Philadelphia: Lippincott Williams & Wilkins.

Therapeutic Interventions: Mental Health (Days 17–19)

Psychiatric Interventions

CHAPTER 12

Regina Parnell, Doreen Head, and Sophia Kimmons

OBJECTIVES

1. Describe the core concepts and assumptions of the psychosocial occupational therapy interventions in various practice settings.
2. Understand and apply knowledge of mental health diagnoses.
3. Define and understand the definition of client-centered therapy.
4. Demonstrate knowledge of common pharmacological treatment used with individuals with mental illness.
5. Review and reinforce indications and any precautions or contraindications that are associated with psychosocial interventions.
6. Demonstrate knowledge of selected occupational therapy intervention methods.
7. Apply knowledge of occupational therapy interventions into practical, clinical scenarios.

Table 12-1 Key Terms

Terms	Definitions
Adaptive behavior	Bruce & Borg, 2002, p.133
Behavioral contract	Bruce & Borg, 2002, p.146
Behavioral excess	Bruce & Borg, 2002, p.133
Behavioral rehearsal	Bruce & Borg, 2002, p.135
Corrective learning	Bruce & Borg, 2002, p.135
Habit maps	Bruce & Borg, 2002, p. 216
Maladaptive behavior	Bruce & Borg, 2002, p.134
Medical model	Bruce & Borg, 2002, p. 57
Performance deficit	Bruce & Borg, 2002, p.133
Psychotropic medication	Early, 2009, p. 217

(continues)

Table 12-1 Key Terms *(continued)*

Terms	Definitions
Recovery	Early, 2009, p. 257
Side effects	Early, 2009, p. 219
Skill deficit	Bruce & Borg, 2002, p. 133
Splinter skill	Bruce & Borg, 2002, p. 136
Wellness model	Crepeau, Cohn, & Schell, 2009, p. 618

INTRODUCTION

Welcome to Days 17 and 18 of your study guide. This chapter will review the content area of occupational therapy psychosocial interventions. Psychiatric treatment occurs in a number of settings. Some interventions can be limited by the type of setting where treatment is provided, and other intervention strategies can be utilized across settings. This chapter will provide an in-depth review of the primary treatment environments for clients who are diagnosed with mental health disorders. Use the outline to gather pertinent information and complete the corresponding work sheets to reinforce your understanding of the key points and application of knowledge.

OUTLINE

1. Client-centered clinical reasoning

Persons diagnosed with mental health disorders maintain their unique personhood despite any health condition label. Core personality characteristics often remain intact and manifest in treatment as individual strengths and challenges and personal likes and dislikes. It is important to approach intervention planning with this in mind. Individuals with mental health disorders make the greatest and most meaningful gains when treatment approaches are based on their unique characteristics and not solely on the symptoms of the disorder.

2. Treatment settings

Individuals with mental health disorders may receive treatment in a variety of psychosocial healthcare settings. These settings are broadly divided into two categories: traditional and community. Traditional settings are typically based on the medical model where the individual is defined as a patient. They include inpatient and outpatient models and often are affiliated with a hospital. Community settings are also called nontraditional sites. These venues view individuals as clients or consumers. Generally, they are not directly under the auspices of any hospital but may have an ongoing relationship with a medical facility to provide care as needed for the clients. Some settings are treatment based; some are focused on supporting the resumption of developing the skills necessary to live independently.

   a. Traditional inpatient setting
      i. Long term

      (Early, 2009, p. 187)
         Facilities that provide long-term care for individuals with mental illness often treat inpatients for extended periods of time. They comprise a full medical team including a psychiatrist, internist, psychologist, nurse, occupational therapist, social worker, and various support personnel. They typically offer specialized treatment based on age (e.g., adolescent or geriatric), diagnoses, or both. Currently, long-term care facilities are limited in number because the majority of these facilities have been closed in most major cities.

    I.   Facility intervention
- **a.** Medication
- **b.** Psychotherapy
- **c.** Medical model

    II. Psychosocial intervention
- **a.** Work
- **b.** ADL and IADL
- **c.** Social skills training
- **d.** Behavior management
- **e.** Leisure
- **f.** Group sessions
- **g.** Milieu therapy
- **h.** Communication skills
- **i.** Community reintegration

ii. Short term

(Early, 2009, pp. 189–190)

Facilities that provide short-term care for individuals with mental illness often treat inpatients ranging from a number of days to a few weeks. They also comprise a full complement of medical staff. These facilities tend to not specialize in particular treatment populations but may segregate patients based on client factors.

    I.   Facility intervention
- **a.** Medication
- **b.** Psychotherapy
- **c.** Medical and crisis model

    II. Psychosocial intervention
- **a.** Counseling
- **b.** Self-care
- **c.** Social skills training
- **d.** Group sessions
- **e.** Milieu therapy

b. Community outpatient settings

(Early, 2009, pp. 192–195)

i. Community mental health clinic

Large agencies that provide a wide range of services offer transitional housing, day treatment, and supportive skills training.

    I.   Facility intervention
- **a.** Medication
- **b.** Psychotherapy
- **c.** Wellness and crisis model

    II. Psychosocial intervention
- **a.** Counseling
- **b.** Self-care
- **c.** Social skills training
- **d.** Exercise
- **e.** Life skills training
- **f.** Group sessions
- **g.** Stress management
- **h.** Chemical dependence and other supports
- **i.** Resources

ii. Day treatment

(Early, 2009, pp. 194–196)

Facilities that provide day treatment offer services during daytime working hours. Each day, clients travel to the facility and attend sessions that are therapeutic in scope, and they return to their homes in the evening. Some clients commute to and from day treatment programs independently, and others depend on transportation arrangements. Clients in day treatment programs have access to paraprofessionals and have their medications and behaviors monitored in that setting.

    I.   Facility intervention
- **a.** Medication
- **b.** Psychotherapy
- **c.** Wellness model

    II.   Psychosocial intervention
- **a.** Counseling
- **b.** Self-care
- **c.** Social skills training
- **d.** Exercise
- **e.** Life skills training
- **f.** Group sessions
- **g.** Coping skills

iii.   Consumer-run facilities (e.g., clubhouses)

(Early, 2009, pp. 196–201)

These facilities are run and sometimes owned and operated by individuals with histories of mental illness. They are based on a self-help model. Fountain House (http://www.fountainhouse.org/) is the premier model in the United States for this approach. The goals are for members to assist each other with reentry into society, promote members' rights, and challenge social stigma. Consumer-run programs offer clients the opportunity to practice social, work, and leisure skills in a supportive peer environment. Members often remain a part of the clubhouse program even after they have returned to independent or semi-independent productive living.

    I.   Facility intervention
- **a.** Independent medication management
- **b.** Independent community mobility
- **c.** Wellness model

    II.   Psychosocial intervention
- **a.** Peer counseling
- **b.** ADL and IADL
- **c.** Social participation
- **d.** Leisure
- **e.** Life skills training
- **f.** Work groups and individuals
- **g.** Staff as a resource
- **h.** Paraprofessional job training and transitional employment
- **i.** Support groups
- **j.** Community resources

c. Community residential settings

(Early, 2009, p. 199)

    i.   Halfway house

These facilities are designed to help individuals who are recovering from various addictions and to facilitate their ongoing recovery. Residents must adhere to rules and make changes that are necessary to avoid relapses and ensure advancement toward a healthy and independent lifestyle. Time at the halfway house provides the person who is recovering from addiction with an opportunity to put into practice new habits and life patterns devoid of substance abuse.

    I.   Facility intervention
- **a.** Supportive medication management
- **b.** Supported group therapy
- **c.** Wellness model

    II.   Psychosocial intervention
- **a.** Nutrition
- **b.** ADL and IADL support
- **c.** Vocational skills and community resources
- **d.** Leisure
- **e.** Socialization
- **f.** Stress management

ii.   Adult foster care

(Early, 2009, p. 203)

These are facilities designed as housing for adults who require some assistance with activities of daily living (ADL). Staff members provide supervision as needed with personal care; however, nursing services are excluded.

iii.   Semi-independent living

(Early, 2009, pp. 203–204)

These are facilities that provide assistance for adolescents who are preparing for independent living. Residents are given assistance with accessing education, employment, and other community services.

iv.   Home health care

(Early, 2009, p. 201)

These services provide intervention in the natural environment that involves the family and the client in a collaborative relationship.

    I.   Transfer skills from inpatient to outpatient
    II.   ADL and IADL
    III.   Solve routine household issues
    IV.   Coping strategies
    V.   Crisis management
    VI.   Cognitive training or retraining
    VII.   Stress management

d. Supportive employment settings
    i.   Transitional employment program (TEP)

(Early, 2009, pp. 200–201)

These programs help individuals with a history of mental illness, developmental disabilities, or both develop work-related skills. Program staff members work with community businesses to employ individuals in the TEP for 6-month intervals. Individuals in this program have an opportunity to get real-world work experience in a competitive but supportive environment, a work reference, and develop a recent and successful work history.

    I.   Counselors
    II.   Job coach
    III.   Placement into part-time job

ii.   Prevocational and vocational rehabilitation program

(Early, 2009, pp. 200–201)

These programs are designed to help individuals develop skills that are necessary for jobs and joblike situations.

> **I.** Help acquire work skills
> **II.** Reinforce work behaviors
> **III.** Train in a particular job function

3. **Client-centered treatment planning**

(Early, 2009, pp. 38–51)

a. Data gathering

Key data includes basic demographic information and a medical history, including current diagnosis.

b. Assess client strengths and challenges or weaknesses

Based on a specific set of assessments utilized in the evaluation process, assessments may focus on client factors and their occupational performance, as well as environmental or contextual factors.

c. Precautions and contraindications

Safety precautions and risk factors are determined by examining a combination of factors. Some diagnoses have inherent deficits associated with the progression of the disorder (e.g., Alzheimer disease). Sometimes precautions are based on the setting in which treatment is provided; for example, an inpatient setting versus a community setting.

Contraindications may arise due to the nature of the intervention, such as a client with poor impulse control on a community outing. The assessment of safety risks should always be based on the unique characteristics and behaviors of the individual in treatment.

4. **OT practice framework intervention strategies**

Five basic intervention strategies are outlined in this chapter, which are discussed next. Each of these intervention strategies requires knowledge of human development, specific disease processes, and an appreciation for human resilience and potential.

a. Create and promote

When the goal of the intervention is to create and promote skills, the underlying assumption is that a skill set has failed to develop; for example, a developmental delay occurs, and as a result the person has minimal ability in communication and social participation.

b. Establish and restore

This is appropriate when the loss of function has occurred. The client may have some previous experience with a skill set and needs assistance with restoration of function.

c. Maintain

This approach is appropriate when a client has the potential to experience a loss of function if certain behaviors, practices, or disease processes continue.

d. Modify

This is appropriate when some functional ability has been permanently lost or diminished.

e. Prevention

This intervention approach is often used to prevent acquired health conditions. This is an appropriate intervention strategy when an individual has an identified risk factor for injury, illness, or disease. This approach also encourages individuals to modify their environments and behaviors to minimize the risk of injury or acquiring a particular health condition.

5. **Interventions**

a. Therapeutic use of self (Early, 2009, pp. 265–281)

(American Occupational Therapy Association [AOTA], 2008, p. 653)

The practitioner's planned use of his or her insights, personality, and judgments are part of the therapy process.

b. Therapeutic use of groups

c. Therapeutic use of occupations and activities

The selection of occupations and activities to meet therapeutic goals:

i. Occupation based: Client engages in client-centered occupations that match goals (e.g., apply for a job)

ii. Purposeful: Specifically selected activity that allows the client to develop skills (e.g., practice folding clothes)

iii. Preparatory method: Selection of methods and techniques (e.g., rhythmic breathing)
   I. Physical
   II. Motor
   III. Cognitive
   IV. Activities of daily living (ADL)
   V. Instrumental activities of daily living (IADL)
   VI. Work
   VII. Play or leisure
   VIII. Medication management
   IX. Emotional regulation
   X. Social participation
   XI. Communication and socialization
   XII. Habits and routines

iv. Precautions and contraindications

v. Consultations
   I. Patient education

6. **Psychosocial outcomes**
   a. Occupational performance
   b. Client satisfaction
   c. Role competence
   d. Adaptation
   e. Health and wellness
   f. Prevention
   g. Quality of life

7. **Pharmacology treatment**

(Early, 2009, pp. 217–229)

a. Antipsychotic medications
   i. Psychotic disorders
   ii. Chemically induced psychotic disorder
   iii. Medically induced psychotic disorder

b. Anti-Parkinsonian medications
   i. Medication side effects
   ii. Movement disorder

c. Antianxiety medications
   i. Reduce stress of nonpsychotic disorder
   ii. Reduce emotions noted with personality disorder

d. Antidepressant medications
   i. Elevate mood

e. Antimanic medications
   i. Control mania symptoms
   ii. Reduce intensity of mood

f. Attention deficit disorder
   i. Stimulate and increase mental activity
   ii. Minimize hyperactivity

g. Side effects and occupational therapy adaptation and interventions

    i.   Teach management skills

    ii.   Help identify, tolerate, and adapt to side effects

    iii. Observe and report side effects to doctor or team

    iv. Encourage medication compliance

    v.   Help with activity selection

    vi. Avoid activities that prolong sitting

    vii. Avoid use of unsafe objects

    viii. Incorporate gross motor activity

    ix. Teach compensatory techniques

    x.   Educate on mixture of medication and other chemicals (e.g., alcohol and illicit drugs)

WORK SHEETS

Work Sheet 12-1. Practice Setting Review Activity

(Bruce & Borg, 2002, pp. 2–17)

Table 12-2 Practice Setting Review Activity

Psychosocial	Population	Key Features
Long-term setting		
Short-term setting		
Medical model		
Traditional model		
Community model		
Day treatment		
Adult foster care		
Semi-independent living		
Inpatient		
Halfway house		
TEP		
Outpatient		
Home health		
Vocational		

Work Sheet 12-2. Psychosocial Intervention Selection Learning Activity

(Bruce & Borg, 2002, pp. 28–30)

Table 12-3 Psychosocial Intervention Selection Learning Activity

Signs and Symptoms	Treatment Approaches
Impaired cognition	
Impaired perception	
Psychomotor retardation	
Impaired social skills	
Impulse control	
Substance use	
Impaired ADL	

Work Sheet 12-3. Psychosocial Intervention Occupational Therapy Practice Framework: Domain and Process 2nd Edition (OTPF) and Setting Activity

(Bruce & Borg, 2002, pp. 2–17)

(AOTA, 2008, p. 628)

Table 12-4 Psychosocial Intervention OTPF Framework and Setting Activity

Psychosocial Practice Setting	Intervention Strategies	OTPF Areas and Skills
Long-term setting		
Short-term setting		
Medical model		
Traditional model		
Community model		
Day treatment		
Adult foster care		
Semi-independent living		
Inpatient		
Halfway house		
TEP		
Outpatient		
Home health		
Vocational		

Work Sheet 12-4. Psychosocial Intervention OTPF and Activities Selection Activity

(AOTA, 2008, p. 658)

Identify an activity that coincides with the occupation and skill, for example, an ADL such as dressing.

Table 12-5 Psychosocial Intervention OTPF Framework and Activities Selection Activity

Signs and Symptoms	OTPF Occupations and Skills	Intervention Activities
Impaired cognition		
Impaired perception		
Psychomotor retardation		
Impaired social skills		
Impulse control		
Impaired memory		
Substance use		
Eating disorder		
Elevated mood		
Decreased mood		
Phobia		
Social anxiety		
Impaired ADL		
Acutely ill		
Chronically ill		
Hyperactivity		
Maladaptive communication		
Maladaptive conduct		
Anger		
Impaired boundaries		

Work Sheet 12-5. Psychosocial Intervention Medication Management Learning

(Early, 2009, pp. 217–229)

Table 12-6 Psychosocial Intervention Medication Management Learning Activity

Side Effects	Occupational Therapy, Adaptation, and Interventions
Impaired concentration	
Impaired visual perception	
Psychomotor retardation	
Psychomotor hyperactivity	
Impaired fine motor	
Motor tremors	
Substance use	
Postural hypotension	
Dry mouth	
Weight gain	

REFERENCES

American Occupational Therapy Association. (2008). Occupational therapy practice framework: Domain and process 2nd edition. *American Journal of Occupational Therapy, 62*(6), 625–683.

Bruce, M. A., & Borg, B. (2002). *Psychosocial frames of reference: Core for occupation-based practice* (3rd ed.). Thorofare, NJ: Slack.

Crepeau, E., Cohn, E., & Schell, B. (Eds.). (2009). *Willard & Spackman's occupational therapy* (11th ed.). Philadelphia: Lippincott Williams & Wilkins.

Early, M. B. (2009). *Mental health techniques and concepts for the occupational therapy assistant* (4th ed.). Philadelphia: Lippincott Williams & Wilkins.

Intervention-Group Dynamics

Sophia Kimmons, Doreen Head, and Regina Parnell

OBJECTIVES

1. Describe the scope and limits of group activities and skills through the lenses of theory and evidence-based practice.
2. Identify group leadership guidelines by drawing from occupational therapy frames of reference and the Occupational Therapy Practice Framework: Domain and Process 2nd Edition (OTPF).
3. Demonstrate knowledge of key principles, roles, and functions of the occupational therapist (OT) in program planning and intervention in accordance with the American Occupational Therapy Association's (AOTA) standards of practice.
4. Apply knowledge of occupational therapy assessments and interventions for therapeutic groups that maximize health and wellness of the group and its members.

Table 13-1 Key Terms

Terms	Definitions
Activity analysis	Cole, 2005, p. 7
Client centered	Cole, 2005, pp. 74–75
Counter transference	Hagedorn, 2000, p. 60
Group dynamics	Cole, 2005, pp. 25–48
Group interaction (development) skills	Cole, 2005, pp. 99–101
Group roles	Cole, 2005, pp. 40–41
Occupational Therapy Practice Framework (OTPF)	AOTA, 2008, pp. 625–683
Occupations	AOTA, 2008, p. 658
Therapeutic use of self	AOTA, 2008, pp. 625–683
Transference	Hagedorn, 2000, p. 60

INTRODUCTION

Welcome to Day 19 of your study guide. This chapter will review modes for guiding occupational therapy practice and will cover the following topics:

- Group guidelines
- Group dynamics
- Group design
- Interventions
- Clinical reasoning
- Safety

Use the outline to review key concepts and gather pertinent information. Be sure to complete the corresponding work sheets to reinforce your understanding of topics such as effective group leadership skills and program planning, as well as ways to foster your self-awareness for the development of therapeutic use of self.

OUTLINE

1. **Group guidelines:** This section will address client-centered models of practice, occupational therapy frames of reference, and various group models. These concepts help guide, define, and validate evidence-based occupational therapy practice.
   a. **Client-centered models:** The client is the center and primary focus of client-centered models.
      i. Canadian Occupational Performance Model (COPM): This model was developed to guide service delivery to a diverse group of clients/patients and health care settings; also is referred to as an "open-system model" (Sladyk & Ryan, 2005, p. 78).
      ii. Model of Human Occupation (MOHO): This model asserts that human beings possess an innate drive to explore and master their environments (Cole, 2005, pp. 263–272).
      iii. Frames of reference: These present human functioning on a continuum (i.e., from dysfunctional to functional) and postulate ways occupational therapists can assist clients in ameliorating dysfunction to optimize independence, health, and well-being.
      iv. Sensory Integration (SI): SI theory asserts that the human brain seeks out stimulation that is organized and beneficial for individuals' sensory systems (Cole, 2005, pp. 239–242).
      v. Cognitive Disabilities: This model postulates that a person's ability to use mental energy to guide motor and speech performances will help to predict his or her functioning (Cole, 2005, pp. 177–193).
      vi. Cognitive Behavioral: This model is most often used in psychiatric settings; for example, therapists encourage clients to use their own cognitive abilities to dispute non-productive patterns of thinking (Cole, 2005, pp. 153–158).
      vii. Psychodynamic: The central tenet asserts that a person is capable of developing an increased understanding of self and others, recognizing the causal relationship between behaviors and their outcomes (i.e., cause and effect), and learning from experiences to gain important insights (Cole, 2005, pp. 109–121).
   b. Group models: The group is the structure and focus for each of the following group models:
      i. Task-oriented group: The purpose of the task-oriented group is to provide members a shared working experience (e.g., publishing an electronic newsletter). Collaboration results in an environment where clients' productive and nonproductive behaviors can be observed and addressed. Through their shared experiences, group members begin to recognize the relationship between thinking, feeling, and behavior. Shared experiences also reinforce the notion that one's behavior often has an affect on others, as well as the accomplishment of group tasks and goals. Alternatives

to non-productive behaviors can be identified, tested, and reinforced. This process strengthens members' egos and leads to improved functioning of the group and its members (Cole, 2005, p. 371).

    ii. Developmental group: This group hypothesizes that occupational therapy treatment should be a "recapitulation of ontogenesis." In other words, group processes can repeat the normal course of development, allow opportunities for the individual to return to the earliest developmental lag, and progress until the person reaches the expected developmental level. The model further indicates that one's successful participation in group interaction skill building is related to successfully living in his or her community (Sladyk & Ryan, 2005, pp. 386–387).

    iii. Directive group: This group is designed to provide consistent and structured experiences for individuals who are minimally functioning and acutely mentally ill. Group levels include the following: exploration, competence, and achievement (Cole, 2005, pp. 270–272).

    iv. Integrative group: This group features a five-stage format that is designed to stimulate the senses, encourage movement, and facilitate adequate social interaction, competency, and preferred occupational behaviors (Cole, 2005, pp. 243–248).

  c. OTPF: This framework presents a group of domains and aspects designed to guide occupational therapy practice in all settings while serving any given population.

Table 13-2 Occupational Therapy Practice Framework Domains and Aspects

Areas of Occupation

Activities of daily living (ADL)

Instrumental activities of daily living (IADL)

Rest and sleep

Education

Work

Play

Leisure

Social participation

Performance Skills	**Client Factors**	**Performance Patterns**
Sensory perception	Values	Habits
Motor and praxis	Beliefs	Roles
Emotional regulation	Spirituality	Routines
Cognitive	Body functions	Rituals
Communication and social	Body structure	

Performance and Environment	**Activity Demands**
Cultural	Objects used and their properties
Personal	Social demands
Physical	Sequencing and timing
Social	Required actions
Temporal	Required body functions
Virtual	Required body structures
	Space demands

Source: American Occupational Therapy Association, 2008, p. 628

2. Overview of group dynamics

Occupational therapy intervention may be implemented with clients individually or within a group or both. This section will address the following: group development, group types, group norms, member roles, and decision making and communication.

a. Group development: Tuckman (1965) and Yalom (1995) (cited in Cole, 2005, pp. 29–32) each described stages of group development, regardless of the duration of the group.

   i. Tuckman's four stages of group development

(Cole, 2005, pp. 29–30)

      I. Forming: Involves orientation and testing of the group's task with a high level of dependency on the group's leader.

      II. Storming: As the word implies, this stage involves conflict among the group's members as they challenge the group's task, rules, and leaders.

      III. Norming: In this stage, cohesion and harmony versus discord triumphs and the group's members become accepting and trusting of one another; members actively avoid conflicts.

      IV. Performing: In the last stage, group members work together to openly discuss and resolve conflicts.

   ii. Yalom's three stages of group development

(Cole, 2005, pp. 31–32)

      I. Orientation: Hesitance with regard to participation stems from an individual's need to see how the group can assist him or her in achieving a set of predetermined goals. During this stage, members "size each other up in order determine whether or not they belong as they search for acceptance and approval" (Cole, 2005 p. 31).

      II. Conflict: As members acclimate to the group and compete for power and control, they begin to feel comfortable with contributing personal comments and criticism. Dominance, rebellion, differences, and conflicts arise within the group during this phase of the group's development.

      III. Cohesiveness: Group solidarity results from members resolving initial conflicts and is punctuated by a shared sense of closeness, trust, and support.

   iii. How groups reach maturity

   iv. Maturity: The final stage occurs when "both negative and positive can be freely expressed" by the group's members (Cole, 2005 p. 32).

      I. Focus: The leader helps guide the group toward a predetermined focus.

      II. Attend to feelings: Explore and express personal issues and emotions.

      III. Actively participate: Take an active role; engage in the activity and process.

      IV. Give feedback: Provide honest assessment, both negative and positive, being careful not to single out or belittle.

      V. Be open to feedback: Manage one's emotions and be mindful of such defenses as rationalizing, withdrawing, denying, and/or internalizing the comment(s).

      VI. Take responsibility: Accurately assess situation(s) and take steps to improve the group as needed.

b. Group structures and purpose

   i. Therapeutic groups

      I. Groups are practical and cost-effective.

      II. Through self-disclosure, a person can learn to develop relationships and trust others.

      III. The feedback and support each member gives to one another is of great value.

      IV. Yalom's five factors of therapeutic groups

(Early, 2009, p. 342)

      a. Installation of hope: The positive expectations that members have at the onset of the group

      b. Universality: The sense of relief when one finds that he or she is not the only one with the problem

      c. Altruism: The concept of giving leads to intrinsic benefits.

      d. Group cohesiveness: The sense of camaraderie shared by each group member

      e. Interpersonal learning: The relationship of giving and taking emotionally and socially to enhance one's self or members of the group

ii. The structure of the activity group

(Cole, 2005, pp. 289–294)

    I. Group protocol extensive and detailed plan

      a. Identify population.

      b. Select a frame of reference.

      c. Select a focus of intervention.

      d. Write group intervention plan outline.

      e. Plan sessions.

iii. Selection method

(Early, 2009, pp. 450–452)

    I. After choosing a theory or model of practice, choose the method or the activity/occupation, environment, and therapeutic approach.

    II. *Activities* are the required task behaviors or actions

      a. Choose based on the issue or goal to reach; if following rules is the issue, choose an activity that requires multiple rules.

      b. Choose activities or occupations that are pleasurable and reinforce or enhance the participants' skills.

      c. Choose activities or occupations that are challenging and attainable.

      d. Choose activities or occupations according to the domain areas of occupation; for example, grooming (activities of daily living), medication management (instrumental activities of daily living), social participation or social conduct, and work or job interview.

    III. Environment consists of the physical and social settings.

      a. Environmental demands will evoke expected behaviors or acts.

      b. Environmental support encourages or assists in the performance of a particular behavior or action.

      c. Use the actual environment or simulate the environment when possible.

      d. Modify the environment to encourage successful completion of targeted behaviors or actions or both.

    IV. Therapeutic approach and the conceptual mode (Early, 2009, p. 354)

iv. The success of a group can depend on the kind of preparations the leader has made.

v. There are four areas to consider when preparing for a group:

    I. Knowledge: How well the leader understands and can analyze the various factors of the group; for example, the members, group dynamics, activity/occupation, environment, and their own abilities to successfully lead a group

    II. Space: The preparation of the area in which the group will meet—arrangement of furniture, needed supplies, placement, mix of participants, and social norms

    III. Materials: Ensure equipment, tools and materials, handouts, and samples are ready and available for the group in advance.

    IV. Paperwork: Any documents that will be required, such as attendance sheets, group protocols, session plans, and work sheets; however, with the exception of taking attendance or completing a work sheet, the leader should avoid writing during a session.

Table 13-3 Group Norms

Norms	Criteria
Explicit	Consistent rules **a.** Social: Confidentiality, waiting turns, discussions remain in the group, supportive and nonjudgmental **b.** Punctuality: Begin and end the group on time, arrive and leave at designated times **c.** Work related: Carry out task as directed or instructed **d.** Group organization: Behavior management, rules, disruptive behaviors (i.e., ask person to leave after three disruptions)
Implicit	Indirectly implied evolving rules based on observations of nonverbal behavioral observations **a.** Give permission to behave emotionally with acceptance and offering support. **b.** Imitation of acts through social reinforcement **c.** Adapt behaviors based on nonverbal act (i.e., extinction of negative behaviors and acknowledgment of positive behaviors).
Positive	Acts that create cohesiveness and trust **a.** Negotiate **b.** Compromise
Negative	Acts that create dissension **a.** Interrupting or disrupting group in process **b.** Subgrouping **c.** Avoiding topics or becoming directly involved **d.** Criticizing or blaming others

Source: Cole, 2005, p. 37

    c. Group goals
        i. The purpose for which the group is meeting
        ii. Provides direction and reason for being together; without it groups may fall apart
        iii. Provides task or activity to work toward or to accomplish
        iv. Establish a commonality between group members
    d. Group norms: The rules of behavior, attitudes, and expectations of the group. These norms may be viewed as explicit, implicit, positive, or negative.
    e. Group member roles: The roles that each member assumes based on past experiences and social skills that are consistent with the adaptive-maladaptive continuum. This area will cover adaptive and maladaptive group roles and maladaptive behaviors often displayed in group settings.
        i. Roles are interchangeable.
        ii. Healthy individuals will assume many roles.
        iii. Leaders can enhance group functioning by supporting role formation and modeling adaptive and functional behaviors.
        iv. Adaptive group roles
            I. Task roles

        (Cole, 2005, pp. 40–41)

            a. Initiator-contributor: Individual suggests new ideas.
            b. Information seeker: Individual asks for facts.

    c. Opinion seeker: Individual asks for feelings about issues.

    d. Information giver: Individual provides facts.

    e. Opinion giver: Individual expresses feelings not necessarily based on facts.

    f. Elaborator: Individual spells out suggestions and gives examples.

    g. Coordinator: Individual pulls ideas together.

    h. Orienter: Individual focuses on goals.

    i. Energizer: Individual prods or arouses.

    j. Procedural technician: Individual performs tasks.

    k. Recorder: Individual writes down key points.

II. Maintenance roles

(Cole, 2005, p. 41)

    a. Encourager: Individual praises and accepts others.

    b. Harmonizer: Individual settles differences.

    c. Compromiser: Individual gives in to disputes.

    d. Gatekeeper: Individual keeps communication going.

    e. Standard setter: Individual expresses norms.

    f. Observer: Individual records and offers record to group for feedback.

    g. Follower: Individual goes along with the mood and decisions of the group.

v. Maladaptive group roles and problem behaviors

    I. Antigroup (egocentric) roles

(Cole, 2005, p. 41)

    a. Aggressor: Individual belittles or attacks others.

    b. Blocker: Individual prevents progression.

    c. Recognition seeker: Individual calls attention to him- or herself.

    d. Self-confessor: Individual expresses personal problems.

    e. Playboy: Individual is disruptive and disinterested.

    f. Dominator: Individual controls, manipulates, or interrupts others.

    g. Help seeker: Individual tries to get sympathy and views him- or herself as being victimized.

    h. Special-interest pleader: Individual pretends to speak on behalf of others to express his or her own biases.

    II. Problem behaviors

(Cole, 2005, pp. 41–47)

    a. Monopolist: The person who takes over and dominates the group

    b. Silent member: The person who sits quietly and does not actively engage or participate in the group process

    c. Attention-getter: The person who will use any means to divert attention from others and onto themselves (e.g., self-deprecating, help rejecting, or self-love)

    d. Psychosis: The person who is out of touch with reality

f. Group decision making and communication: This course of action will require the therapist to become self-aware and self-accepting while maintaining and/or developing some key qualities, such as therapeutic use of self. To facilitate this process, the therapist will need to use and/or develop the following eight therapeutic qualities:

    i. Eight therapeutic qualities:

(Early, 2009, pp. 268–270)

    I. Empathy: The ability to understand how the other person feels

    II. Sensitivity: The alertness to a person's needs and awareness of your effect upon that person

    III. Respect: The ability to recognize others as unique individuals with interests and values; to interact with others and allow freedom of choice

    IV. Warmth: The sense of friendliness, interest, and enthusiasm displayed by the therapist

    V. Genuineness: The ability to be oneself; the therapist must be comfortable with him- or herself

    VI. Self-disclosure: The practice of revealing issues about oneself

    VII. Specificity: The art of stating issues simply, directly, and concisely

    VIII. Immediacy: The practice of giving feedback right after the related event

  ii. The eight qualities required to develop therapeutic use of self

(Early, 2009, p. 271)

    I. Ask trusted friends and peers as well as clients for feedback.

    II. Process feedback through the acronym ALOR:

      a. **A**sk open-ended questions.

      b. **L**isten to response.

      c. **O**bserve behaviors and nonverbal actions.

      d. **R**eflect on and consider responses.

3. Group design

Group design is the format used for group sessions. Although there are many designs available, this section discusses three forms of design for the occupational therapy group and exploring the use of therapeutic media.

  a. Classification of activity groups (Hagedorn, 2000, p. 114): The activity is the central and essential component to the group. Mosey's classifications are evaluation, thematic, topical, task oriented, developmental, and instrumental (1973).

  b. Five group interaction skills: Mosey (1973) (cited in Cole, 2005, pp. 99–100) indicates that to effectively facilitate the progression and development of the person's skill levels, people are placed one level above their performance. The designation of interaction skills groups are as follows: parallel, project, egocentric-cooperative, cooperative, and mature.

  c. Seven-step format for group leadership: According to Cole (2005), the seven-step group can be used with the highest level groups and may be easily adapted for other groups. The seven steps are the following: introduction, activity, sharing, processing, generalizing, application, and summary (pp. 3–11).

  4. Occupational therapy intervention may be implemented by an individual therapist or by cotherapists. According to Hagedorn (2000), there are four essential core processes that define the unique contribution of occupational therapy in health care.

Table 13-4 Classification of Activity Groups

Classification	Description
Evaluation	Assess aspects of client performance or ability to function in a group.
Thematic	Gain knowledge, skills, and attitudes needed for mastery of components and aspects of occupational performance (i.e., ADL skills).
Topical	Discussion group that focuses on participation in activities that take place outside of the group (e.g., medication management)
Task oriented	Awareness of members' needs values, ideas, and feelings as they influence actions
Developmental	Meeting a client's needs on different developmental levels of social skills
Instrumental	Meeting health needs and maintaining function and well-being

Table 13-5 Five Group Interaction Skills

Group skills	Description
Parallel	Individuals work or play in the presence of others.
Project	Members involved in short-term task cooperatively or competitively
Egocentric–cooperative	Members jointly decide on long-term activity and carry it through until completion.
Cooperative	Individuals have common interests, concerns, and values, and activity is of little importance.
Mature	Individuals of different backgrounds, ages, interests, and ideas take on roles for task development and group member satisfaction.

Table 13-6 Seven-Step Format for Group Leadership

Seven Steps	Description
Introduction	• OT introduction (name, title, group topic) • Members greet group by saying their name (acknowledge members, help members learn each others' names). • Friendly "hello" when members are late entering the group • Utilize a warm-up activity if necessary (observe receptivity of the members: alertness, preoccupation, mood); may be in the form of a discussion or an activity • Set the mood (environment, facial expressions, and body language, media used, lighting, reduce clutter, and have equipment ready) • Therapeutic use of self (be a role model, explain the purpose of the group, and provide a brief outline of the session) • Brief outline of the activity
Activity	• Consider many factors (knowledge of clients: health conditions, corresponding dysfunctions, assessments). • Intervention planning, activity analysis, and synthesis • Clinical reasoning (therapeutic goals, apply knowledge of their abilities and disabilities, knowledge and skill of the leader and adaptation of activity) • Timing of the group (keep fairly simple and short, activity no longer than one-third of the total session) • Be aware of the behaviors of group members, such as wandering or being preoccupied, being disruptive, or monopolizing. • Meet the needs of most of the group members.
Sharing	• After completing an activity, each member is asked to share the experience with the group (varies with each experience). • Make sure each of the members' contributions are verbally or nonverbally acknowledged. • Be supportive and provide encouragement and reassurance, as well as a role model sharing process.

(continues)

Table 13-6 Seven-Step Format for Group Leadership *(continued)*

Seven Steps	Description
Processing	• This step reveals important and relevant information about the client and encourages members to express their feelings. • Feelings are easy to express if they reflect positive experiences. • Feelings are difficult to express if they reflect negative experiences. • The OTPF helps therapists identify issues that encourage or discourage "engagement in occupation" or emotions that facilitate or present "barriers to participation" (AOTA, 2002).
Generalizing	• Address the cognitive learning aspects of the group. • Sum up the group members' responses into a few general principles. • Look at patterns, opinions, commonalities, disagreements, and conflicts among the group's members. • Make this activity exciting and interesting.
Application	• Help the group understand how the principles learned during the group session can be applied to everyday life. • OTPF application addresses how the group members' learning will facilitate their participation in life (AOTA, 2002).
Summary	• Purpose is to verbally emphasize the most important aspects of the group so that the members will be understood and remembered • Points to emphasize should come from the group • Take about 5 minutes to review the goals, the content, and the process of the group.

   a. Core processes to occupational therapy intervention

(Hagedorn, 2000, pp. 60, 62–63)

      i. Therapeutic use of self
          I. The ability of the therapist to communicate with the client and develop a therapeutic alliance through a conscious and planned use of self
          II. The therapist's flexibility and adaptability to modify his or her behavior to meet the needs of the client and to modify the environment
          III. The therapist's ability to manage the group process, assist the client in developing interactive skills, help alleviate his or her fears, provide reassurance, and model desired behaviors
          IV. The negative effect of the therapeutic use of self is that it may facilitate unacceptable boundaries.
      ii. Assessment of individual
          I. Obtain a clear and accurate assessment of an individual's actual and potential abilities using the three methods shown in **Table 13-7**.
      iii. Analysis and adaptation of occupation
          I. Occupations are everyday or day-to-day activities and tasks that a person engages in. The breaking down of these activities to their varying details is called analysis. Analysis takes place on the three levels shown in **Table 13-8**.
              a. Tasks are sequences of performances with a clear purpose and product that take 3 to 10 minutes to complete. Longer chains fall under the term "activity analysis" (Hagedorn, 2000, p. 191).
              b. Task analysis is focused on what is done and the circumstances while doing it.
              c. Six-question system

Table 13-7 Assessment of Individual

Three Methods	Definitions
Objective	Therapist uses observation and/or standardized and nonstandardized testing to assess abilities.
Functional	Therapist assesses through observation in relationship to occupations (i.e., ADL activities).
Subjective	The individual reports past and current history, thoughts, feelings, motivations, interests, and aptitudes.

Table 13-8 Analysis and Adaptation of Occupation

Three Levels	Definitions
Developmental	Breaks down task into smallest units of performance by observing, recording, and analyzing elements of the client's behavior or performance
Effective	Integrates performances in different areas (e.g., work, leisure, and self-care)
Organizational	Understands the complexity of occupational behaviors across the person's life and lifespan; interactions between occupational roles and social roles and their relationships

    II.   Activity analysis is the process of breaking down an activity into its components and matching those component parts with human skills and abilities.

    III.   Adaptation is the ability to change one's activities and occupations to meet a therapeutic aim or to facilitate performance by matching needs and altering sequence, timing, structure, or complexity of the activity.

    IV.   Therapeutic media or occupation

        a. Materials and activities that are used to facilitate change that have meaning, symbolism, context, and purpose (Hagedorn, 2000, p. 7).

        b. When choosing a therapeutic medium, it is important to understand what should and should not be used in occupational therapy practice.

            i. Therapeutic media range from simple to very complex.

            ii. Media that require certifications or additional training or both should not be used until the therapist has successfully completed the appropriate requirements.

            iii. Groups that employ a traditional psychotherapy format should not be used.

            iv. Media may include activities generally used in day-to-day performance of occupations as guided by the OTPF, chosen conceptual models, and frames of reference.

            v. Examples of therapeutic media are arts and crafts, life skills, grooming and hygiene, routine functional tasks (e.g., managing a checkbook), and cooking, to name a few.

    iv. Analysis and adaptation of the environment

        I. Observations of the physical and social environments and the process of altering these environments to meet the needs of the individual and the group

            a. The physical environment includes the physical setting and the objects within the environment (AOTA, 2008, p. 653).

      b. The social environment includes environmental demands, such as people, culture, and rules of behavior (AOTA, 2008, p. 653).

b. Therapist's leadership style

    i. Guidelines for the leader

(Cole, 2005 pp. 60–64)

      I. One's leadership style is determined by the goals of the group, the characteristics of the group members, and the leader's therapeutic use of self.

      II. It is important for the therapist to understand the needs of the client.

      III. The leader should maintain client-centered group goals and activities that are safe, meaningful, and age appropriate.

      IV. The leader should maintain an awareness of his or her strengths and weaknesses and model acceptable and desired behaviors.

      V. The leader should provide nonjudgmental and unconditional positive regard for every person in the group.

      VI. The group leader guides the client through the group experience and encourages members to reflect and learn about the process by doing or directing the group or both.

      VII. The leader is the gatekeeper and needs to control the direction of the group to match the clients' needs and the type of group selected.

    ii. Leadership styles: The style the therapist chooses to exhibit will be influenced, in part, by the conceptual models used. There are three leadership styles, as shown in **Table 13-9**, according to Cole (2005, pp. 13–15).

Table 13-9 Leadership Styles

Autocratic	Democratic	Laissez-faire
The leader has complete control and facilitates vis-à-vis aggression. • Authoritative: Dictatorial and commanding of obedience • Authoritarian: Leader makes independent decisions and is not responsive to the group members.	Input or feedback and the freedom of choice help facilitate group cohesiveness.	Leader deliberately refrains from interfering in the process and does not direct behavior or rules. Guidance or structure is developed by the group members. The leadership style requires the leader to possess a higher cognitive and social level to help ensure that group members make and carry out moral decisions.
Used when group members are functioning at a lower level and require increased structure—an active and attentive leader. This style is most effective when used with the application of cognitive disability concepts.	The leader guides the individual in reaching his or her highest level or potential and acts as a participating member of the group. This style requires that group members function at high cognitive levels and is most effective when used in conjunction with the following client-centered approaches: Model of Human Occupation (MOHO), psychodynamic, and cognitive-behavioral concepts.	Therapist offers guidance as needed or requested. This style is most effective with the humanistic, MOHO, and psychodynamic concepts.

iii. Leadership roles

    I.   Roles in therapeutic relationships

(Early, 2009, pp. 267–268)

        a. Instructor: Someone who educates others on a particular subject

        b. Coach: Someone who trains others on how to deal with emotional challenges and interpersonal relationships

        c. Supervisor: Somebody whose job is to oversee and guide the work or activities of a group

        d. Role model: A worthy person who demonstrates traits and characteristics that can be copied or serve as an example for others

        e. Problem solver: Someone who identifies the problem within the context of a situation and strives to accomplish a successful resolution or minimize the negative consequences of the issue at hand

        f. Environmental manager: Someone who is responsible for directing and controlling the social environment, including group members, emotional climate, physical environment or setting, and other nonhuman elements within the group

        g. Group member: Someone who actively participates in the group activity or task

    II.   Leader's role in the termination of a group

(Cole, 2005, p. 48)

        a. Reviews the experiences and goals of the group members, as well as the learning that took place

        b. Reviews concerns of the group members and their feelings toward being separated from the group

        c. Uses empathy or confrontation skills to address members' behaviors or feelings or both

        d. Addresses unfinished business by bringing up past conflicts to obtain closure

        e. Gives feedback on skills learned

        f. Helps to generalize learning by discussing how various skills learned can be used elsewhere

iv. Skills required to conduct an activity group

(Hagedorn, 2000, p. 114)

    I.   Develop a repertoire of skills in a variety of creative, recreational, and social activities.

    II.   Organize and plan how to manage groups.

    III. Develop a repertoire of leadership styles to accommodate different circumstances.

    IV. Be self-motivated and develop facilitation skills.

    V.   Monitor activities and behaviors and influence them to achieve therapeutic benefits.

    VI. Develop an ability to judge how best to involve each group member.

    VII. Foster group cohesion.

v. Coleadership: Group sessions that are led by two or more practitioners.

    I.   Advantages of coleadership

(Cole, 2005, p. 16)

        a. Mutual support: Provides greater opportunities to complete tasks, meet the needs of group members or the group leader or leaders or both

  b. Increased objectivity: Allows for the comparison of observations and feedback for greater understanding, which can lead to successful goal attainment

  c. Collective knowledge: Provides more knowledge and experience for the task, group facilitation, and participants

  d. Modeling: Leans toward the demonstration and development of different coleadership styles

  e. Different roles: The therapist's ability to play different roles helps to strengthen group processes during facilitation and management of group activities

 II. Disadvantages of coleadership

(Cole, 2005, p. 21)

  a. Competition may occur when a therapist seeks to establish him- or herself as a competent therapist.

  b. Unequal contribution occurs when one leader perceives that he or she does more of the work than the other.

5. Clinical reasoning

 a. Rogers (1983) lists three questions to consider as identified in the Eleanor Clarke Slagle Lecture, when determining which concept, technique, method, or focus to address.

  i. Focus of clinical inquiry

(Early, 2009, p. 390)

  I. What is the person's status? Develop an understanding of who the person is.
   a. What are the client's occupational roles?
   b. What are his or her challenges or problems?
   c. What are his or her strengths?
   d. What is he or she motivated to try?

  II. What are the available options?
   a. What therapeutic approaches are available?
   b. What outcomes and results can be expected?
   c. How much time is needed for a group member to reach his or her objectives?

  III. What ought to be done?
   a. Which options are consistent with the person's values?
   b. Has the person been informed of the potential consequences of the prospective intervention options and been allowed to choose from them?
    i. The types of clinical reasoning are shown in **Table 13-10**.

Table 13-10 Types of Clinical Reasoning

Reasoning	Definition
Procedural	Focuses on the disability and intervention options
Interactive	Focuses on understanding and relating to the person as an individual
Narrative	Creates a vision of hope and sharing through storytelling
Pragmatic	Focuses on getting things done, thinking through problems
Conditional	Focuses on how condition could be altered to form a new condition
Scientific	Uses applied logic and science, such as hypothesis testing
Diagnostic	Analyzes cause or nature of condition
Ethical	Analyzes ethical dilemmas; systematic approach to moral conflict

Source: Crepeau, Cohn, & Schell, 2009, p. 319

6. **Safety**
   a. Universal precautions

(Cole, 2005, pp. 325–335)

   i. Procedures recommended by various government and health agencies to prevent the spread of diseases and infections
   ii. Observe infection control protocols with all clients at all times.
      I. Wash hands with soap and water (preferred method) or use hand sanitizer.
      II. Use protective barriers, such as gloves or a mask or both, when handling or being exposed to bodily fluids.
   b. Controlling the environment
      i. Keep track of keys and sharps, such as scissors, pens, and pencils.
      ii. Ensure restricted items are not taken to the ward; for example, items that can be used as weapons or to deface property.
      iii. Prepare the treatment area before the client enters the room.
      iv. Do not leave a client unattended.
      v. Be selective about who comes to occupational therapy.
      vi. Alert the client to potential dangers related to planned activities.
      vii. Follow safety precautions for hazards and toxins.
      viii. Do not substitute or recycle containers; use original containers with labels.
      ix. Have knowledge of and use proper safety equipment.
      x. Provide structure and manage the group to maintain emotional and physical safety.
      xi. Attend to and take all threats, medical complaints, and emergencies seriously.
   c. Fire precautions

(Hagedorn, 2000, p. 294)

      i. Ensure that all flammable items are stored properly.
      ii. Ensure that all fire exits are clearly marked, unrestricted, and easily accessible.
      iii. Ensure that fire alarms are conveniently located.
      iv. Ensure that fire extinguishers are accessible, suitable, and in good working order.
   d. Incident reports
      i. Record and report any incidents of unsafe situations, assaults, slips, and falls according to applicable policies and procedures.

WORK SHEETS

These work sheets are designed to assess your retention of the information provided in this chapter. Read the directions and the information contained within the work sheets carefully before providing an answer.

Attempt to complete the work sheets without or before returning to the chapter to search for the answers. The following work sheets are included:

- Therapeutic use of self
- Group and activity
- Frames of reference
- Activity Group
- Activity Group Protocol
- Role identification
- Activity selection

Work Sheet 13-1. Therapeutic Use of Self

(Cole, 2005, p. 37)

Choose if the therapist's response would have a positive or negative effect on an individual, a group of individuals, and/or the group process.

Directions:

- Read the therapist's response.

- Place a check in the applicable column.

Table 13-11 Therapeutic Use of Self

Therapist Response	Positive effect	Negative effect
1. The therapist verbally reassures a patient who expressed fear.		
2. The therapist ignores a group's request for help.		
3. The therapist allows a person to cry and offers the individual a tissue before continuing with the group.		
4. The therapist allows an aggressive group member to attack another more passive group member who does not respond.		
5. The therapist allows an individual to choose an activity that is well above the individual's skill level.		
6. An individual attends a group session and sits quietly observing the others, and the therapist asks the person to leave if he or she is not willing to actively engage in the activity.		
7. The therapist notices that the fire extinguisher box door is open; she closes the door and proceeds with the day's activities.		
8. An individual who frequently disrupts the group process raises his hand and asks that the group consider a different activity. The therapist ignores the request and informs the person that he will be asked to leave the group if he interrupts the process again.		
9. The therapist noticed in a previous session that two peers frequently argue with each other or come together and harangue other peers. When the two sit together in another session, the therapist does not seat them apart or address the behaviors.		
10. The therapist does not redirect or correct an individual who continuously refers to her as "auntie."		
11. The therapist sets the behavioral expectations of the group during the introduction of a hygiene group session.		
12. The therapist stands in the corner of the room while the group members are sitting down and provides the introductions and directions for a leisure group. When the group starts the activity, the therapist sits near the door and watches the group members interact and engage in the activity while jotting down notes.		
13. A therapist expresses that one of the patients reminds her of her goddaughter and admits to treating the patient differently than she treats the other members of the group.		
14. The therapist notices a spill on the hallway floor on her way to the clinic area. The therapist does not clean up the spill, nor does she call for someone to clean up the spill.		

Work Sheet 13-2. Group and Activity

(Cole, 2005, pp. 99–102)

Directions:

- Briefly define the different developmental interaction skills.

- Provide a purposeful activity or occupation that best fits the interaction skill.

Table 13-12 Group and Activity

Group	Definition	Activity Example
Parallel		
Project		
Egocentric–cooperative		
Cooperative		
Mature		

Work Sheet 13-3. Frames of Reference

(Cole, 2005, pp. 109–121, 239–242, 369–374)

(Crepeau, et al., 2009, p. 319)

Directions:

- Identify the clinical reasoning style that best fits the different frames of reference.
- Briefly provide the rationale for choosing the clinical reasoning style that you selected in the second column.
- Provide an example of an activity or occupation to use with the chosen frame of reference and clinical reasoning style.

Table 13-13 Frames of Reference

Frame of Reference	Clinical Reasoning	Activity Example
Psychodynamic		
Behavioral–cognitive		
Allen cognitive disabilities		
Developmental		
Sensorimotor		
Model of Human Occupation		

Work Sheet 13-4. Activity Group

(AOTA, 2008, p. 625)

(Crepeau, et al., 2009, p. 319)

(Early, 2009, pp. 267–268)

(Hagedorn, 2000, p. 115)

Directions:

- Provide the purpose for each group type.
- Identify the clinical reasoning style that is best suited for the group type.
- Identify the area of occupation, performance skill, performance pattern, and client factor that may be positively affected by using the identified group and clinical reasoning style.
- Identify the role of the therapist in this type of group.
- Provide an example of a purposeful activity or occupation to use with the group type.

Table 13-14 Activity Group

Type of Group	Purpose	Clinical Reasoning	OTPF Domains and Aspects	Role of Therapist	Activity Example
Evaluation group					
Thematic group					
Topical group					
Task-oriented group					
Developmental group					
Egocentric cooperative group					
Instrumental group					

Work Sheet 13-5. Activity Group Protocol

(Cole, 2005, pp. 3–11, 13–15)

Directions:

- Identify Cole's seven steps of writing a protocol.
- Briefly describe each step.
- Identify the leadership style best used for each step.

Table 13-15 Activity Group Protocol

Seven Steps	Description	Cole's Leadership Style
1.		
2.		
3.		
4.		
5.		
6.		
7.		

Work Sheet 13-6. Role Identification

(Cole, 2005, pp. 41–47, 13–15)

(Early, 2009, pp. 268–270)

Directions:

• Describe the primary behavior of each member's role.

• Choose the best leadership style to manage the desired role behavior.

• Choose one of the eight qualities that are best suited for that role.

Table 13-16 Role Identification

Member Role	Description	Lewin's/Cole's Leadership Style	Eight Qualities
Aggressor			
Information seeker			
Opinion seeker			
Information giver			
Harmonizer			
Compromiser			
Gatekeeper			
Psychotic			
Follower			
Blocker			
Recognition seeker			
Help seeker			
Special interest pleader			
Monopolist			

Work Sheet 13-7. Activity Selection

(Early, 2009, pp. 450–452)

Directions:

- Choose an activity that is ideally suited for facilitating or promoting functional ability.

- Identify or simulate an environment or both to perform an activity within an acute care mental health unit in a community hospital.

- Identify a therapist role to facilitate change.

Table 13-17 Activity Selection

Domains and Aspects	Activity	Environment	Therapist Role
ADL			
IADL			
Rest and sleep			
Social participation			
Work			
Leisure			
Education			
Spirituality			
Memory			
Sensory perception			
Roles			
Social environment			
Physical motor			
Values			
Emotional regulation			

REFERENCES

American Occupational Therapy Association. (2002). Occupational therapy practice framework: Domain and process. *American Journal of Occupational Therapy, 56,* 609–629.

American Occupational Therapy Association. (2008). Occupational therapy practice framework: Domain and process, 2nd edition. *American Journal of Occupational Therapy, 62*(6), 625–683.

Cole, M. B. (2005). *Group dynamics in occupational therapy: The theoretical basis and practice application of group intervention* (3rd ed.). Thorofare, NJ: Slack.

Crepeau, E., Cohn, E., & Schell, B. (Eds.). (2009). *Willard & Spackman's occupational therapy* (11th ed.). Philadelphia: Lippincott Williams & Wilkins.

Early, M. B. (2009). *Mental health techniques and concepts for the occupational therapy assistant* (4th ed.). Philadelphia: Lippincott Williams & Wilkins.

Hagedorn, R. (2000). *Tools for practice in occupational therapy: A structured approach to core skills and processes.* London: Churchill Livingstone.

Mosey, A. C. (1973). *Activity therapy.* New York: Raven Press.

Rogers, J. C. (1983). Clinical reasoning: The ethics, science, and art. *The American Journal of Occupational Therapy, 37,* 601–616.

Sladyk, K., & Ryan, S. (Eds.). (2005). *Ryan's occupational therapy assistant: Principles, practice issues, and techniques* (4th ed.). Thorofare, NJ: Slack.

Therapeutic Specialized Pediatric Assessments and Interventions (Days 20–25)

Pediatric Conditions

Nancy Vandewiele Milligan

OBJECTIVES

1. Describe the common signs and symptoms associated with health conditions.
2. Cite the precautions and contraindications for each condition that a therapist must be aware of prior to treatment intervention.
3. Apply the knowledge of conditions into intervention strategies.

Table 14-1 Key Terms

Case-Smith, 2005, pp. 160–201	Case-Smith, 2005, pp. 457–460
Cardiopulmonary dysfunctions	Anxiety disorders
Developmental disabilities	Attention-deficit/hyperactivity disorder
Diabetes	Mood disorders
Infectious conditions	Pervasive developmental disorders
Musculoskeletal disorders	
Neoplastic disorders	
Neuromuscular disorders	
Toxic agents	
Traumatic brain injuries	

INTRODUCTION

Welcome to Day 20 of your study guide. In this chapter you will review common medical diagnoses that affect children and adolescents. Although some of these conditions may also be seen in adults, the signs, symptoms, precautions, and contraindications may differ for the pediatric population. Work through the outline to review the conditions and then complete the work sheets after each section to assist you in highlighting the major aspects of each condition.

OUTLINE

1. Cardiopulmonary dysfunctions

(Case-Smith, 2005, pp. 160–167)

a. Congenital heart disease
  i. Chromosomal abnormalities
  ii. Increased pulmonary blood flow
   I. Patent ductus arteriosus (PDA)
   II. Atrial septal defects (ASDs)
   III. Ventricular septal defects (VSDs)
  iii. Decreased pulmonary blood flow
   I. Tetralogy of Fallot (TOF)
    a. Symptoms
    b. Medical management
  iv. Obstructed blood flow
  v. Mixed blood flow
   I. Transposition of the great vessels (TGV)
    a. Symptoms
    b. Medical management
b. Dysrhythmias
  i. Bradydysrhythmia
   I. Atrioventricular (AV) block
  ii. Tachydysrhythmia
   I. Supraventricular tachycardia (SVT)
c. Respiratory problems
  i. Respiratory distress syndrome
  ii. Bronchopulmonary dysplasia (BPD)
  iii. Asthma
  iv. Cystic fibrosis
d. Hematologic disorders
  i. Sickle cell anemia
  ii. Hemophilia

Work Sheet 14-1. Cardiopulmonary Dysfunctions

Table 14-2 Cardiopulmonary Dysfunctions

Condition	Etiology & Pathology	Signs & Symptoms	Precautions	Application to the Occupational Therapy Practice Framework: Domain and Processes 2nd Edition (OTPF)
Congenital heart disease				
Chromosomal abnormalities				

Work Sheet 14-1. Cardiopulmonary Dysfunctions *(continued)*

Table 14-2 Cardiopulmonary Dysfunctions

Condition	Etiology & Pathology	Signs & Symptoms	Precautions	Application to the Occupational Therapy Practice Framework: Domain and Processes 2nd Edition (OTPF)
PDA				
ASD				
VSD				
TOF				
TGV				
Bradydysrhythmia				
Tachydysrhythmia				
SVT				
Respiratory distress syndrome				

(continues)

Work Sheet 14-1. Cardiopulmonary Dysfunctions *(continued)*

Table 14-2 Cardiopulmonary Dysfunctions

Condition	Etiology & Pathology	Signs & Symptoms	Precautions	Application to the Occupational Therapy Practice Framework: Domain and Processes 2nd Edition (OTPF)
BPD				
Asthma				
Cystic fibrosis				
Sickle cell anemia				
Hemophilia				

2. **Musculoskeletal disorders**

(Case-Smith, 2005, pp. 167–175)

    a. Congenital anomalies
       i. Osteogenesis imperfecta (OI)
      ii. Marfan syndrome (arachnodactyly)
    iii. Achondroplasia
      iv. Multiplex congenital
     v. Congenital clubfoot (talipes equinovarus)
     vi. Congenital club hand
    vii. Congenital hip dislocation
    b. Limb deficiencies
      i. Polydactyly
     ii. Syndactyly
    iii. Bradydactyly
    iv. Microdactyly
    c. Juvenile rheumatoid arthritis (JRA)
      i. Pauciarticular
     ii. Polyarticular

        iii. Systemic (Still disease)
            I. Symptoms
            II. Medical management
    d. Soft tissue injuries
        i. Contusions
        ii. Crush injuries
        iii. Dislocation
        iv. Sprain
    e. Fractures
        i. Compound (open) fracture
        ii. Closed fracture
        iii. Greenstick fracture
        iv. Comminuted fracture
            I. Symptoms
            II. Medical management
  f. Curvature of the spine
        i. Lordosis
        ii. Kyphosis
        iii. Scoliosis

Work Sheet 14-2. Musculoskeletal Disorders

Table 14-3 Musculoskeletal Disorders

Condition	Etiology & Pathology	Signs & Symptoms	Precautions	Application to the OTPF
Congenital Anomalies				
OI				
Marfan syndrome				
Achondroplasia				
Multiplex congenital				
Congenital clubfoot				

(continues)

Work Sheet 14-2. Musculoskeletal Disorders *(continued)*

Table 14-3 Musculoskeletal Disorders

Condition	Etiology & Pathology	Signs & Symptoms	Precautions	Application to the OTPF
Congenital club hand				
Congenital hip dislocation				
Limb Deficiencies				
Polydactyly				
Syndactyly				
Bradydactyly				
Microdactyly				
Juvenile Rheumatoid Arthritis (JRA)				
Pauciarticular				
Polyarticular				
Systemic (Still disease)				

Work Sheet 14-2. Musculoskeletal Disorders *(continued)*

Table 14-3 Musculoskeletal Disorders

Condition	Etiology & Pathology	Signs & Symptoms	Precautions	Application to the OTPF
Soft Tissue Injuries				
Contusions				
Crush injuries				
Dislocation				
Sprain				
Fractures				
Compound (open) fracture				
Closed fracture				
Greenstick fracture				
Comminuted fracture				
Curvature of the Spine				
Lordosis				

(continues)

Work Sheet 14-2. Musculoskeletal Disorders (continued)

Table 14-3 Musculoskeletal Disorders

Condition	Etiology & Pathology	Signs & Symptoms	Precautions	Application to the OTPF
Kyphosis				
Scoliosis				

3. Neuromuscular disorders

(Case-Smith, 2005, pp. 175–188)

- **a.** Cerebral palsy
    - **i.** Tone classifications

    (Case-Smith, 2005, pp. 177–179)

    - **ii.** Limb involvement
        - **I.** Hemiplegia
        - **II.** Tetraplegia
        - **III.** Quadriplegia
        - **IV.** Diplegia
    - **iii.** Complications
    - **iv.** Medical management
- **b.** Epilepsy
- **c.** Seizure disorders
    - **i.** Generalized seizures
        - **I.** Tonic-clonic
        - **II.** Absence
        - **III.** Atypical absence
        - **IV.** Myoclonic
        - **V.** Atonic forms
    - **ii.** Partial seizures
        - **I.** Simple
        - **II.** Complex
    - **iii.** Mixed seizure disorder
    - **iv.** Medical management
        - **I.** Emergency treatment of seizures

        (Case-Smith, 2005, p. 183)

- **d.** Muscular dystrophies

    (Case-Smith, 2005, p. 183)

    - **i.** Limb-girdle
    - **ii.** Facioscapulohumeral
    - **iii.** Congenital

  iv. Duchenne
  v. Medical management
e. Neural tube defects
  i. Encephalocele
  ii. Anencephaly
  iii. Spina bifida

  (Case-Smith, 2005, p. 186)

  I. Spina bifida occulta
  II. Meningocele
  III. Myelomeningocele
  iv. Complications
  v. Medical management
f. Hydrocephalus
  i. Clinical signs
  ii. Complications
  iii. Medical management
g. Peripheral nerve injuries
  i. Brachial plexus lesions
    I. Erb-Duchenne palsy
    II. Klumpke palsy
  ii. Traumatic injury of peripheral nerves

Work Sheet 14-3. Neuromuscular Disorders—Cerebral Palsy

Table 14-4 Neuromuscular Disorders—Cerebral Palsy

Cerebral Palsy Classifications	Tone Quality & Distribution	ROM	Quality of Movement	Reflexes & Reactions	Oral Motor	Associated Problems	Personality Characteristics
Severe spasticity							
Moderate spasticity							
Mild spasticity							
Pure athetosis							

(continues)

Work Sheet 14-3. Neuromuscular Disorders—Cerebral Palsy *(continued)*

Table 14-4 Neuromuscular Disorders—Cerebral Palsy

Cerebral Palsy Classifications	Tone Quality & Distribution	ROM	Quality of Movement	Reflexes & Reactions	Oral Motor	Associated Problems	Personality Characteristics
Athetosis with spasticity							
Athetosis with tonic spasms							
Choreo-athetosis							
Flaccid							
Ataxia							

Work Sheet 14-4. Neuromuscular Disorders

Table 14-5 Neuromuscular Disorders

Condition	Etiology & Pathology	Signs & Symptoms	Precautions	Application to the OTPF
Cerebral palsy • Hemiplegia • Tetraplegia • Quadriplegia • Diplegia				
Epilepsy				
Seizure disorders • Tonic-clonic • Absence • Atypical absence • Myoclonic • Atonic forms			See Case-Smith, 2005, p. 183, Box 6-1	
Partial seizures • Simple • Complex				

Work Sheet 14-4. Neuromuscular Disorders *(continued)*

Table 14-5 Neuromuscular Disorders

Condition	Etiology & Pathology	Signs & Symptoms	Precautions	Application to the OTPF
Muscular dystrophies • Limb-girdle • Facioscapulo-humeral • Congenital • Duchenne				
Neural tube defects • Encephalocele • Anencephaly				
Spina bifida • Spina bifida occulta • Meningocele • Myelomen-ingocele				
Hydrocephalus				
Peripheral nerve injuries • Brachial plexus lesions • Erb-Duchenne palsy • Klumpke palsy • Traumatic injury of peripheral nerves				

4. **Traumatic brain injuries**

(Case-Smith, 2005, pp. 188–189)

   a. Glasgow Coma Scale

(Pendleton & Schultz-Krohn, 2006, p. 843, Table 34-1)
(Radomski & Latham, 2008, p. 1047, Table 39-1)

Work Sheet 14-5. Traumatic Brain Injuries

Table 14-6 Traumatic Brain Injuries

Condition	Etiology & Pathology	Signs & Symptoms	Precautions	Application to the OTPF
Traumatic brain injuries		Glasgow Coma Scale		

5. **Developmental disabilities**

(Case-Smith, 2005, pp. 189–200)

    a. Mental retardation

    b. Pervasive developmental disorders

        i. Autism

        ii. Atypical autism

        iii. Rett syndrome

        iv. Asperger syndrome

        v. Pervasive developmental disorder—unspecified

    c. Attention-deficit/hyperactivity disorder

    d. Learning disabilities

    e. Tourette syndrome

    f. Genetic and chromosomal abnormalities

        i. Cri du chat syndrome

        ii. Klinefelter syndrome

        iii. Fragile X syndrome

        iv. Prader-Willi syndrome

        v. Peripheral neurofibromatosis

        vi. Central neurofibromatosis

        vii. Williams syndrome

    g. Inborn errors of metabolism

        i. Tay-Sachs disease

        ii. Phenylketonuria (PKU)

        iii. Galactosemia

        iv. Lesch-Nyhan syndrome

    h. Developmental coordination disorder

(Case-Smith, 2005, pp. 77–79)

        i. Sensory integrative processing disorder

(Case-Smith, 2005, pp. 365–366)

Work Sheet 14-6. Developmental Disabilities

Table 14-7 Developmental Disabilities

Condition	Etiology & Pathology	Signs & Symptoms	Precautions	Application to the OTPF
Mental retardation				
Pervasive developmental disorders • Autism • Atypical autism • Rett syndrome • Asperger syndrome • Pervasive developmental disorder— unspecified				
Attention-deficit/ hyperactivity disorder				
Learning disabilities				
Tourette syndrome				
Genetic and chromosomal abnormalities • Cri du chat syndrome • Fragile X syndrome • Prader-Willi syndrome				
Inborn errors of metabolism • Tay-Sachs disease • Phenylketonuria (PKU)				

(continues)

Work Sheet 14-6. Developmental Disabilities *(continued)*

Table 14-7 Developmental Disabilities

Condition	Etiology & Pathology	Signs & Symptoms	Precautions	Application to the OTPF
Developmental coordination disorder				
Sensory integrative processing disorder				

Work Sheet 14-7. Diabetes

Table 14-8 Diabetes

Condition	Etiology & Pathology	Signs & Symptoms	Precautions	Application to the OTPF
Diabetes Type I				
Diabetes Type II				

⊷ 6. Diabetes

(Case-Smith, 2005, pp. 200–201)

    a. Type I

    b. Type II

7. Toxic agents

(Case-Smith, 2005, pp. 201–203)

    a. Drugs
    b. Chemicals

Work Sheet 14-8. Toxic Agents

Table 14-9 Toxic Agents

Substance	Effect on Fetus or Child	Application to the OTPF
Drugs		
Alcohol		
Aspirin		
Cortisone		
Caffeine		
Dilantin		
Heroin, codeine, morphine		
LSD		
Tetracycline		
Thalidomide		
Tobacco		
Tranquilizers		
Radiation therapy		
Chemicals		
Methylmercury		
Pesticides		
Lead		

8. Infectious conditions

(Case-Smith, 2005, pp. 203–206)

    a. Maternal infections

    (Case-Smith, 2005, p. 204)

    b. Acquired immunodeficiency syndrome (AIDS)

9. Neoplastic disorders

(Case-Smith, 2005, pp. 206–208)

    a. Leukemia
    b. Brain tumors
    c. Hodgkin disease
    d. Bone tumors

Work Sheet 14-9. Intrauterine Infections (STORCH)

Table 14-10 Intrauterine Infections (STORCH)

Infection	Cause	Type	Effect on Fetus	Application to the OTPF
Syphilis				
Toxoplasmosis				
Rubella				
Cytomegalovirus				
Herpes				

Work Sheet 14-10. Neoplastic Disorders

Table 14-11 Neoplastic Disorders

Condition	Etiology & Pathology	Signs & Symptoms	Precautions	Application to the OTPF
Leukemia				
Brain tumors				
Hodgkin disease				
Bone tumors				

Work Sheet 14-11. Burns

Table 14-12 Burns

Condition	Etiology & Pathology	Signs & Symptoms	Precautions	Application to the OTPF
Burns		See Pendleton & Schultz-Krohn, p. 1062, Rule of nines		
Superficial burns				
Partial-thickness burns				
Full-thickness burns				

10. Burns

(Case-Smith, 2005, pp. 208–211)

    a. Rule of nines
    b. Superficial burns
    c. Partial-thickness burns
    d. Full-thickness burns

11. Visual impairment

(Case-Smith, 2005, pp. 858–862)

    a. Blindness
    b. Myopia
    c. Hyperopia
    d. Cataracts
    e. Glaucoma
    f. Neurologic visual impairment (NVI)
    g. Cortical visual impairment (CVI)
    h. Retinopathy of prematurity (ROP)

Work Sheet 14-12. Visual Impairment

Table 14-13 Visual Impairment

Condition	Etiology & Pathology	Signs & Symptoms	Precautions	Application to the OTPF
Blindness		See Case-Smith, 2005, p. 859, Box 23A-1, Gradations of acuity 20/20–20/70 20/70–20/100 20/100–20/200 20/200–20/1000 Greater than 20/1000		
Myopia				
Hyperopia				
Cataracts				
Glaucoma				
NVI				
CVI				
ROP				

Work Sheet 14-13. Hearing Impairment

Table 14-14 Hearing Impairment

Condition	Etiology & Pathology	Signs & Symptoms	Precautions	Application to the OTPF
Hearing Loss				
Conductive				
Sensorineural				
Classifications				
Mild loss (25–40 dB)				
Moderate loss (55–70 dB)				
Moderate to severe loss (70–90 dB)				
Severe loss (70–90 dB)				
Profound loss (90 dB or greater)				

12. **Hearing impairment**

(Case-Smith, 2005, pp. 863–867)

    a. Conductive
    b. Sensorineural

13. **Visual perception**

(Case-Smith, 2005, pp. 412–446)

    a. Visual-perceptual problems
        i. Visual fixation

    ii. Visual pursuit
    iii. Saccadic eye movement
    iv. Acuity
    v. Accommodation
    vi. Binocular fusion
    vii. Stereopsis
    viii. Convergence and divergence
b. Visual attention
    i. Alertness
    ii. Selective attention
    iii. Vigilance
    iv. Divided attention
c. Visual memory
d. Visual discrimination
e. Object perception
    i. Form consistency
    ii. Visual closure
    iii. Figure ground
f. Spatial perception
    i. Position in space
    ii. Depth perception
    iii. Topographic orientation
    iv. Visual imagery

Work Sheet 14-14. Visual Perception

Table 14-15 Visual Perception

Visual Function	Definition	Impact on Function Application to the OTPF
Visual-perceptual problems • Visual fixation • Visual pursuit • Saccadic eye movement • Acuity • Accommodation • Binocular fusion • Stereopsis • Convergence and divergence		
Visual attention • Alertness • Selective attention • Vigilance • Divided attention		
Visual memory		
Visual discrimination		

Work Sheet 14-14. Visual Perception *(continued)*

Table 14-15 Visual Perception

Visual Function	Definition	Impact on Function Application to the OTPF
Object perception • Form constancy • Visual closure • Figure ground		
Spatial perception • Position in space • Depth perception • Topographic orientation • Visual imagery		

Work Sheet 14-15. Mental Disorders

Table 14-16 Mental Disorders

Condition	Etiology & Pathology	Signs & Symptoms	Precautions	Application to Practice Framework
Mood disorders				
Anxiety disorders				
Obsessive-compulsive disorder				
Attention-deficit/ hyperactivity disorder				
Pervasive developmental disorder				

14. **Mental disorders commonly affecting children and adolescents**

(Case-Smith, 2005, pp. 457–460)

    a. Mood disorders
    b. Anxiety disorders
        i. Obsessive-compulsive disorder (OCD)
    c. Attention-deficit/hyperactivity disorder (ADHD)
    d. Pervasive developmental disorder

CASE STUDIES

Case Study 14-1. Justin is a 4-year-old client with cerebral palsy. He displays near normal tone at rest, but it increases whenever he attempts to move his extremities or becomes excited. Justin's tone would be classified as:

    A. Choreoathetosis
    B. Ataxic
    C. Pure athetosis
    D. Moderate spasticity

Case Study 14-2. Bella is a 4-week-old infant who was delivered breech. She demonstrates a weak to absent reflexive grasp in her right hand. It appears that Bella may have a brachial plexus lesion. This condition is known as:

    A. Duchenne muscular dystrophy
    B. Erb-Duchenne palsy
    C. Hydrocephalus
    D. Congenital muscular dystrophy

Case Study 14-3. Emma is a 7-year-old child who displays difficulties in school and at home in social interactions, problems with tolerating changes in her routine, and some deficits in her sensory processing skills. Emma's developmental impairment would most likely be termed as:

    A. Rett syndrome
    B. Mental retardation
    C. Asperger syndrome
    D. Attention-deficit/hyperactivity disorder

Case Study 14-4. Levi is a 10-year-old child who has been referred to a pediatric vision clinic for evaluation. Levi's teacher has noted that he holds his books and papers close to his face in school. He also complains of blurred vision. Levi does not presently wear glasses. Levi's visual impairment most likely is:

    A. Myopia
    B. Hyperopia
    C. Amblyopia
    D. Astigmatism

REFERENCES

Case-Smith, J. (Eds.). (2005). *Occupational therapy for children* (5th ed.). St. Louis, MO: Mosby.

Pendleton, H. M., & Schultz-Krohn, W. (Eds.). (2006). *Pedretti's occupational therapy: Practice skills for physical dysfunction* (6th ed.). St. Louis, MO: Mosby.

Radomski, M. V., & Latham, C. A. T. (Eds.). (2008). *Occupational therapy for physical dysfunction* (6th ed.). Philadelphia: Lippincott Williams & Wilkins.

CASE STUDY RATIONALE

Case Study 14-1. **Correct answer: D.** The quality of tone of moderate spasticity is described as "moderately increased tone [that is] near normal at rest but increases with excitement, movement attempts, effort, emotion, speech, [and] sudden stretch" (Case-Smith, 2005, p. 177).

Case Study 14-2. **Correct answer: B.** Erb-Duchenne palsy is often caused by breech deliveries with after-coming arms, which may cause brachial plexus lesions. "These infants may demonstrate weakness or wasting of the small muscles of the hands and sensory diminution in the area of the hand and arm served by the plexus" (Case-Smith, 2005, p. 187).

Case Study 14-3. Correct answer: C. "Asperger syndrome can be distinguished from autism by the fact that they do not exhibit clinically significant delays in language skills," but they do display significant sustained impairment in social interaction and the development of restricted, repetitive patterns of behavior, interests, and activities (Case-Smith, 2005, p. 193).

Case Study 14-4. Correct answer: A. "A child with myopia, or nearsightedness, sees most clearly at close range and much less efficiently at a distance" (Case-Smith, 2005, p. 859). A child with myopia may have blurred vision and often holds printed material close to the eyes (Case-Smith, 2005, p. 859).

Exhibit 1-1 Stress Vulnerability Scale

In modern society, most of us can't avoid stress. But we can learn to behave in ways that lessen its effects. Researchers have identified a number of factors that affect one's vulnerability to stress—among them are eating and sleeping habits, caffeine and alcohol intake, and how we express our emotions. The following questionnaire is designed to help you discover your vulnerability quotient and to pinpoint trouble spots. Rate each item from 1 (always) to 5 (never), according to how much of the time the statement is true of you. Be sure to mark each item, even if it does not apply to you—for example, if you don't smoke, circle 1 next to item six.

		Always	Sometimes			Never
1.	I eat at least one hot, balanced meal a day.	1	2	3	4	5
2.	I get 7–8 hours of sleep at least four nights a week.	1	2	3	4	5
3.	I give and receive affection regularly.	1	2	3	4	5
4.	I have at least one relative within 50 miles on whom I can rely.	1	2	3	4	5
5.	I exercise to the point of perspiration at least twice a week.	1	2	3	4	5
6.	I limit myself to less than half a pack of cigarettes a day.	1	2	3	4	5
7.	I take fewer than five alcohol drinks a week.	1	2	3	4	5
8.	I am the appropriate weight for my height.	1	2	3	4	5
9.	I have an income adequate to meet basic expenses.	1	2	3	4	5
10.	I get strength from my religious beliefs.	1	2	3	4	5
11.	I regularly attend club or social activities.	1	2	3	4	5
12.	I have a network of friends and acquaintances.	1	2	3	4	5
13.	I have one or more friends to confide in about personal matters.	1	2	3	4	5
14.	I am in good health (including eyesight, hearing, and teeth).	1	2	3	4	5
15.	I am able to speak openly about my feelings when angry or worried.	1	2	3	4	5
16.	I have regular conversations with the people I live with about domestic problems—for example, chores and money.	1	2	3	4	5
17.	I do something for fun at least once a week.	1	2	3	4	5
18.	I am able to organize my time effectively.	1	2	3	4	5
19.	I drink fewer than three cups of coffee (or other caffeine-rich drinks) a day.	1	2	3	4	5
20.	I take some quiet time for myself during the day.	1	2	3	4	5

Exhibit 1-1 Stress Vulnerability Scale *(continued)*

Scoring Instructions: To calculate your score, add up the figures and subtract 20.

Score Interpretation:
A score below 10 indicates excellent resistance to stress.
A score over 30 indicates some vulnerability to stress.
A score over 50 indicates serious vulnerability to stress.

Self-Care Plan: Notice that nearly all the items describe situations and behaviors over which you have a great deal of control. Review the items on which you scored three or higher. List those items in your self-care plan. Concentrate first on those that are easiest to change—for example, eating a hot, balanced meal daily and having fun at least once a week—before tackling those that seem difficult.

Source: Exhibit courtesy Copyright 2009 Stress Directions, Inc., Lyle H. Miller and Alma Dell Smith, Boston, MA
www.stressdirections.com

Exhibit 5-1 Reflection Question Journal

1. What? (What have I accomplished? What have I learned?)

2. So what? (What difference did it make? Why should I do it? How is it important? How do I feel about it?)

3. Now what? (What's next? Where do we go from here?)

Source: Exhibit courtesy of Live Wire Media.

Specialized Pediatric Assessments

Robin Mercer and Beth Angst

OBJECTIVES

1. Understand core concepts of pediatric assessments, including the purpose and appropriate methods.
2. Review standardized evaluation tools as well as skilled observation methods and interviews and determine relevant information obtained from each.
3. Demonstrate knowledge of developmental sequence in areas including gross and fine motor development, feeding, sensory processing, and visual motor control.
4. Apply knowledge of assessments into practical, clinical scenarios.

KEY TERMS

Table 15-1 Key Terms

Case-Smith, 2005, pp. 218, 278; Mulligan, 2003, pp. 110, 123	Case-Smith, 2005, pp. 356, 412, 481, 521, 587; Mulligan, 2003, pp. 112, 135
Arena assessments	ADL for pediatrics
Criterion-referenced measures	Feeding evaluation
Developmental sequence	Fine motor development
Interview	Handwriting components
Norm-referenced measures	Sensory processing
Postural control	Visual perception
Skilled observations	
Standardized tests	

INTRODUCTION

Welcome to Days 21 and 22 of your study guide. This chapter reviews the important aspects of evaluations in pediatrics. The underlying theory is the same as with the adult population in that the purpose of a pediatric evaluation is to obtain a sense of problems, strengths, weaknesses, and functional goals. The evaluation of children requires that you have a strong understanding of typical development as well as knowledge of the different assessments available. It also relies more on an ability to use other means of gathering information, such as interviewing the parents or caregivers and using skilled observations because children are not always willing or able to cooperate with standardized testing. Use the outline to gather pertinent information and complete the corresponding work sheets to reinforce your understanding of the key points and application of knowledge.

OUTLINE

1. Assessment process

(American Occupational Therapy Association, 2002)
(Case-Smith, 2005, pp. 219, 222, 233–237)
(Mulligan, 2003, pp. 6, 8, 22)

  a. Assessment purpose
    i. The purpose of a pediatric evaluation is to assess what the child wants and needs to do, what strengths support, and what weaknesses or problems interfere with childhood occupations. Childhood occupations include play, school activities, and self-help skills.
    ii. A comprehensive evaluation is completed to determine eligibility, assist with diagnosis, plan intervention, and reevaluate, as well as contributing to clinical research.
    iii. The evaluation may be conducted in one of a variety of settings depending on the initial concerns and the reason for the assessment. These typically include educational, outpatient (e.g., mental health facilities), and inpatient settings.
  b. Assessment participation
    i. Follow a client-centered practice model. For children, this will involve play and observation in the environment where the child is having difficulty, if possible. This may include the home, classroom, or playground, but observation may also have to be completed in a hospital setting with a simulation of typical activities.
    ii. Include parents or caregivers. They may give you pertinent information about history as well as information on their perception of the child's difficulties and how these challenges impact family life. Parents may assist in getting the child to participate in the evaluation process to help determine if the performance is typical.

2. Assessment methods

(Case-Smith, 2005, pp. 224, 233–237, 241–245, 249–254)
(Mulligan, 2003, pp. 155–163)

  a. Standardized assessments: The choice of which test to give is based on a number of issues, including the reason for the referral, availability of tests, and the therapist's level of competence in conducting them. Standardized tests must be administered according to the test protocol using the standardized test materials for the scores to be valid.
    i. Calculate chronological age and adjust for prematurity.
    ii. Norm-referenced compares the child's score to that of a sample group that was assessed when the test was developed. Common pediatric assessments that are norm-referenced include, but are not limited to the following.

Work Sheet 15-1. Assessment

Fill in the chart with the missing information.

Table 15-2 Assessment A

Test Name	Author(s)	Age Ranges	What It Tests
Battelle Developmental Inventory	Newborg, J. (1988)	Birth to 8 years	Personal social skills, adaptive behavior (self-help), psychomotor, communication, and cognition
Bayley Scales of Infant Development	Bayley, N. (1993)	1–42 months	Cognitive and motor development
Beery-Buktenica Developmental Test of Visual Motor Integration (VMI)	Beery, K. E., Buktenica, N. A., & Beery, N. A. (2004)	~~3–18 months~~ Short form: 2-8 yrs. Long form: up to 100 yrs.	Visual motor integration deficits
Bruininks-Oseretsky Tests of Motor Skills, second edition	Bruininks, R. (2005)	4.5 years to 14.5 years	Gross motor, upper limb, and fine motor proficiency
DeGangi-Berk Test of Sensory Integration	Berk R. A., & DeGangi, G. A. (1983)	3–5 years	Sensory processing difficulties
Developmental Test of Visual Perception (DTVP-2)	Hammill, D. D., Pearson, N. A., & Voress, J. K. (1993)	4–10 years	Visual perceptual and visual motor integration
Miller Assessment for Preschoolers (MAP)	Miller, L. J. (1988)	2 years 9 months to 5 years 8 months	Sensory motor foundations, motor coordination, verbal and nonverbal skills, and performance on complex tasks
Motor-Free Visual Perception Test (MVPT-3)	Colarusso, R. R., & Hammill, D. D. (1995)	4–70 years	Visual perceptual abilities that do not require motor involvement
Peabody Developmental Motor Scales, second edition (PDMS-2)	Folio, M. R., & Fewell, R. R. (2000)	Birth–5 years	Gross and fine motor skills
Sensory Integration and Praxis Test	Ayres, J. (1989)	4–9 years	Sensory integration processes
Test of Visual Motor Skills—Revised	Gardner, M. F. (1995)	3–13 years	Eye–hand coordination skills needed to copy geometric designs
Test of Visual Perceptual skills (TVPS-R)	Gardner, M. F. (1996)	4–13 years	Visual perceptual skills

---

Work Sheet 15-2. Assessment Methods

1. Describe the difference between norm-referenced measures and criterion-referenced measures and give three examples of each type of measure.

2. Determine which assessment method would be the best given the scenario described.

SA = standardized assessment, **SO** = skilled observations, **I** = interview,
AA = arena assessments using transdisciplinary model

AA **A.** You are looking for the best approach for an infant who comes in to the early intervention setting with concerns about gross motor skills, fine motor skills, and language development.

SO **B.** You need to determine the type of splint that would be most beneficial to prevent a contracture.

SA **C.** You need to determine a developmental level to determine if the child qualifies for services.

SO **D.** You need to assess tone and posture.

I **E.** You want to determine if the child's behavior during the session was typical.

I **F.** You are in a clinic or school setting and you want to understand how the child functions at home.

AA **G.** You have a child with feeding difficulties and you are asked to evaluate as part of a team that includes a dietitian and a nurse.

SA ~~SO~~ **H.** You want to determine how the child is functioning in relation to a normative group.

I **I.** You want to know the parents' main concerns and their perception of the child's abilities.

SO **J.** You want to determine the effect the environment has on the child's behavior.

AA **K.** You want to observe the child in a play session along with other professionals and develop team recommendations according to IDEA requirements.

I **L.** You want your teenage client's perspective on his or her disability.

Work Sheet 15-3. Assessment

Fill in the chart with the missing information.

Table 15-3 Assessment B

Test Name	Ages	What It Tests
Hawaii Early Learning Profile	Infants, toddlers, and young children	Developmental needs, intervention goals, and track progress
School Function Assessment (Costner, et al.)	Kindergarten through grade 6	Student's level of participation, supports needed, and activity performance on specific school tasks
Evaluation Tool of Children's Handwriting (ETCH) (Amundson)	Grades 1–6	Manuscript and cursive handwriting skills
Gross Motor Function Measure revised (GMFM)	Children whose motor skills are at or below a 5-year-old level	Gross motor function in children with cerebral palsy and Down syndrome

iii. Criterion-referenced measures group skills into functional or developmental areas, generally by age level. Common pediatric assessments that are criterion-referenced include, but are not limited to the following.

b. Skilled observation is essential to the pediatric occupational therapist. Children do not always comply with standardized testing, often making the scores invalid. Children act differently in different environments and with different people. Important information can be gathered through skilled observation that is not covered on a standardized developmental assessment, including tone, strength, posture, and overall cooperation.

    i. Some assessments are set up as observational tools and include but are not limited to the following:

        I. Childhood Autism Rating Scale (CARS) (Schopler, Reichler, & Renner, 2002): Two or more years to distinguish children with autism from children with developmental delays without autism

        II. Erhardt Developmental Prehension Assessment (Revised) (Erhardt, 1994): Looks at components of arm and hand development in children with cerebral palsy or other neurological impairments

        III. Knox Preschool Play Scale (Revised) (Parham & Fazio, 1997, pp. 35–51): Birth to 6 years; assesses play behaviors

        IV. WeeFIM (Hamilton & Granger, 1991): Six months to 6 years; looks at self-care, mobility, and cognitive skills to determine amount of caregiver assistance required

    ii. Skilled observation of neuromotor status

c. Conduct interviews with the child if appropriate, with the referral source (e.g., physician, school teacher or psychologist, clinic staff), and with the parents or caregivers. This gives background information as well as validation of information gathered through more formal assessments. Assessments that are set up as questionnaires will assist with the interview process. They include, but are not limited to, the following:

    i. Sensory Profile (Dunn, 2002): Three to 12 years, caregiver questionnaire. There is also an adolescent/adult sensory profile for ages 11 and older (Brown & Dunn, 2002).

    ii. Ages and Stages Questionnaire (Bricker, Squires, & Mounts, 1995): Birth to 5 years, including communication, gross motor, fine motor, problem solving, personal-social

    iii. Canadian Occupational Performance Measure (Law, 1994): Helps identify family priorities for children with special needs.

    iv. Pediatric Evaluation of Disability Inventory (PEDI) (Haley, Coster, Ludlow, Haltiwanger, & Andrellos, 1992): Six months to 7.5 years. Measures capabilities and performance in self-care, mobility, and social function.

d. Arena assessments

3. Specific assessment areas

(Case-Smith, 2005, pp. 289–290, 705–707)
(Mulligan, 2003, pp. 122–125)

    a. Evaluation of the neonate

    b. Reflex testing

        i. Primitive reflexes

        ii. Righting reactions assessed through handling

        iii. Equilibrium reactions

        iv. Protective reactions

Work Sheet 15-4. Postural Control

Match the stimulus with the reflex or automatic righting, equilibrium, or protective reaction you would be observing.

Table 15-4 Postural Control

A. Body on body righting	_G_	1. Child sits. Displace the child forward so he or she could possibly fall.	_G_
B. Moro reflex	_F_	2. Place your finger into a newborn's palm.	_F_
C. Symmetrical tonic neck	_H_	3. In supine, rotate infant's head and observe either log rolling or segmental rolling.	_H_
D. Rooting	_J_	4. Child is in a supported position sitting on a ball. Displace the child gently and watch the trunk and head.	_I_
E. Asymmetrical tonic neck	_C_	5. A 5-month-old is in prone position over your lap. Flex or extend the head and observe extremities.	_C_
F. Palmar grasp	_D_	6. Stroke the side of a 2-month-old's cheek. Observe head turning toward stimulus.	_D_
G. Protective reaction	_I_	7. Tilt 7-month-old while in supported sitting position and observe head movement in opposite direction to maintain alignment with body.	_I_
H. Neck on body righting	_E_	8. In supine position, turn the head of a 2-month-old to one side. Observe the extension of the arm on the face side and the flexion of the arm on the skull side.	_E_
I. Equilibrium reactions	_B_	9. Support a full-term newborn in a semireclined position and release the head support momentarily. Observe the arm movements.	_B_
J. Head righting	_A_	10. In supine position, rotate an infant's hips to one side. Observe upper body rotating or segmental rolling.	_A_

---

   c. Muscle tone: The evaluation of tone is a skilled observation that involves handling the child and observing his or her functional movement patterns.

(Case-Smith, 2005, pp. 177–179, 292–293)
(Mulligan, 2003, p. 58)
(Radomski & Trombly, 2008, pp. 193–194)

     i. Hypotonia
     ii. Hypertonia: Can be more formally documented using the Modified Ashworth Scale
   d. Motor development: The developmental sequence is based on developing mobility or stability or both in weight bearing, then mobility and stability in nonweight bearing for increased skill level.

(Case-Smith, 2005, p. 280)
(Mulligan, 2003, pp. 126–127)

     i. Prone development
     ii. Supine development
     iii. Sitting/quadraped development
     iv. Standing development

Work Sheet 15-5. Developmental Sequence

Arrange the following in proper sequence by numbering 1–4 or 5 depending on the area. Provide an age range for when the skill typically develops.

Prone development:

_4_ Hand propping with extended elbows. Able to roll prone to supine. *4-6*

_2_ Shoulder girdle begins to protract, weight bearing is through lower body. Able to lift head and *2-3* maintain posture.

_1_ Clears head, majority of weight bearing is through chest. *0-2*

_5_ Can assume quadraped position and begin to rock, may crawl. *6-8*

_3_ Head and neck dissociated from lower trunk. Weight bearing on forearms or hands. *3-4*

Supine development:

_4_ Able to roll to prone with rotation.

_2_ Able to maintain head in neutral and can get some neck flexion in pull to sit. Visually tracks and can get hands to mouth.

_3_ Midline play with arms over chest and play with feet. Can roll to side lying.

_1_ Unable to maintain supine position, head falls to either side and body follows.

Sitting/quadraped development:

_4_ Creeps well.

_1_ Unable to sit unsupported, rounded back in supported sit.

_3_ Moves in and out of sitting, sits well, beginning to creep.

_2_ Can sit with hand support to front or sides. Can momentarily free a hand. Can weight bear in quadraped position. Pivots in prone or may scoot backwards.

Standing development:

_5_ Walks independently.

_4_ Full weight bearing, takes steps when hands held.

_3_ Pulls self to stand, cruises on furniture.

_1_ Stepping reflexes when held in standing.

_2_ Partial weight bearing in supported standing.

e. Play skills are generally assessed through clinical observations, although there are criterion-referenced measures available. The purpose of assessing play skills is usually to observe specific skills, developmental level, social interactions, and general cognitive functioning.

(Case-Smith, 2005, pp. 575–576)

f. Fine motor: It is generally accepted that motor skill development occurs from proximal to distal; however, new theories such as the systems theory of motor development have presented an alternative viewpoint. Irrespective of this ongoing debate, evaluation of fine motor skills should incorporate an evaluation of overall postural control; for example head control, balance, tone, and strength. Fine motor skills may also be impaired due to sensory impairments such as, tactile, proprioceptive, and visual deficits.

(Case-Smith, 2005, pp. 304–328)
(Mulligan, 2003, pp. 135–137)

Work Sheet 15-6. Fine Motor Skills

Match the grasp pattern with the functional description.

Hook grasp

Pincer (two-point, pad to pad)

Lateral pinch

Power grasp

Three jaw chuck (three-point pinch)

Spherical grasp

Cylindrical grasp

Throwing a tennis ball – *spherical*

Picking up a cube for stacking – *3 jaw chuck*

Using a key in a lock – *lateral*

Carrying a briefcase – *hook*

Holding a microphone – *cylindrical*

Pulling the string for lacing – *pincer*

Using a knife for cutting – *power*

Given the activity, decide what component of hand skills you would be assessing: reach, grasp/release, in-hand manipulation, bilateral hand skills, or tool use.

1. Ability to bat at suspended toy while in supine – *tool*
2. Scribbling with crayon – *tool use*
3. Throwing ball – *grasp/release*
4. Holding paper while cutting – *bilateral*
5. Rotate pencil to use eraser – *in hand*
6. Handwriting – *tool use*
7. Putting a coin from palm in a bank – *in hand*
8. Stacking blocks – *reach, grasp/release*
9. Put raisin in bottle – *reach*
10. Stabilize paper with nondominant hand while coloring – *bilateral*

---

    i. Reach
    ii. Grasp and release
    iii. In-hand manipulation
    iv. Bilateral hand use
    v. Tool use

g. Visual motor/visual perception: Visual acuity, visual fields, and oculomotor control may require an evaluation by an optometrist or ophthalmologist; however, as the occupational therapist, you can perform a functional assessment to determine if a referral for further testing is appropriate. Review the standardized tests that assess visual spatial and visual motor functioning.

(Case-Smith, 2005, p. 428)
(Mulligan, 2003, p. 52)

    i. Visual acuity
    ii. Visual tracking/oculomotor control
    iii. Functional vision
    iv. Sensitivity to visual stimuli
    v. Form perception
    vi. Spatial perception
    vii. Visual motor integration

Work Sheet 15-7. Feeding Evaluation

Answer yes or no to the following questions, assuming the children are developing typically.

1. Can a 10-month-old use a fork? N

2. Can a 28-week gestation newborn drink from a breast or bottle? N

3. Should you give a 4-month-old a cracker? N

4. Can a 9-month-old feed herself using her fingers? Y

5. Should you offer a fork to a 2-year-old? Y

6. Can a 6-month-old handle pureed foods? Y

7. Should you expect a 12-month-old to self-feed cereal with milk from a spoon? N

8. Can a 9-month-old have mashed table foods? Y

9. Can you offer a 5-month-old cereal from a spoon? Y

10. Can an 18-month-old chew table food? Y

11. Can a 1-month-old chew? N

12. Should a newborn, at 30 weeks gestation, have a coordinated, nutritive suck/swallow/breathe pattern? n

13. Should you position a child so the neck is hyperextended to facilitate swallowing? N

14. When evaluating feeding, are tone and posture important? Y

15. If a child is tube fed for prolonged periods, should you expect oral defensiveness? Y

16. Can you tell the difference between aspiration and penetration without a videofluoroscopic swallow study (modified barium swallow)? N

17. Are gagging and head turning signs of oral defensiveness? Y

---

h. Feeding: This requires input from family members in addition to the information gathered from an evaluation. The time it takes to complete a meal, the diets appropriate for nutrition, the diet appropriate for the child's culture, and the stress involved in getting the child to participate are all important aspects that are not directly found by conducting an oral motor assessment.

(Case-Smith, 2005, pp. 486–498)

   i. Developmental sequence of eating
   ii. Physical aspects, including positioning and oral motor skills
   iii. Sensory aspects, including environment as well as individual responses to the sensation of the food presented

i. Activities of daily living (ADL): Need to take into account the context of the task as well as where the task is being carried out (e.g., home, school, community), the developmental level of the child, and the social environment, including cultural differences in expectations.

(Case-Smith, 2005, pp. 527, 543, 547)

   i. Feeding (previously discussed)
   ii. Toileting
   iii. Dressing

Work Sheet 15-8. Pediatric ADL Skill Development

Answer yes or no to the following questions, assuming the children are developing typically.

1. Can an 18-month-old sit on a potty chair for short periods? *Y*
2. Can a 13-month-old remove his socks? *Y*
3. Can a 30-month-old zip her jacket? *n*
4. Can a 3-year-old tell someone he needs to go to the bathroom? *Y*
5. Would you expect an 18-month-old to be toilet trained? *n*
6. Can a 2.5-year-old unbutton large buttons? *Y*
7. Can a 4-year-old lace shoes? *Y*
8. Can a 3-year-old dress unsupervised? *n*
9. Can a 2-year-old remove a pullover shirt? *n*
10. Can a 14-month-old cooperate with dressing by pushing arms through sleeves? *Y*
11. Would you expect a 3-year-old to be mostly toilet trained during the day? *Y*
12. Can a 4-year-old button a series of three to four buttons? *Y*
13. Can a 42-month-old snap in the front? *Y*
14. Should you expect complete toilet training (bowel and bladder) between 4–5 years of age? *Y*
15. Would you expect a 36-month-old to engage a separating zipper? *n*

---

   j. Strength and range of motion: Not different in theory from adults but may require skilled observation because the child cannot always follow specific instructions for a manual muscle test.

(Case-Smith, 2005, p. 224)

     i. Observe functional strength and range by noting ability to complete an activity and also monitoring endurance. Can he or she reach against gravity to get a toy? Can the motion be repeated several times? Is it a smoother motion when they are in side lying, reaching with gravity eliminated, or are they able to reach over their head in sitting?

     ii. Specific range of motion measurements are valuable, in particular, for children with cerebral palsy or other disorders that result in increased tone as well as with children who have been burned. The treatment will be designed to maintain or increase the range of motion, so specific measurements will assist with monitoring progress.

   k. Sensory: A clear understanding of the many aspects of sensory processing is necessary to properly evaluate sensory problems. This includes an understanding of modulation, registration, defensiveness, discrimination, and proprioception, as well as motor planning or praxis.

(Case-Smith, 2005, pp. 374–387)
(Mulligan, 2003, pp. 58–59)

     i. Formal assessments, including interviews and questionnaires
     ii. Informal observations, including clinical observations

   l. Handwriting

(Case-Smith, 2005, pp. 590–596)

     i. Domains of handwriting
       I. Writing alphabet, upper- and lowercase
       II. Copying, near and far point

Work Sheet 15-9. Sensory Integration

Match the concept on the left with the definition on the right.

Table 15-5 Sensory Integration

Concept	Answer	Definition
A. Adaptive response	K	Pertaining to receptors and organs that detect head position, movement, and gravity
B. Body scheme	H / A	Ability to generate a response that is appropriately proportionate to the incoming sensory stimuli
C. Perception	J / B	Referring to the handling of sensory information by neural systems
D. Praxis	G	Organization of sensation for use
E. Ideation	B	The brain's map of body parts and how they interrelate
F. Sensory defensiveness	D	The ability to conceptualize, organize, and execute nonhabitual motor tasks
G. Sensory integration	C	The organization of sensory data into meaningful units
H. Sensory modulation	L	Pertaining to the tactile and proprioceptive systems
I. Sensory registration	F	Characterized by overresponsivity in one or more sensory systems
J. Sensory processing	E	The ability to conceptualize a new action to be performed in a given situation
K. Vestibular	A	A successful response to an environmental challenge
L. Somatosensory	I	Process by which the central nervous system attends to stimuli

III. Manuscript to cursive translation
IV. Writing from dictation
V. Writing from an original thought
ii. Legibility
iii. Speed
iv. Ergonomic factors, including posture, overall tone and stability, and pencil grip
v. Visual motor control

Work Sheet 15-10. Handwriting

1. Katie can form all letters correctly, but she presses hard, slumps while writing, and although it takes her longer than her peers, she can complete the assignment in the allotted time. This is a problem with:

   A. Her ability to copy
   B. Her overall posture and tone
   C. Her speed
   D. B and C

2. You are working with Sally, an 8-year-old female who has been referred to you to assist with her handwriting. While observing her writing her name on the paper, you notice that parts of her fingers are blanching due to how tightly she is holding her pencil. You have her put the pencil down and instruct her to relax while you passively move her fingers, wrist, elbow, forearm, and shoulder through their range of motion. During this assessment you find that there is not much resistance felt in her muscles as you move them. Based on this information, you decide that:

   A. She needs a harder surface to write on.
   B. She is holding the pencil tightly because her tone is increased in her arms and hands.
   C. She holds the pencil tightly because she is fixating or blocking due to decreased tone in her arms and hands.
   D. She needs a word processor.

3. Which of the following contributes to overall legibility of handwriting?

   A. Letter formation
   B. Alignment
   C. Sizing and spacing
   D. None of the above
   E. All of the above

4. You are asked by the classroom teacher to evaluate Jim, a third grader with mild cerebral palsy. The first thing you should do is:

   A. Gather handwriting samples and talk to his teacher about her concerns
   B. Evaluate Jim's muscle tone
   C. Give a standardized writing test, such as the ETCH
   D. Give a standardized visual motor test

5. You have looked at the samples and interviewed the teacher, and now you are going to do a direct observation of Emma's writing. What will you be able to tell through observation?

   A. If there are any avoidance behaviors
   B. Ability to form letters
   C. Posture and pencil grip
   D. B and C only
   E. A, B, and C

6. You are asked to evaluate the pencil grip of a sixth grader. According to the teacher, the grip appears to be awkward. When you see the child, you find he does not use a dynamic tripod grasp, but more of a lateral quadruped grip (thumb slightly wrapped, pencil stabilized at tips of all four fingers). His writing is legible, and he has no complaints of fatigue. What do you do next?

   A. Instruct him on how to change his grip to a dynamic tripod.
   B. Give him a home program to work on in hand manipulation skills.
   C. Nothing, this is an acceptable grip pattern.
   D. Give him a pencil with a pencil grip to pattern his hand.

7. You are called in to observe a kindergartner who is having difficulty with writing skills. During your observation, you notice that she is wiggling in her seat with her feet dangling, often stands up to write, or kneels on her chair. What may help improve the situation?

   A. Giving her something for under her feet to stabilize her
   B. Giving her an incentive program for increasing her attention span
   C. Making sure the table/desk is at the right height so she can see what she's doing
   D. All of the above
   E. A and C

REFERENCES

American Occupational Therapy Association. (2002). Occupational therapy practice framework: Domain and process. *American Journal of Occupational Therapy, 56,* 609–639.

Bricker, D., Squires, J., & Mounts, L. (1995). *Ages and stages questionnaires: A parent-completed, child-monitoring system* (2nd ed.). Baltimore: Brookes.

Brown, C., & Dunn, W. (2002). *Adolescent/adult sensory profile: User's manual.* San Antonio, TX: Psychological Corporation.

Case-Smith, J. (Ed.). (2005). *Occupational therapy for children* (5th ed.). St. Louis, MO: Mosby.

Dunn, W. (2002). *Sensory profile: User's manual.* San Antonio, TX: Psychological Corporation.

Erhardt, R. P. (1994). *Erhardt developmental prehension assessment (revised).* San Antonio, TX: Psychological Corporation.

Haley, S. M., Coster, W. J., Ludlow, L. H., Haltiwanger, M. A., & Andrellos, P. J. (1992). *Pediatric evaluation of disability inventory.* San Antonio, TX: Psychological Corporation.

Hamilton, B. B., & Granger, C. U. (1991). *Functional independence measure for children (WeeFIM).* Buffalo, NY: Research Foundation of the State University of New York.

Parham L. D., & Fazio, L. S. (Eds.). (1997). *Play in occupational therapy for children.* St. Louis, MO: Mosby.

Law, M., Baptiste, S., Carswell, A., McColl, M. A., Polatajko, H., & Pollock, N. (1994). *Canadian occupational performance measure* (2nd ed.). Ottawa, Ontario: Canadian Association of Occupational Therapy Publications.

Mulligan, S. (2003). *Occupational therapy evaluation for children: A pocket guide.* Philadelphia: Lippincott Williams & Wilkins.

Radomski, M. V., & Latham, C. A. T. (Eds.). (2008). *Occupational therapy for physical dysfunction* (6th ed.). Philadelphia: Lippincott Williams & Wilkins.

Schopler, E., Reichler, R. J., & Renner, B. R. (2002). *Childhood autism rating scale.* Los Angeles: Western Psychological Services.

WORK SHEET ANSWERS

Work Sheet 15-2. Assessment Methods

1. Describe the difference between norm-referenced measures and criterion-referenced measures and give three examples of each type of measure.

   (Case-Smith, 2005, pp. 233, 241–243, 254)

   Correct Answer: Norm-referenced tests have been standardized on a sample population, and the results are based on the performance as compared to the normative sample. Examples include Battelle Developmental Inventory, Bruininks-Oseretsky Test of Motor Proficiency, Developmental Test of Visual Perception, Beery Test of Visual Motor Integration, and many others.

   Criterion-referenced measures look at a specific skill set, generally grouped by developmental level. The child's performance is compared to the criteria set forth by the test and gives an indication of the child's developmental level. Examples include HELP (Hawaii Early Learning Profile), ETCH (Evaluation Tool of Children's Handwriting), LAP (Learning Accomplishment Profile), and Erhardt Developmental Prehension Assessment.

2. Determine which assessment method would be the best given the scenario described.

   SA = standardized assessment, **SO** = skilled observations, **I** = interview, **AA** = arena assessments using transdisciplinary model

   A. You are looking for the best approach for an infant who comes in to the early intervention setting with concerns about gross motor skills, fine motor skills, and language development.

   Correct Answer: AA. (Case-Smith, 2005, p. 237). This will address all areas of concern and fits with IDEA standards.

   B. You need to determine the type of splint that would be most beneficial to prevent a contracture.

   Correct Answer: SO. (Case-Smith, 2005, pp. 224, 234). There is no standardized test that will provide you with the information you need, and your professional input is needed over input gained from an interview.

   C. You need to determine a developmental level to determine if the child qualifies for services.

   Correct Answer: SA. (Case-Smith, 2005, p. 222). One of the reasons for completing a standardized assessment is to determine eligibility.

   D. You need to assess tone and posture.

   Correct Answer: SO. (Case Smith, 2005, p. 224). This cannot be fully assessed through either standardized assessment or interview.

   E. You want to determine if the child's behavior during the session was typical.

   Correct Answer: I. (Case Smith, 2005, p. 235). This information could only come from interviewing someone who is familiar with the child.

   F. You are in a clinic or school setting and you want to understand how the child functions at home.

   Correct Answer: I. (Case-Smith, 2005, p. 224). Most likely you would not have the opportunity to evaluate the child at home, but the information would be key to your understanding of the problems and would help you better determine a treatment plan.

   G. You have a child with feeding difficulties and you are asked to evaluate as part of a team that includes a dietitian and a nurse.

   Correct Answer: AA. (Case-Smith, 2005, p. 237). You may be part of a team, and you may give parts of a standardized assessment, but one person would take the lead.

   H. You want to determine how the child is functioning in relation to a normative group.

   Correct Answer: SA. (Case-Smith, 2005, p. 233). Norm-referenced assessments provide this information.

   I. You want to know the parents' main concerns and their perception of the child's abilities.

   Correct Answer: I. (Case-Smith, 2005, p. 235). Only an interview with parents could provide this information.

Work Sheet 15-2. Assessment Methods *(continued)*

J. You want to determine the effect the environment has on the child's behavior.

Correct Answer: SO. (Case-Smith, 2005, pp. 234–235).

K. You want to observe the child in a play session along with other professionals and develop team recommendations according to IDEA requirements.

Correct Answer: AA. (Case-Smith, 2005, p. 237). Most evaluations that involve a team would fall under arena assessments, and IDEA is a clue for use of an arena assessment.

L. You want your teenage client's perspective on his or her disability.

Correct Answer: I. (Case-Smith, 2005, p. 235). Only an interview could give you this information.

Work Sheet 15-4. Postural Control

Match the stimulus with the reflex or automatic righting, equilibrium, or protective reaction you would be observing.

Table 15-6 Postural Control Answer Key

A. Body on body righting	_G_	1.	Child sits. Displace the child forward so he or she could possibly fall.
B. Moro reflex	_F_	2.	Place your finger into a newborn's palm.
C. Symmetrical tonic neck	_H_	3.	In supine, rotate infant's head and observe either log rolling or segmental rolling.
D. Rooting	_J_	4.	Child is in a supported position sitting on a ball. Displace the child gently and watch the trunk and head.
E. Asymmetrical tonic neck	_C_	5.	A 5-month-old is in prone position over your lap. Flex or extend the head and observe extremities.
F. Palmar grasp	_D_	6.	Stroke the side of a 2-month-old's cheek. Observe head turning toward stimulus.
G. Protective reaction	_I_	7.	Tilt 7-month-old while in supported sitting position and observe head movement in opposite direction to maintain alignment with body.
H. Neck on body righting	_E_	8.	In supine, turn the head of a 2-month-old to one side. Observe the extension of the arm on the face side and the flexion of the arm on the skull side.
I. Equilibrium reactions	_B_	9.	Support a full-term newborn in a semireclined position and release the head support momentarily. Observe the arm movements.
J. Head righting	_A_	10.	In supine position, rotate an infant's hips to one side. Observe upper body rotating or segmental rolling.

Work Sheet 15-5. Developmental Sequence

Arrange the following in proper sequence by numbering 1–4 or 5 depending on the area. Provide an age range for when the skill typically develops. **Answers are bold.**

Prone development:

4. Hand propping with extended elbows. Able to roll prone to supine. **(4–6 months without rotation, 6–8 months with rotation)**

2. Shoulder girdle begins to protract, weight bearing is through lower body. Able to lift head and maintain posture. **(2–3 months)**

1. Clears head, majority of weight bearing is through chest. **(0–2 months)**

5. Can assume quadruped position and begin to rock, may crawl. **(6–8 months)**

3. Head and neck dissociated from lower trunk. Weight bearing on forearms or hands. **(3–4 months)**

Supine development:

4. Able to roll to prone with rotation. **(6–9 months)**

2. Able to maintain head in neutral and can get some neck flexion in pull to sit. Visually tracks and can get hands to mouth. **(2–4 months)**

3. Midline play with arms over chest and play with feet. Can roll to side lying. **(4–6 months)**

1. Unable to maintain supine position, head falls to either side and body follows. **(0–2 months)**

Sitting/quadruped development:

4. Creeps well. **(8–10 months)**

1. Unable to sit unsupported, rounded back in supported sit.

3. Moves in and out of sitting, sits well, beginning to creep. **(6–8 months)**

2. Can sit with hand support to front or sides. Can momentarily free a hand. Can weight bear in quadruped position. Pivots in prone or may scoot backwards. **(4–6 months)**

Standing development:

5. Walks independently. **(12–14 months)**

4. Full weight bearing, takes steps when hands held. **(6–8 months)**

3. Pulls self to stand, cruises on furniture. **(9–13 months)**

1. Stepping reflexes when held in standing. **(0–3 months)**

2. Partial weight bearing in supported standing. **(4–6 months)**

Work Sheet 15-6. Fine Motor Skills

Match the grasp pattern with the functional description.

Hook grasp	Throwing a tennis ball
Pincer (two-point, pad to pad)	Picking up a cube for stacking
Lateral pinch	Using a key in a lock
Power grasp	Carrying a briefcase
Three jaw chuck (three-point pinch)	Holding a microphone
Spherical grasp	Pulling the string for lacing
Cylindrical grasp	Using a knife for cutting

Answers: Hook = briefcase, pincer = lacing, lateral = key, power = knife, three jaw chuck = blocks (this could be two point, but pulling string is not three point), spherical = tennis ball, cylindrical = microphone.

Given the activity, decide what component of hand skills you would be assessing: reach, grasp/release, in-hand manipulation, bilateral hand skills, or tool use. **Answers are bold.**

1. Ability to bat at suspended toy while in supine: **reach**

2. Scribbling with crayon: **tool use**

3. Throwing ball: **grasp/release**

4. Holding paper while cutting: **bilateral hand use**

5. Rotate pencil to use eraser: **in-hand manipulation**

6. Handwriting: **tool use**

7. Putting a coin from palm in a bank: **in-hand manipulation**

8. Stacking blocks: **grasp/release**

9. Put raisin in bottle: **grasp/release**

10. Stabilize paper with nondominant hand while coloring: **bilateral hand use**

Work Sheet 15-7. Feeding Evaluation

Answer yes or no to the following questions, assuming the children are developing typically. **Answers are bold.**

1. Can a 10-month-old use a fork? **No**
2. Can a 28-week gestation newborn drink from a breast or bottle? **No**
3. Should you give a 4-month-old a cracker? **No**
4. Can a 9-month-old feed herself using her fingers? **Yes**
5. Should you offer a fork to a 2-year-old? **Yes**
6. Can a 6-month-old handle pureed foods? **Yes**
7. Should you expect a 12-month-old to self-feed cereal with milk from a spoon? **No**
8. Can a 9-month-old have mashed table foods? **Yes**
9. Can you offer a 5-month-old cereal from a spoon? **Yes**
10. Can an 18-month-old chew table food? **Yes**
11. Can a 1-month-old chew? **No**
12. Should a newborn, at 30 weeks gestation, have a coordinated, nutritive suck/swallow/breathe pattern? **No**
13. Should you position a child so the neck is hyperextended to facilitate swallowing? **No**
14. When evaluating feeding, are tone and posture important? **Yes**
15. If a child is tube fed for prolonged periods, should you expect oral defensiveness? **Yes**
16. Can you tell the difference between aspiration and penetration without a videofluoroscopic swallow study (modified barium swallow)? **No**
17. Are gagging and head turning signs of oral defensiveness? **Yes**

Work Sheet 15-8. Pediatric ADL Skill Development

Answer yes or no to the following questions, assuming the children are developing typically. **Answers are bold.**

1. Can an 18-month-old sit on a potty chair for short periods? **Yes**
2. Can a 13-month-old remove his socks? **Yes**
3. Can a 30-month-old zip her jacket? **No**
4. Can a 3-year-old tell someone he needs to go to the bathroom? **Yes**
5. Would you expect an 18-month-old to be toilet trained? **No**
6. Can a 2.5-year-old unbutton large buttons? **Yes**
7. Can a 4-year-old lace shoes? **Yes**
8. Can a 3-year-old dress unsupervised? **No**
9. Can a 2-year-old remove a pullover shirt? **No**
10. Can a 14-month-old cooperate with dressing by pushing arms through sleeves? **Yes**
11. Would you expect a 3-year-old to be mostly toilet trained during the day? **Yes**
12. Can a 4-year-old button a series of three to four buttons? **Yes**
13. Can a 42-month-old snap in the front? **Yes**
14. Should you expect complete toilet training (bowel and bladder) between 4–5 years of age? **Yes**
15. Would you expect a 36-month-old to engage a separating zipper? **No**

Work Sheet 15-9. Sensory Integration

Match the concept on the left with the definition on the right.

Table 15-7 Sensory Integration Answer Key

A. Adaptive response	_K_	Pertaining to receptors and organs that detect head position, movement, and gravity
B. Body scheme	_H_	Ability to generate a response that is appropriately proportionate to the incoming sensory stimuli
C. Perception	_J_	Referring to the handling of sensory information by neural systems
D. Praxis	_G_	Organization of sensation for use
E. Ideation	_B_	The brain's map of body parts and how they interrelate
F. Sensory defensiveness	_D_	The ability to conceptualize, organize, and execute nonhabitual motor tasks
G. Sensory integration	_C_	The organization of sensory data into meaningful units
H. Sensory modulation	_L_	Pertaining to the tactile and proprioceptive systems
I. Sensory registration	_F_	Characterized by overresponsivity in one or more sensory systems
J. Sensory processing	_E_	The ability to conceptualize a new action to be performed in a given situation
K. Vestibular	_A_	A successful response to an environmental challenge
L. Somatosensory	_I_	Process by which the central nervous system attends to stimuli

---

Work Sheet 15-10. Handwriting

1. Katie can form all letters correctly, but she presses hard, slumps while writing, and although it takes her longer than her peers, she can complete the assignment in the allotted time. This is a problem with:

   A. Her ability to copy
   B. Her overall posture and tone
   C. Her speed
   D. B and C

   Correct Answer: B. Her posture and tone are causing her decreased speed. Speed is an issue only when work cannot be completed within the parameters set in class, not necessarily when compared to peers (Case-Smith, 2005, pp. 594–595).

2. You are working with Sally, an 8-year-old female who has been referred to you to assist with her handwriting. While observing her writing her name on the paper, you notice that parts of her fingers are blanching due to how tightly she is holding her pencil. You have her put the pencil down and instruct her to relax while you passively move her fingers, wrist, elbow, forearm, and shoulder through their range of motion. During this assessment you find that there is not much resistance felt in her muscles as you move them. Based on this information, you decide that:

   A. She needs a harder surface to write on.
   B. She is holding the pencil tightly because her tone is increased in her arms and hands.
   C. She holds the pencil tightly because she is fixating or blocking due to decreased tone in her arms and hands.
   D. She needs a word processor.

   Correct Answer: C. Increased tone in her arms and hands would be revealed during range of motion. She is compensating for decreased shoulder stability by fixating. Giving her a harder surface would not change her performance, and whether or not a keyboard would improve her performance cannot be determined from passive range of motion.

3. Which of the following contributes to overall legibility of handwriting?

   A. Letter formation
   B. Alignment
   C. Sizing and spacing
   D. None of the above
   E. All of the above

   Correct Answer: E (Case-Smith, 2005, p. 593)

4. You are asked by the classroom teacher to evaluate Jim, a third grader with mild cerebral palsy. The first thing you should do is:

   A. Gather handwriting samples and talk to his teacher about her concerns
   B. Evaluate Jim's muscle tone
   C. Give a standardized writing test, such as the ETCH
   D. Give a standardized visual motor test

   Correct Answer: A. You need to know what the specific concerns are before you can decide if a standardized test is necessary. Evaluation of tone may be part of your assessment at some point, but it would not be the first thing you would do (Case-Smith, 2005, p. 590).

5. You have looked at the samples and interviewed the teacher, and now you are going to directly observe Emma's writing. What will you be able to tell through observation?

   A. If there are any avoidance behaviors
   B. Ability to form letters
   C. Posture and pencil grip
   D. B and C only
   E. A, B, and C

   Correct Answer: E (Case-Smith, 2005, p. 592)

Work Sheet 15-10. Handwriting *(continued)*

6. You are asked to evaluate the pencil grip of a sixth grader. According to the teacher, the grip appears to be awkward. When you see the child, you find he does not use a dynamic tripod grasp, but more of a lateral quadruped grip (thumb slightly wrapped, pencil stabilized at tips of all four fingers). His writing is legible, and he has no complaints of fatigue. What do you do next?

   A. Instruct him on how to change his grip to a dynamic tripod.
   B. Give him a home program to work on in hand manipulation skills.
   C. Nothing, this is an acceptable grip pattern.
   D. Give him a pencil with a pencil grip to pattern his hand.

   Correct Answer: C (Case-Smith, 2005, pp. 591–592)

7. You are called in to observe a kindergartener who is having difficulty with writing skills. During your observation, you notice that she is wiggling in her seat with her feet dangling, often stands up to write, or kneels on her chair. What may help improve the situation?

   A. Giving her something for under her feet to stabilize her
   B. Giving her an incentive program for increasing her attention span
   C. Making sure the table/desk is at the right height so she can see what she's doing
   D. All of the above
   E. A and C

   Correct Answer: E. She may not be able to steady herself or see her work, so she may be standing or kneeling to compensate, not because of decreased attention span (Case-Smith, 2005, p. 595).

Specialized Pediatric Interventions

Beth Angst and Robin Mercer

OBJECTIVES

1. Describe the core concepts and assumptions of intervention strategies and approaches used in the pediatric population.
2. Investigate clinical reasoning skills used by occupational therapists in providing intervention to the pediatric population.
3. Investigate the basic principles of providing intervention services to the pediatric population in common pediatric clinical settings.
4. Apply knowledge of the intervention strategies and approaches used in the pediatric population into clinical case scenarios.
5. Demonstrate basic competence in intervention strategies and approaches used in the pediatric population.

KEY TERMS

Table 16-1 Key Terms

Case-Smith, 2005, pp. 278, 304, 688	Case-Smith, 2005, pp. 356, 795
Adaptive response	Adaptive responses
Balance	Dyspraxia
Dexterity	Inclusion
Equilibrium	Individualized education program (IEP)
Fine motor coordination	Individuals with Disabilities Education Act (IDEA)
In-hand manipulation	Overresponsiveness
Nonnutritive sucking	Praxis
Nutritive sucking	Proprioception
Protective reactions	Sensation seeking
Righting reactions	Sensory discrimination
Visual–motor integration	Sensory modulation
	Sensory registration
	Underresponsiveness

INTRODUCTION

Welcome to Days 23 and 24 of your study guide. This chapter will help you review the exciting area of pediatric intervention. Although some intervention strategies that you may have learned with the adult population can be used in pediatrics with modification for age, size, cognitive status, etc., intervention strategies in the pediatric population do produce unique challenges. This outline will help you gather information to investigate pediatric intervention techniques in more detail. Work through the outline to gather pertinent information on the various interventions, and then complete the work sheets to help you assess your understanding of the material.

OUTLINE

1. Intervention settings

(Case-Smith, 2005, pp. 688–793, 795–826, 868–893)
(Crepeau, Cohn, & Schell, 2009, pp. 592–613)
(Pendleton & Schultz-Krohn, 2006, pp. 42–49)

- **a.** Early intervention services
  - **i.** Definition
  - **ii.** Individualized family service plan (IFSP)
- **b.** School-based services
  - **i.** Definition
  - **ii.** Individualized education plan (IEP)
  - **iii.** Goal writing
  - **iv.** Intervention strategies when consulting
- **c.** Hospital-based services
  - **i.** Acute care
  - **ii.** Outpatient
  - **iii.** Neonatal intensive care unit (NICU)
    - **I.** Light modifications
    - **II.** Sound modifications
    - **III.** Caregiver modifications
    - **IV.** Supplemental sensory stimulation

2. Specific intervention strategies
- **a.** Handling

(Case-Smith, 2005, pp. 280–283, 297–298, 330–331, 718–726, 767–769)
(Pendleton & Schultz-Krohn, 2006, pp. 740–742)

- **i.** Developmental positioning: Work in various developmental positions is very important in the pediatric population. Weight bearing provided through developmental positions works to improve strength in the shoulder girdle and the upper extremities. Facilitation of weight shift in various developmental positions increases the development of proximal stability and postural control. Static weight bearing in developmental positions can provide an inhibitory effect on tone, and dynamic weight shift over a stable base in developmental positions can provide a facilitory effect on tone.
  - **I.** Specifics of developmental positioning with neonatal population
  - **II.** Principles for general pediatric populations
    - **a.** Supine
    - **b.** Prone
    - **c.** Side lying
    - **d.** Side sitting
    - **e.** Four-point, quadruped

Work Sheet 16-1. Settings

Define which specialized pediatric setting would be most appropriate for intervention services for the patients in the following case scenarios. Choose from the following possible intervention settings:

A. Early intervention
B. School based
C. Hospital-based acute
D. Hospital-based outpatient

Case One: Alonzo is a child with Down syndrome who has an active IFSP. Where would Alonzo most likely receive services? _____

Case Two: Jennifer is a 3-year-old with spastic diplegia whose family is concerned about her development. Her upper extremity tone and strength is within normal limits. Who would be most appropriate to provide consultative services? _____

Case Three: Jonathan is an 8-year-old boy who is demonstrating handwriting difficulties and fine motor delays that are interfering with his ability to produce written work at a pace equal to his peers. He may benefit from assistive technology. Where would he most likely be referred for an evaluation for occupational therapy services? _____

Case Four: Tyrone is a 10-year-old boy status postfracture to his radius and is having difficulty with writing postsurgery. Where would he most likely be referred for evaluation for occupational therapy services? _____

Case Five: Julie is a 6-year-old female with left hemiparesis due to a stroke. She demonstrates significant range and strength limitations and increased tone in her left hand. She is able to self-ambulate around the school environment. She uses classroom tools appropriately. Where would she most likely receive therapy services? _____

Case Six: Natasha is a 5-year-old with a history of a brain tumor whose parents are concerned about her IEP. She has endurance and coordination issues. She frequently drops objects and has difficulty with her dressing and feeding skills. Which setting would help the parents address these issues? _____

Case Seven: Michael is a 13-year-old male who was involved in a motor vehicle accident in which he sustained a concussion and a fractured femur. Michael and his parents are concerned about him being able to perform lower extremity dressing and carry his books at school due to his external fixator. Where would Michael most likely be referred to help his family address their concerns? _____

Work Sheet 16-2. Developmental Positions # 1

Developmental positions are frequently used in intervention with the pediatric population to help develop desired strength, proximal stability, and skill. Match the developmental position with the skills it helps to facilitate.

Table 16-2 Developmental Positions #1

Position	Answer	Skill
A. Supine	F	Facilitates the development of head control, muscles of the trunk, back and hips, and balance.
B. Prone	A	Encourages hands to reach and engage and encourages midline activities. Facilitates development of stomach muscles through body flexion in older infants. Facilitates extension in premature infants. Easy visual attention.
C. Side lying	E	Develops muscles of the trunk, back, and hips. Strengthens muscles of the arm. Allows the child to accept body weight to one side.
D. Prone on elbows	B	Facilitates head control and helps develop muscles of the shoulders, arms, back, and hips. Facilitates hand-to-mouth activities. Facilitates development of flexor tone in premature infants.
E. Side sitting	C	Facilitates hands together and makes it easier to touch or hold a toy. Facilitates hand and head at midline. Relaxes the child and requires less effort to move the body. Encourages extremity flexion and adduction. Develops the rib cage. Encourages rolling when reaching for toys.
F. Ring sitting	G	Helps develop muscle control and strength in the shoulders, arms, hips, legs, and back. Helps to facilitate balance with weight shifting.
G. Four point, quadruped	D	Facilitates the development of muscles of the shoulders, arms, and back; head control; and the ability to weight shift when reaching.

Work Sheet 16-3. Developmental Positions #2

List the advantages and disadvantages of each developmental position.

Table 16-3 Developmental Positions #2

	Advantages	Disadvantages
Supine		
Prone		
Side lying		
Sitting		
Standing		

  ii. Proximal stability/postural control: Appropriate proximal stability and postural control provide the basis from which gross motor and fine motor skills develop, including the ability to isolate oral movements required during eating. If proximal stability and postural control are inadequate, the child will develop compensatory strategies and inefficient movement patterns. This will greatly affect the child's ability to progress through developmentally appropriate areas of occupation. Early facilitation of appropriate postural control and proximal stability through therapeutic handling are imperative to allow the child to progress through all areas of development with the most efficient patterns possible.

   I. Progression of motor development

    a. Prone antigravity development

    b. Supine antigravity development

    c. Sitting antigravity development

   II. Facilitating antigravity movement

   III. Facilitating postural reactions

 b. Strengthening: Just as in the adult population, a pediatric patient with decreased strength in areas such as trunk, upper extremity, and/or facial musculature can experience a significant loss in functional skills. Unlike the adult population, however, addressing decreased strength in the pediatric group, especially those less than approximately 6 years of age, can test the therapist's ability to embed therapeutic activities into occupations. A young pediatric patient cannot be expected to complete a rote exercise program with any amount of success. Strengthening activities for young children must be incorporated into occupational tasks, such as lifting a weighted ball up onto a slide for it to roll down and knock over bowling pins, pushing a toy grocery cart with weights inside, completing activities with wrist weights on, and finding items that have been buried in theraputty.

(Case-Smith, 2005, pp. 292–293, 346–348, 900–901, 903)

(Radomski & Latham, 2008, pp. 1029–1030)

  i. Impact on postural control

  ii. Constraint-induced therapy

  iii. Preventing secondary deformities

  iv. Basic rehabilitation strategies

 c. Muscle tone: Abnormal muscle tone needs to be addressed as soon as possible in the pediatric population. Abnormal tone leads to the development of abnormal movement patterns resulting in high energy, inefficient patterns that impact all areas of function. It is important to use therapeutic techniques to help the child normalize tone so that he or she develops movement patterns that are as normal, fluid, and efficient as possible.

(Case-Smith, 2005, pp. 180–181, 331–332, 347–350, 718)

(Radomski & Latham, 2008, pp. 440–441, 452–455, 651–654, 692–697)

  i. Managing increased tone

   I. Spasticity management

    a. Medications

     i. Oral medications

     ii. Baclofen pump

     iii. Neural blocks (Botox)

    b. Orthopedic surgeries (tendon lengthening)

    c. Rhizotomy

   II. Improving postural tone and control

   III. Inhibition

   IV. Serial casting

   V. Splinting

    a. Air splint

      b. Antispasticity

      c. Neoprene

      d. Weight bearing

  ii. Managing low tone

      I. Hypotonia in premature infants

      II. Facilitation

      III. Orthotics: Splints and orthotics are generally thought of for use in children with increased tone. Children with low tone, however, can benefit greatly from specialized trunk and extremity supports that provide deep pressure, assist with proprioception, and result in improved support and stability. These garments may be used in therapy, at home, and in school environments.

        a. Benik vests (www.benik.com)

        b. TheraTogs (www.theratogs.com)

Work Sheet 16-4. Tone Questions

1. Pick the statement that best describes normal postural tone.

  A. It must be high enough to withstand gravity.

  B. It provides the background on which movement is based.

  C. Easy movement is only available if postural tone is low enough to allow it to happen.

  D. All of the above

2. Which statement is *not* true about muscle tone?

  A. Tone is highly influenced by gravity.

  B. Your emotional state can influence your muscle tone.

  C. Muscle tone allows movement against an outside source.

  D. Tone allows smooth, coordinated movements.

3. If the child you are treating has increased tone in the flexor muscles of the arm resulting in severe elbow flexion, you would expect that:

  A. The extensor muscles are also tight.

  B. The extensor muscles are overstretched and weak.

  C. The extensor muscles have not been affected because they are innervated differently.

  D. All of the above

4. You are working with a 4-year-old male who has increased tone in the muscles of his upper arm. This tone is noted to increase with participation in all functional activities. Which technique would be the best idea to help decrease the tone?

  A. Tap the muscle belly to inhibit or deactivate the muscle.

  B. Use quick stroking movements along the muscle with the muscle on stretch.

  C. Cast the arm for stretch and neutral warmth.

  D. Provide slow, firm massage strokes with stretch.

5. Evan is a 3-year-old male with a history of cerebral palsy. He has significantly increased tone in his right upper extremity. He is holding his right upper extremity in elbow and wrist flexion. You know that his increased tone is interfering with his ability to participate in occupations. During treatment the best thing you could do would be which of the following?

  A. Place the child in supported sitting and slowly stretch and move his right upper extremity through full range.

  B. During home program instruction encourage the parents to hand him things to his left upper extremity.

  C. Position him in right side sitting with support at his elbow and have him shoot baskets with his left hand.

  D. Provide vibration to the right upper extremity.

(continues)

Work Sheet 16-4. Tone Questions *(continued)*

6. You are working with the family of a 5-year-old child with cerebral palsy who has increased extensor tone. The family has difficulty getting this patient from supine to sitting after changing his diaper. Which of the following statements best describes how you would teach the parents to bring their child from the supine to the sitting position?

   A. Tell them to place their hand behind his head and slowly push him up into a sitting position because hip flexion helps to break up tone.

   B. Tell them it would be easiest to hold him by his hands and slowly pull him into a sitting position.

   C. Tell them to hold his upper arms and gently lift and turn the shoulders to rotate the trunk slightly and then come up.

   D. Tell them to flex his legs and knees so they face up in the air and use your body to hold his legs in this position; then, holding his upper arms near the shoulders, gently lift his shoulders up and toward you as you use your body to push his legs back so that he ends up in a sitting position.

7. Alex is a 4-year-old male with a history of hypotonia. He sits with a forward posture with his ribs resting on his hip bones. He can use his upper extremities in activities within his base of support and below his center of gravity but without crossing midline. The best activity to improve the overall tone and help increase his trunk stability to free his upper extremities for improved use would be which of the following?

   A. Position him in sitting on a platform swing and have him throw beanbags into a basket while slowly swinging in wide, full circles.

   B. Position him in sitting on a therapy ball and support him on the lateral sides of his trunk to facilitate appropriate trunk alignment and provide firm, quick pressure into the ball; then have him shoot beanbags into a basket that is above his head and off to the left.

   C. Position him in sitting on a therapy ball and support him on the lateral sides of his trunk to facilitate appropriate trunk alignment and provide firm, quick pressure into the ball; then have him place beanbags into a basket that is at his shoulder height and in front of him.

   D. Have him shoot baskets at shoulder level while he is sitting stable on the ground in tailor sitting and you are providing slow stroking to his extensor and abdominal muscles to increase his trunk stability.

---

    d. Sensory integration (SI): Not all pediatric therapists have the opportunity to work in a facility that is set up for the sole purpose of sensory integrative treatment. These facilities differ significantly from the multiple-purpose treatment environments in which many pediatric therapists provide their services. This does not mean, however, that pediatric therapists who do not have access to specific sensory integrative gyms will not use sensory integrative techniques in their treatment sessions. In fact, all pediatric therapists should have knowledge of these techniques because they are an invaluable tool in helping to address many of the treatment needs of the pediatric population and can be adapted for use in all treatment environments. An understanding of the sensory processing needs of the patient and acknowledging and addressing these needs appropriately in the treatment session can often increase the success of the session when standard treatment approaches alone may not achieve the desired result.

(Case-Smith, 2005, pp. 356–403)

    i.   Define
    ii.   Adaptive response: Active, comes from within child
    iii.   Sensory modulation disorders
        I.   Sensory registration disorders
        II.   Sensory seeking behaviors
        III.   Overresponsiveness
            a. Tactile defensiveness
            b. Gravitational insecurity

iv. Sensory discrimination and perception problems
   I. Tactile discrimination
   II. Proprioceptive problems
   III. Visual perceptual problems
v. Visual proprioceptive problems
vi. Praxis problems
   I. Dyspraxia
   II. Somatodyspraxia
vii. Guiding principles of SI treatment
viii. Classic SI treatment
   I. Individualized
   II. Balance of structure and freedom
   III. Inner drive and active participation
   IV. Appropriate setting
ix. Compensatory skill development
x. Consultation
xi. Outcomes

Work Sheet 16-5. Sensory Integration #1

Match the sensory modulation disorder with the appropriate description.

Table 16-4 Sensory Integration #1

A. Gravitational insecurity	B	Patient reacts defensively to ordinary sensory input. Often demonstrates activation of sympathetic nervous system.
B. Hyperresponsivity	F	Disorder used interchangeably with hyperresponsivity.
C. Hyporesponsivity	G	Disorder used interchangeably with hyporesponsivity.
D. Sensory seeking	B E	Patient tends to react negatively to clothing, dislikes having shoes off, and has tendency to weight bear on fingertips rather than palms.
E. Tactile defensiveness	D	Patient searches out specific sensory input at higher frequency and/or intensity.
F. Overresponsiveness	A	Patient reacts negatively to movement, especially when head is moving backward.
G. Underresponsiveness	C	Patient tends to ignore sensory stimuli that would be responded to by most individuals.

Work Sheet 16-6. Sensory Integration #2

Listed below are several treatment strategies that could be used in addressing disorders of sensory integration. Match the treatment strategy with the primary type of sensory integration disorder that it could be used to address the following:

TD = Tactile defensiveness

TDD = Tactile discrimination disorders

PPD = Poor proprioceptive discrimination

GI = Gravitational insecurity

PBI = Poor bilateral integration

(continues)

Work Sheet 16-6. Sensory Integration #2 *(continued)*

Table 16-5 Sensory Integration #2

Sensory Integration Disorder	Possible Treatment Strategy
TD	Begin with vestibular and proprioceptive input, continue with deep pressure and end with touch if tolerated.
GI	Respect the child's fears, do not force movement.
PBI PPD	On swing in prone and propelling self with hands on floor.
PPD PBI	Play tug-of-war games.
GI	Start with anterior–posterior trunk movements; progress to lateral and then rotational.
TD	Avoid light touch.
PPD TD	Use blow toys and resistive chewing activities.
TD	Respect child's personal space, do not impose.
PBI	Catching a ball.
TD	Reduce sensory overload in the environment, lower voice, use natural light, work in small spaces.
PPD	Have patient push and pull bolsters, wedges, mats, etc. to help set up obstacle courses/treatment area.
TDD	Place small stickers of various sizes on child's arms, legs, and feet and have the child find them with eyes open and with eyes closed.
GI	Work with child near the ground, maintain feet on floor.
PBI	Pulling hand over hand on rope.
PPD	Have child push a toy grocery cart with weights in it to go shopping for toys.
GI	Use swings attached to two suspension points to gain more linear movement.
TDD TD	Have the child dip his or her finger in shaving cream and then write letters on his or her arm/hand and your arm/hand.

Note: PPD activities can also be used to provide basis for GI, TD, and TDD activities because proprioception also helps to modulate tactile and vestibular input.

Tactile defensiveness
Tactile discrim disorder
Poor prop discrim
Gravitational insecurity
Poor bilateral integration

Work Sheet 16-7. Sensory Integration #3

Listed below are some statements that a parent might make during your treatment session to describe their child's behavior in the home and community environment. Next to each statement place the initials of the most appropriate type of sensory integrative disorder this type of statement might describe.

TD = Tactile defensiveness

TDD = Tactile discrimination disorders

PPD = Poor proprioceptive discrimination

GI = Gravitational insecurity

PBI = Poor bilateral integration

TDD — Jeffrey is constantly touching everything. I can't take him to a store with delicate items because I am afraid he will want to touch everything and end up breaking something.

TD — Johnny cries and becomes upset every time he is put in the bathtub. After he is there for a while he calms down but then gets upset when he is taken out again.

PBI — Theresa's teacher told me that she is having a very difficult time with learning how to cut with scissors. She said that she doesn't seem to be able to get the hand holding the paper and the hand holding the scissors to work together.

PPD — The other day Tony was trying to put a dime in the gum ball machine at the grocery store, and he must have dropped that dime 10 times before I finally helped him put the dime in the slot.

GI — I have become very good at changing Jerry's diaper while he is standing up because every time I try to lie him down to change his diaper he cries.

PPD — Jenny complained that her teacher always puts her at the end of the line in school. When I asked the teacher about this, she said that she does this because when Jenny is between other students in line she tends to bump into the other kids or stand really close to them, and this upsets the other children.

TD — If someone lightly bumps into or touches Katie, she hits herself wherever she was touched, and she hits herself pretty hard.

PPD — Luke prefers to sit and play by himself. If you take him to the playground, all the other kids will be running, climbing, and playing, but Luke will stay on the sidelines, mostly just standing and watching.

TDD — Shelly is very hard on her toys. I just bought her a new doll the other day and she already broke the arm off the poor doll.

TD — Keisha is very happy when I hold her, but when her grandma tries to touch or hold her she becomes very upset.

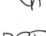

e. Fine motor

(Case-Smith, 2005, pp. 309–317, 322–341, 787, 812)

    i.   Grasp patterns
- **I.** Hook
- **II.** Power
- **III.** Lateral pinch
- **IV.** Pad to pad, two-point pinch
- **V.** Tip pinch
- **VI.** Ulnar–palmar grasp
- **VII.** Radial–digital grasp
- **VIII.** Spherical grasp
- **IX.** Cylindrical grasp
- **X.** Disc grasp

ii.   Development of grasp patterns
iii.   Problems that affect hand skills
iv.   Isolating arm and hand movements
v.   Enhancing reach
vi.   Facilitating grasp skills
vii.   Facilitating release
viii. In-hand manipulation skills
    I.   Types of patterns
        a. Translation
        b. Shift
        c. Simple rotation
        d. Complex rotation
    II.   Prerequisite motor skills
    III. Patterns observed when skills limited
    IV.   Facilitating in-hand manipulation skills
ix.   Fine motor and manipulative hand function
x.   Activities to improve fine motor skills

Work Sheet 16-8. Facilitating In-Hand Manipulation

Intervention for enhancing a child's in-hand manipulation skills needs to be embedded into everyday play activities. Match the treatment activity with the type of in-hand manipulation skill it would help to facilitate. After identifying the skill, place an "S" next to the ones that would be completed with stabilization.

In-hand manipulation skills:

A. Shift
B. Translation (fingers to palm)
C. Translation (palm to fingers)
D. Rotation (may be simple or complex depending on object's orientation)

Treatment Activity:

Table 16-6 Facilitating In-Hand Manipulation

 1. You are playing a basketball game where you are having the child crumple up sheets of paper and then throw them in a container.

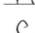 2. You are playing a game of Uno and having the child pick up and deal the cards one at a time from the deck sitting on the table.

 3. You are completing a puzzle that is made of colored blocks. The blocks have different colors on each of their sides. You are placing the blocks into the palm of the child's hand, and the child needs to turn them until he or she finds the right side to put in.

 4. During a coloring activity, what in-hand manipulation skill is used when removing a crayon from the box and preparing to color with it?

 5S. The child is holding fabric in one hand while trying to button with the other.

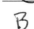 6S. You are having the child hold pennies in one hand and move them one at a time to place them in a bank.

 7S. In preparation for placing the pennies into a bank, you are having the child pick five pennies up from the palm of your hand, one at a time.

 8. You are having the child string beads.

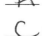 9. You are working on a cutting task. To move the paper in the nonpreferred hand during cutting, what type of in-hand manipulation skill is used?

 10. You are placing a fish cracker into the palm of the child's hand and allowing the child to eat the cracker.

Work Sheet 16-9. Handwriting

Each of the following activities can be completed to help improve the handwriting skills of your patients/students. For each activity listed, identify what portion of the handwriting process that activity can help to address (e.g., strengthening, posture, visual motor, manipulation, tripod grasp, letter forming, spacing).

1. Present the child with theraputty, Play-Doh, or clay that has small beads or objects hidden inside. *S* Have the child remove all of the objects and then replace them for the next child to find.

2. Practice dot-to-dot pictures and letters. *V M*

3. Have a child help you set up an obstacle course in the gym. Have the child practice moving through the obstacle course from front to back and back to front, timed and untimed. *S|P*

4. Build with magnet toys or small LEGOs. *M*

5. Complete a board game in prone on elbows. *S|P*

6. Use putty or clay to create letters and words. *If*

7. Have the child place pennies in a horizontal slot then move it to be vertical. *V M*

8. Draw two lines across a sheet of paper then trace them with glue and let them dry. Have the child practice writing words and letters on this paper. *If*

9. Have the child prone over a therapy ball and extend up to draw on a mirror with shaving cream. *S|P*

10. Use clothespins and a clothesline to clip 3 × 5 cards with letters on them to the clothesline to spell words, or have a prepared set already clipped to the line and have the child match the letters that are there. *Tg*

---

f. Handwriting

(Case-Smith, 2005, pp. 590–604, 812)

  i. Activities to promote handwriting readiness
  ii. Mature pencil grasps
   a. Dynamic tripod
   b. Lateral tripod
   c. Dynamic quadruped
   d. Lateral quadruped
  iii. Intervention approaches
   I. Neurodevelopmental
   II. Acquisitional
   III. Sensorimotor
   IV. Biomechanical
  iv. Strategies for handwriting problems
  v. Preparatory activities for handwriting
g. Coordination

(Case-Smith, 2005, pp. 322–324, 341–343, 346–347, 903)

  i. Problems affecting fine motor coordination
  ii. Bilateral hand usage
  iii. Forced use
  iv. Basic rehabilitation strategies
h. Feeding

(Case-Smith, 2005, pp. 493–518, 728–730, 733–734, 738–740, 788)

  i. Oral motor function and feeding
  ii. Nippling
   I. Nutritive versus nonnutritive sucking

Table 16.7 Nippling

	Nonnutritive Sucking	Nutritive Sucking
Developmental progression		
Rate		
Pattern		
Stimulus		
Arousal		
Feeding		
Suck/swallow/breathe ratio		
Respiration		
Indicator of neurologic impairment		

        II.   Nippling interventions
              a. Manage environment
              b. Infant level of arousal
              c. Postural stability
              d. Positioning
              e. Prep with oral stimulation
              f. Jaw support
              g. Temperature considerations
              h. Flow rate
              i. Respiratory concerns
              j. Increasing sucking strength
              k. Specialty nipples
              l. Timing of feedings
              m. Thickening foods
       III.   Feeding scenarios with premature infants
   iii. Feeding solids
        I.   Appropriate postural alignment
        II.   Feeding positions and positioning devices

Table 16.8 Feeding Solids

Position	Advantage	Disadvantage
Sideways in caregiver's arms		
On caregiver's thighs facing caregiver		
In an infant seat		
In a cradle bouncer		
Foam-filled feeder seat		
Regular car seat		
Wheelchair		
Beanbag chair		
High chair		

III. Handling techniques
  a. Decreasing hypertonicity
  b. Jaw support
  c. Cheek support
  d. Spoon placement
  e. Head position
  f. Food textures
IV. Swallowing problems
  a. Swallowing initiation
  b. Oral transit
  c. Respiration and swallowing
V. Transitioning to oral feedings
VI. Self-feeding issues
  a. Positioning
    i. Tray usage
  b. Handling during self-feeding
  c. Adaptive equipment
VII. Case studies

37 = full term

Work Sheet 16-10. Feeding Scenario

1. Jacob is a 4-week-old infant born at 34 weeks gestational age. He has a diagnosis of bronchopulmonary dysplasia and is currently on oxygen via a nasal cannula. He was referred to occupational therapy for assistance with his nippling skills. The nurses report that he initiates sucking on the nipple but then quickly stops. He loses a lot of the formula from the oral cavity. What intervention strategies should be considered with Jacob?

2. Jennifer is an 8-week-old infant born at 24 weeks gestational age. She has a cardiac abnormality and demonstrates hypotonia throughout her body. She spends much of her day sleeping in a side lying position. When supported in an upright position she tends to demonstrate an open mouth position. When presented with the bottle she demonstrates weak mouth closure and initiates a suck but doesn't seem to obtain much from the bottle. After about 5 minutes of working on the bottle, she tends to become drowsy and wants to fall back to sleep. What intervention strategies should you consider when working with Jennifer?

3. Antoine is a 6-year-old male with a history of cerebral palsy who has been referred to you for treatment for his feeding difficulties. You observe his parents feeding him and note that they hold him in their lap during feedings. Antoine is noted to push into extensor patterns with his trunk, and his arms go into a high guard position (arms abducted to about 90° with elbows flexed) and his neck goes into extension. He almost lies in his parent's lap during feeding. You worry about aspiration in this position due to the neck extension. How would you instruct his parents to position him?

4. Jessica is a 2-month-old female who is on gastric tube (g-tube) feedings due to aspiration noted on her modified barium swallow. Her parents hope to be able to feed her orally in the future. You are working on a program with the family to help Jessica be able to progress from tube feedings to oral feedings. What might you recommend to the family to help Jessica maintain a suck pattern in preparation for later oral feedings?

5. Angelica is a 4-year-old female with low tone of unknown etiology. She demonstrates low tone throughout her trunk, extremities, and facial area. During feeding she tends to demonstrate an open mouth posture and often loses the bolus from the oral cavity. What things might you do in treatment to help decrease her open mouth posture during spoon feedings?

6. John is a 3-year-old male who is having problems transitioning to drinking from a regular cup. When he attempts to drink from the cup, the liquid spills between the cup and his lips. What enters the oral cavity makes him cough and sputter. What can you do to help John learn to transition to a regular cup?

(continues)

Work Sheet 16-10. Feeding Scenario *(continued)*

7. Elijah is a 5-year-old male who demonstrates poor motor control. With UE reaching activities he often demonstrates over- or underreaching of his target. He frequently uses too much force in activities. His parents report that their major concern for him at this time is his inability to scoop food off of his plate. What could you do to help Elijah improve his ability to complete this task?

8. Tiffany is a 4-year-old female who demonstrates a weak gross grasp and poor grip reflex. She attempts to self-feed with a spoon but often ends up dropping the spoon when attempting to scoop the food onto the spoon, bringing the spoon to her mouth, or both. She is becoming very frustrated with the task overall and often refuses to eat unless her parents feed her. What can you do to help Tiffany complete this task more independently?

[handwritten: 33-36 in for doors 17-19 in toilet)]

   i. Activities of daily living (ADL)

(Case-Smith, 2005, pp. 533–554, 903–904)

      i. General information
- **I.** Questions to help plan treatment
- **II.** General approaches to treatment
  - **a.** Addressing performance
  - **b.** Adaptation
    - **i.** Adapting task method
    - **ii.** Adapting task object
    - **iii.** Adapting context
  - **c.** Prevention and education
  - **d.** Basic rehabilitation strategies

      ii. Improving toileting independence
- **I.** Typical problems
- **II.** Compensatory strategies
  - **a.** Social adaptations
  - **b.** Adaptations to environment
  - **c.** Adaptations to toileting process
  - **d.** Adaptations for posture problems

      iii. Improving independence in dressing
- **I.** Addressing cognition and process skills
- **II.** Addressing physical or motor limitations
- **III.** Addressing difficulties in self-dressing skills

      iv. Improving independence in bathing or showering
- **I.** Restore approach
- **II.** Adaptation approach
- **III.** Prevention and education approach

      v. Improving independence in hygiene and grooming

Work Sheet 16-11. ADL

1. You are working with a child and having him place pennies into a penny bank. What ADL skill could you be addressing with this activity?

    A. Tying shoes
    B. Donning shirt
    C. Buttoning
    D. Zipping

2. You are working with a child and are completing an activity where you have the child sitting on a bench and you have placed five hoops around the child's waist. You are having the child take the hoop from around the waist, up over the head, and then trying to throw the hoop onto a post a few feet in front of him or her. What ADL skill could you be addressing with this activity?

    A. Zipping
    B. Donning a shirt
    C. Doffing a shirt
    D. Buttoning

3. You are working with a child and are having the child play tug-of-war with you to help strengthen his or her grasp. What ADL skill could you be addressing with this activity?

    A. Buttoning
    B. Pulling up pants
    C. Zipping
    D. Brushing hair

4. You are working with a child and are having the child grasp a beanbag animal then put his or her arm through a tube (such as an empty oatmeal container with both ends cut off) and then drop the animal into a basket. What ADL skill could you be addressing with this activity?

    A. Buttoning
    B. Donning a shirt
    C. Zipping
    D. Pulling up pants

5. You are working with a child in treatment and begin by having the child pinch and pull theraputty. You then use a pair of plastic, child-size tweezers to pick up small plastic animals placed at arm's length and then sustain the grasp to place them in a small container near the child's body. What ADL skill could you be addressing with this activity?

    A. Zipping
    B. Donning pants
    C. Buttoning
    D. Tying

6. You are working with Tony, a 7-year-old little boy. In treatment, you are having him play Connect Four, a game where you place checkers in slots and see who is the first to get four in a row of a particular color. What ADL skill could you be addressing with this activity?

    A. Feeding skills
    B. Gross grasp skills
    C. Buttoning skills
    D. Bathing skills

7. You are working with a child with mental retardation, and his parents are concerned because he is not yet toilet trained at 4 years of age. What do you tell his parents?

    A. There are larger diapers available and they should call their durable medical equipment (DME) company to get some because it is not likely that he will be toilet trained.
    B. Many children with mental retardation just take longer to potty train and you can help them with some strategies to progress him along.
    C. They should begin to remodel their bathroom because it is likely that he will not be independent with toileting.
    D. Children with mental retardation have difficulty with sequencing activities, and because toileting requires the appropriate sequencing of several tasks, it is unlikely that the child will be able to be toilet trained.

(continues)

Work Sheet 16-11. ADL *(continued)*

8. The child you are trying to dress continues to go into an asymmetric tonic neck reflex (ATNR) pattern. What would be the *best* thing to tell the parents to do to help make dressing the child easier?

   A. Gently roll the baby toward you so that the baby's head comes into midline and his or her arms relax, making dressing easier.
   B. It will be easier to get the shirt on if you dress the extended arm first and then the flexed arm.
   C. It will be easier if you dress the flexed arm first and then the extended arm because the flexed arm is closer to the head and easier to get in.
   D. It would be best to dress the child in a sitting position because this is how a child at that age would be dressing.

9. Your 5-year-old patient, Luke, has decreased upper extremity strength and decreased hand strength. He is having problems with pulling up his pants after they are put on. Your goal is for him to be independent in donning his pants. What would be the *best* activity to use during treatment?

   A. Placing his leg through a ring
   B. Placing rings over his feet
   C. Playing tug of war
   D. Stepping into a box

10. Jennifer is an 8-year-old female with a history of developmental delay. She has difficulty with putting her clothes on in the appropriate order. Which activity would be the *best* to do with her during treatment?

    A. Play games or sing songs that help to identify body parts.
    B. Use a set of sequencing cards that depict a child completing the different stages of dressing.
    C. Change Jennifer's positioning during dressing, such as having her sit supported in the corner to dress.
    D. Provide wrist loops to make it easier for Jennifer to pull up her clothing.

---

    j. Home programs: A large part of success in pediatric intervention is dependent upon the family's ability to help carry over treatment techniques and functional gains into life outside of the therapy room. A child may be positioned to complete an appropriate movement pattern for the 30 to 90 minutes a week he or she is in therapy, but if this is not reinforced at times in the home environment, that leaves 9,990 to 10,050 minutes a week for the child to work on developing inappropriate movement patterns. Therapists, however, need to be prudent in establishing realistic expectations for home programs. Strict home programs that add another task to the already stressful day of the family of a child with an injury or disability are likely not going to be successful. Home program activities need to be embedded in and around the normal daily activities of the family. Appropriate involvement of the families in the therapy goals, good communication with caregivers on a regular basis, and clear, concise, verbal, written, and/or illustrated instructions on ways to help the family integrate therapeutic techniques into everyday activities are all paramount to successful intervention.

(Case-Smith, 2005, pp. 139–145)

        i. Establishing a partnership
        ii. Cultural considerations
        iii. Communication strategies
        iv. Home program considerations

    k. Managing behavior in therapy situations: When encountering behavior difficulties with a patient in the pediatric population, especially in a very young child, the therapist should be asking, What is this child trying to tell me? Children may demonstrate behavioral difficulties for several reasons, including being requested to do an activity that is too difficult, perceiving the activity to be too easy, and/or having a sensory processing disorder that is interfering with their ability to function in the given situation. Identifying the stimulus that resulted in the given behavior will provide the key to managing the behavior during the treatment session.

(Case-Smith, 2005, pp. 473–475, 900–901)

    i.   Intervention in children with social performance problems
   ii.   Rational intervention
  iii.   Behavioral management with TBI

REFERENCES

Case-Smith, J. (Ed.). (2005). *Occupational therapy for children* (5th ed.). St. Louis, MO: Mosby.

Crepeau, E. B., Cohn, E. S., & Schell, B. A. B. (Eds.). (2009). *Willard & Spackman's occupational therapy* (11th ed.). Philadelphia: Lippincott Williams & Wilkins.

Pendleton, H. M., & Schultz-Krohn, W. (Eds.). (2006). *Pedretti's occupational therapy: Practice skills for physical dysfunction* (6th ed.). St. Louis, MO: Mosby.

Radomski, M. V., & Latham, C. A. T. (Eds.). (2008). *Occupational therapy for physical dysfunction* (6th ed.). Philadelphia: Lippincott Williams & Wilkins.

WORK SHEET ANSWERS

Work Sheet 16-1. Settings

Define which specialized pediatric setting would be most appropriate for intervention services for the patients in the following case scenarios. Choose from the following possible intervention settings:

A. Early intervention
B. School based
C. Hospital-based acute
D. Hospital-based outpatient

Case One: Alonzo is a child with Down syndrome who has an active IFSP. Where would Alonzo most likely receive services? **Correct Answer: A.** An IFSP or individualized family service plan is a result of the evaluation completed on an at-risk child that has been referred to early intervention. It is an outline of the family's services and who is providing them.

Case Two: Jennifer is a 3-year-old with spastic diplegia whose family is concerned about her development. Her upper extremity tone and strength is within normal limits. Who would be most appropriate to provide consultative services? **Correct Answer: A.** Jennifer is age 3 years or younger and at risk for developmental delay. She does not currently demonstrate significant tonal involvement that is greatly impacting her function. She would be best served in the least restrictive environment of early intervention services provided in the home or consultative group setting.

Case Three: Jonathan is an 8-year-old boy who is demonstrating handwriting difficulties and fine motor delays that are interfering with his ability to produce written work at a pace equal to his peers. He may benefit from assistive technology. Where would he most likely be referred for an evaluation for occupational therapy services? **Correct Answer: B.** He is school aged, and his delay has a direct impact on his educational performance.

Case Four: Tyrone is a 10-year-old boy status postfracture to his radius and is having difficulty with writing postsurgery. Where would he most likely be referred for evaluation for occupational therapy services? **Correct Answer: D.** Although his difficulty is with writing and may impact his educational performance, it is due to a temporary impairment. School-based therapy services are not provided when a student has a temporary impairment. Rehabilitation is more appropriately addressed in the outpatient therapy setting.

(continues)

Work Sheet 16-1. Settings *(continued)*

Case Five: Julie is a 6-year-old female with left hemiparesis due to a stroke. She demonstrates significant range and strength limitations and increased tone in her left hand. She is able to self-ambulate around the school environment. She uses classroom tools appropriately. Where would she most likely receive therapy services? **Correct Answer: D.** Although she demonstrates significant impairment with the left upper extremity, she is independent in her educational setting and would not qualify for school services.

Case Six: Natasha is a 5-year-old with a history of a brain tumor whose parents are concerned about her IEP. She has endurance and coordination issues. She frequently drops objects and has difficulty with her dressing and feeding skills. Which setting would help the parents address these issues? **Correct Answer: B.** The parent's issue is with the IEP. An IEP is an individualized education plan and is developed in the school system to address the child's present level of performance and how his or her disability impacts the child's function in the school environment and participation in the curriculum.

Case Seven: Michael is a 13-year-old male who is status post-involvement in a motor vehicle accident in which he sustained a concussion and a fractured femur. Michael and his parents are concerned about him being able to dress his lower extremities due to his external fixator and about him being able to carry his books at school. Where would Michael most likely be referred to help his family address their concerns? **Correct Answer: C.** In the acute setting patients are frequently referred to occupational therapy services just prior to discharge. The therapist and family identifies strengths and weaknesses in the discharge environment and develops an intervention plan.

Work Sheet 16-2. Developmental Positions #1

Developmental positions are frequently used in intervention with the pediatric population to help develop desired strength, proximal stability, and skill. Match the developmental position with the skills it helps to facilitate.

Table 16-9 Developmental Positions #1 Answer Key

A. Supine	**F**	Facilitates the development of head control, muscles of the trunk, back and hips, and balance.
B. Prone	**A**	Encourages hands to reach and engage and encourages midline activities. Facilitates development of stomach muscles through body flexion in older infants. Facilitates extension in premature infants. Easy visual attention.
C. Side lying	**E**	Develops muscles of the trunk, back, and hips. Strengthens muscles of the arm. Allows the child to accept body weight to one side.
D. Prone on elbows	**B**	Facilitates head control and helps develop muscles of the shoulders, arms, back, and hips. Facilitates hand-to-mouth activities. Facilitates development of flexor tone in premature infants.
E. Side sitting	**C**	Facilitates hands together and makes it easier to touch or hold a toy. Facilitates hand and head at midline. Relaxes the child and requires less effort to move the body. Encourages extremity flexion and adduction. Develops the rib cage. Encourages rolling when reaching for toys.
F. Ring sitting	**G**	Helps develop muscle control and strength in the shoulders, arms, hips, legs, and back. Helps to facilitate balance with weight shifting.
G. Four point, quadruped	**D**	Facilitates the development of muscles of the shoulders, arms, and back; head control; and the ability to weight shift when reaching.

Work Sheet 16-3. Developmental Positions #2

List the advantages and disadvantages of each developmental position.

Table 16-10 Developmental Positions #2 Answer Key

	Advantages	Disadvantages
Supine	• Recommended position to reduce SIDS • Easy visual exploration • Can help facilitate abdominal muscles in older infants	• Can encourage extensor posturing • May provide too much support and not challenge patient enough • In low tone and weak patients, encourages external rotation positional deformities of arms and legs so need outside positioning assists to decrease this deformity • Greater risk of aspiration than in prone or side lying
Prone	• Facilitates head control • Helps develop muscles of the shoulders, arms, back, and hips • Facilitates development of flexor tone in premature infants • Improves oxygenation and ventilation in premature infants • Reduces reflux, especially if head of surface elevated 30° • Can help reduce hip flexion contractures	• Associated with increased risk of SIDS in infants • Can cause flattened, frog leg positioning if not appropriately positioned • Infants with weak and low tone may not have enough strength to clear airway • Makes visual exploration more difficult • Less face-to-face contact with caregivers
Side lying	• Right side lying can improve gastric emptying • Encourages midline orientation of head and extremities • Allows gravity eliminated positioning of UE so can increase use in weak and low tone patients • Facilitates hand-to-mouth • Facilitates hand-to-hand activity • When positioned appropriately can help decrease a patient's extensor patterning because requires less effort to move	• May be difficult to maintain position of a patient with increased extensor patterning • Left side lying can decrease gastric emptying time

(continues)

Work Sheet 16-3. Developmental Positions #2 *(continued)*

List the advantages and disadvantages of each developmental position.

Table 16-10 Developmental Positions #2 Answer Key

	Advantages	Disadvantages
Sitting	• Facilitates balance • Good alerting posture • Good visual exploration • Encourages social interaction	• May be too difficult for patients with abnormal tone and/or weakness because may have too much difficulty working against gravity • Can cause increased neck flexion and difficulty breathing in patients with poor head control
Standing	• Frees UE for prehension and manipulation • Facilitates higher level neurological integration	• Need good trunk stability or much outside support to facilitate this position

Refer to Case-Smith, 2005, pp. 718–726, 767–769 and Pendleton & Schultz-Krohn, 2006, pp. 740–742 for a full list of advantages and disadvantages to each position.

Work Sheet 16-4. Tone Questions

1. Pick the statement that best describes normal postural tone.

   A. It must be high enough to withstand gravity.
   B. It provides the background on which movement is based.
   C. Easy movement is only available if postural tone is low enough to allow it to happen.
   D. All of the above

   Correct Answer: D.

2. Which statement is *not* true about muscle tone?

   A. Tone is highly influenced by gravity.
   B. Your emotional state can influence your muscle tone.
   C. Muscle tone allows movement against an outside source.
   D. Tone allows smooth, coordinated movements.

   Correct Answer: C. This is the definition of strength. Tone and strength are not the same. Tone is the amount of resistance felt in the muscle during passive movement.

3. If the child you are treating has increased tone in the flexor muscles of the arm resulting in severe elbow flexion, you would expect that:

   A. The extensor muscles are also tight.
   B. The extensor muscles are overstretched and weak.
   C. The extensor muscles have not been affected because they are innervated differently.
   D. All of the above

   Correct Answer: B. Tightness and shortening in the agonist muscle almost always produces weakness and overstretching of the antagonist muscle. Care must be given in treatment to address the tightness, weakness, and shortening of the agonist as well as the lengthening and weakness of the antagonist muscle to provide appropriate biomechanical alignment of the joint and improve functioning.

(continues)

Work Sheet 16-4. Tone Questions *(continued)*

4. You are working with a 4-year-old male who has increased tone in the muscles of his upper arm. This tone is noted to increase with participation in all functional activities. Which technique would be the best idea to help decrease the tone?

   A. Tap the muscle belly to inhibit or deactivate the muscle.
   B. Use quick stroking movements along the muscle with the muscle on stretch.
   C. Cast the arm for stretch and neutral warmth.
   D. Provide slow, firm massage strokes with stretch.

   Correct Answer: C. Tapping and quick stroking are both facilitory and would increase tone. Slow, firm massage strokes can help decrease tone but are more temporary in nature. Casting the arm would provide a prolonged stretch and more long-lasting impact to the tone of the arm.

5. Evan is a 3-year-old male with a history of cerebral palsy. He has significantly increased tone in his right upper extremity. He is holding his right upper extremity in elbow and wrist flexion. You know that his increased tone is interfering with his ability to participate in occupations. During treatment the best thing you could do would be which of the following?

   A. Place the child in supported sitting and slowly stretch and move his right upper extremity through full range.
   B. During home program instruction encourage the parents to hand him things to his left upper extremity.
   C. Position him in right side sitting with support at his elbow and have him shoot baskets with his left hand.
   D. Provide vibration to the right upper extremity.

   Correct Answer: C. Vibration is facilitory and would increase tone. Handing the patient items in the left UE would not help to address the child's increased tone in his or her right UE and would encourage decreased use of the right UE. Weight bearing through right side sitting while facilitating use of the left UE is the best way to inhibit the tone in the right UE.

6. You are working with the family of a 5-year-old child with cerebral palsy who has increased extensor tone. The family has difficulty getting this patient from supine to sitting after completing his diaper changes. Which of the following statements best describes how you would teach the parents to bring their child from the supine to the sitting position?

   A. Tell them to place their hand behind his head and slowly push him up into a sitting position because hip flexion helps to break up tone.
   B. Tell them it would be easiest to hold him by his hands and slowly pull him into a sitting position.
   C. Tell them to hold his upper arms and gently lift and turn the shoulders to rotate the trunk slightly and then come up.
   D. Tell them to flex his legs and knees so they face up in the air and use your body to hold his legs in this position; then, holding his upper arms near the shoulders, gently lift his shoulders up and toward you as you use your body to push his legs back so that he ends up in a sitting position.

   Correct Answer: C. Using rotation of the trunk and bringing him into flexion will help to decrease his extensor tone and mimics the natural progress of coming from supine into sitting. Placing your hand behind the head of someone with extension patterns usually encourages them to push into extension. Pulling the patient into sitting does not encourage active use of the abdominals through normal patterns. Option D does not facilitate the patient to be active in any way, it would be very difficult with a 5-year-old, and it would become more difficult as the child grows.

(continues)

Work Sheet 16-4. Tone Questions *(continued)*

7. Alex is a 4-year-old male with a history of hypotonia. He sits with a forward posture with his ribs resting on his hip bones. He can use his upper extremities in activities within his base of support and below his center of gravity but without crossing midline. The best activity to improve the overall tone and help increase his trunk stability to free his upper extremities for improved use would be which of the following?

A. Position him in sitting on a platform swing and have him throw beanbags into a basket while slowly swinging in wide, full circles.

B. Position him in sitting on a therapy ball and support him on the lateral sides of his trunk to facilitate appropriate trunk alignment and provide firm, quick pressure into the ball; then have him shoot beanbags into a basket that is above his head and off to the left.

C. Position him in sitting on a therapy ball and support him on the lateral sides of his trunk to facilitate appropriate trunk alignment and provide firm, quick pressure into the ball; then have him place beanbags into a basket that is at his shoulder height and in front of him.

D. Have him shoot baskets at shoulder level while he is sitting stable on the ground in tailor sitting and you are providing slow stroking to his extensor and abdominal muscles to increase his trunk stability.

Correct Answer: C. You want to encourage increased trunk tone to provide increased stability for reaching against gravity. Slow swinging in circles in unsupported sitting on the swing would not help to address his decreased tone and trunk stability. Having him reach overhead and off to the side is too much of a challenge at this time given his inability to reach above his center of gravity. Providing slow stroking and keeping him on a static surface would not help to increase his tone and stability.

Work Sheet 16-5. Sensory Integration #1

Match the sensory modulation disorder with the appropriate description.

Table 16-11 Sensory Integration #1 Answer Key

	Answer	Description
A. Gravitational insecurity	B	Patient reacts defensively to ordinary sensory input. Often demonstrates activation of sympathetic nervous system.
B. Hyperresponsivity	F	Disorder used interchangeably with hyperresponsivity.
C. Hyporesponsivity	G	Disorder used interchangeably with hyporesponsivity.
D. Sensory seeking	E	Patient tends to react negatively to clothing, dislikes having shoes off, and has tendency to weight bear on fingertips rather than palms.
E. Tactile defensiveness	D	Patient searches out specific sensory input at higher frequency and/or intensity.
F. Overresponsiveness	A	Patient reacts negatively to movement, especially when head is moving backward.
G. Underresponsiveness	C	Patient tends to ignore sensory stimuli that would be responded to by most individuals.

Work Sheet 16-6. Sensory Integration #2

Listed below are several treatment strategies that could be used in addressing disorders of sensory integration. Match the treatment strategy with the primary type of sensory integration disorder that it could be used to address the following:

TD = Tactile defensiveness

TDD = Tactile discrimination disorders

PPD = Poor proprioceptive discrimination

GI = Gravitational insecurity

PBI = Poor bilateral integration

Table 16-12 Sensory Integration #2 Answer Key

Sensory Integration Disorder	Possible Treatment Strategy
TD	Begin with vestibular and proprioceptive input, continue with deep pressure and end with touch if tolerated.
GI	Respect the child's fears, do not force movement.
PBI	On swing in prone and propelling self with hands on floor.
PPD	Play tug-of-war games.
GI	Start with anterior–posterior trunk movements; progress to lateral and then rotational.
TD	Avoid light touch.
PPD	Use blow toys and resistive chewing activities.
TD	Respect child's personal space, do not impose.
PBI	Catching a ball.
TD	Reduce sensory overload in the environment, lower voice, use natural light, work in small spaces.
PPD	Have patient push and pull bolsters, wedges, mats, etc. to help set up obstacle courses/treatment area.
TDD	Place small stickers of various sizes on child's arms, legs, and feet and have the child find them with eyes open and with eyes closed.
GI	Work with child near the ground, maintain feet on floor.
PBI (also PPD but using alternating hands also addresses bilateral integration)	Pulling hand over hand on rope.
PPD	Have child push a toy grocery cart with weights in it to go shopping for toys.
GI	Use swings attached to two suspension points to gain more linear movement.
TDD	Have the child dip his or her finger in shaving cream and then write letters on his or her arm/hand and your arm/hand.

Note: PPD activities can also be used to provide basis for GI, TD, and TDD activities because proprioception also helps to modulate tactile and vestibular input.

Work Sheet 16-7. Sensory Integration #3

Listed below are some statements that a parent might make during your treatment session to describe their child's behavior in the home and community environment. Next to each statement place the initials of the most appropriate type of sensory integrative disorder this type of statement might describe.

TD = Tactile defensiveness

TDD = Tactile discrimination disorders

PPD = Poor proprioceptive discrimination

GI = Gravitational insecurity

PBI = Poor bilateral integration

Answers are bold.

___TDD___ Jeffrey is constantly touching everything. I can't take him to a store with delicate items because I am afraid he will want to touch everything and end up breaking something. **Children with tactile discrimination disorders are hyporesponsive to touch and tend to seek out many touch experiences.**

___TD___ Johnny cries and becomes upset every time he is put in the bathtub. After he is there for a while he calms down but then gets upset when he is taken out again. **He doesn't tolerate the temperature change.**

___PBI___ Theresa's teacher told me that she is having a very difficult time with learning how to cut with scissors. She said that she doesn't seem to be able to get the hand holding the paper and the hand holding the scissors to work together. **Children with poor bilateral coordination skills have difficulty using their two hands together in a coordinated manner, especially when each hand is doing a different task.**

___TDD___ The other day Tony was trying to put a dime in the gum ball machine at the grocery store, and he must have dropped that dime 10 times before I finally helped him put the dime in the slot. **Children with tactile discrimination disorders tend to have difficulty with tasks that require in-hand manipulation skills. Due to their hyporesponsiveness to touch they tend to not be aware of where objects are in their hands.**

___GI___ I have become very good at changing Jerry's diaper while he is standing up because every time I try to lie him down to change his diaper he cries. **Children with gravitational insecurity dislike being moved backwards in space.**

___PPD___ Jenny complained that her teacher always puts her at the end of the line in school. When I asked the teacher about this, she said that she does this because when Jenny is between other students in line she tends to bump into the other kids or stand really close to them, and this upsets the other children. **Children with poor proprioceptive discrimination tend to seek out proprioceptive experiences and will often bump into other children, doorways, desks, etc.**

___TD___ If someone lightly bumps into or touches Katie, she hits herself wherever she was touched, and she hits herself pretty hard. **Katie is using deep touch to help modulate her tactile defensiveness.**

___GI___ Luke prefers to sit and play by himself. If you take him to the playground, all the other kids will be running, climbing, and playing, but Luke will stay on the sidelines, mostly just standing and watching. **Children with gravitational insecurity tend to avoid any activities that take their feet off the ground. They are fearful of movement, avoid activities that challenge balance, and often move very carefully.**

___PPD___ Shelly is very hard on her toys. I just bought her a new doll the other day and she already broke the arm off the poor doll. **Children with poor proprioceptive discrimination tend to be very poor at grading the amount of force that they use in tasks.**

___TD___ Keisha is very happy when I hold her, but when her grandma tries to touch or hold her she becomes very upset. **Children with tactile defensiveness tend to be very particular about who they allow to handle them. They learn to accommodate to their primary caregiver's touch but do not adjust well to the touch of other people. It is likely that her mother has learned to handle Keisha with a firmer, more consistent touch.**

Work Sheet 16-8. Facilitating In-Hand Manipulation

Intervention for enhancing a child's in-hand manipulation skills needs to be embedded into everyday play activities. Match the treatment activity with the type of in-hand manipulation skill it would help to facilitate. After identifying the skill, place an "S" next to the ones that would be completed with stabilization.

In-hand manipulation skills:

A. Shift
B. Translation (fingers to palm)
C. Translation (palm to fingers)
D. Rotation (may be simple or complex depending on object's orientation)

Treatment Activity:

Table 16-13 Facilitating In-Hand Manipulation

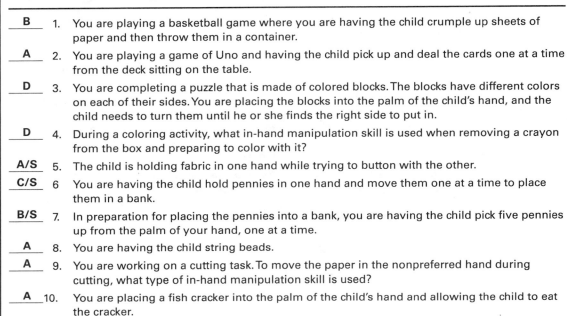

B	1.	You are playing a basketball game where you are having the child crumple up sheets of paper and then throw them in a container.
A	2.	You are playing a game of Uno and having the child pick up and deal the cards one at a time from the deck sitting on the table.
D	3.	You are completing a puzzle that is made of colored blocks. The blocks have different colors on each of their sides. You are placing the blocks into the palm of the child's hand, and the child needs to turn them until he or she finds the right side to put in.
D	4.	During a coloring activity, what in-hand manipulation skill is used when removing a crayon from the box and preparing to color with it?
A/S	5.	The child is holding fabric in one hand while trying to button with the other.
C/S	6	You are having the child hold pennies in one hand and move them one at a time to place them in a bank.
B/S	7.	In preparation for placing the pennies into a bank, you are having the child pick five pennies up from the palm of your hand, one at a time.
A	8.	You are having the child string beads.
A	9.	You are working on a cutting task. To move the paper in the nonpreferred hand during cutting, what type of in-hand manipulation skill is used?
A	10.	You are placing a fish cracker into the palm of the child's hand and allowing the child to eat the cracker.

Work Sheet 16-9. Handwriting

Each of the following activities can be completed to help improve the handwriting skills of your patients/students. For each activity listed, identify what portion of the handwriting process that activity can help to address (e.g., strengthening, posture, visual motor, manipulation, tripod grasp, letter forming, spacing).

1. Present the child with theraputty, Play-Doh, or clay that has small beads or objects hidden inside. Have the child remove all of the objects and then replace them for the next child to find.

   Answer: This activity helps to improve finger strength and manipulation skills. It provides increased proprioceptive awareness to the hand and fingers, and through improved proprioception, the activity can help the child learn to better grade the force used in writing.

2. Practice dot-to-dot pictures and letters.

   Answer: This activity helps with visual–motor and eye–hand control and helps to improve the ability to form letters.

3. Have a child help you set up an obstacle course in the gym. Have the child practice moving through the obstacle course from front to back and back to front, timed and untimed.

   Answer: This activity helps to increase shoulder, arm, hand, and trunk strength. It provides increased proprioceptive input. It helps with directionality concepts and motor planning skills.

4. Build with magnet toys or small LEGOs.

   Answer: This activity helps to increase finger and hand strength. It assists with visual–motor and eye–hand coordination. It helps to improve manipulation skills. It increases proprioceptive input, which can help with grading of force in writing tasks. It can also help to improve strength and movement of the fingers for tripod grasp. It also improves with the concept of coordinating two hands, with one hand stabilizing while the other hand works.

5. Complete a board game in prone on elbows.

   Answer: This activity helps to improve shoulder strength, arm strength, and trunk strength. Proprioception to forearm and shoulders is provided. It can help to improve overall proximal stability and impact sitting posture during writing.

6. Use putty or clay to create letters and words.

   Answer: This activity helps to improve motor planning and perceptual skills. It helps to improve manipulation skills and increases proprioceptive input to the fingers.

7. Have the child place pennies in a horizontal slot then move it to be vertical.

   Answer: This activity works to improve in-hand manipulation. Having the child hold multiple pennies in the hand while completing the activity works on using the ulnar side of the hand for stabilization while having movement on the radial side, which is what is done during writing. Changing the slot from horizontal to vertical increases wrist rotation and movement.

8. Draw two lines across a sheet of paper then trace them with glue and let them dry. Have the child practice writing words and letters on this paper.

   Answer: The glue drying on the sheet produces raised lines that help to provide input during writing. It provides cues to the child to help with spacing and alignment of letters.

9. Have the child prone over a therapy ball and extend up to draw on a mirror with shaving cream.

   Answer: This activity helps to increase strength in the back and upper trunk. It helps to work on sustained neck and trunk extension to help improve posture during writing tasks. Drawing in the shaving cream helps to increase input to the fingers to improve awareness to assist with in-hand manipulation skills.

10. Use clothespins and a clothesline to clip 3 × 5 cards with letters on them to the clothesline to spell words, or have a prepared set already clipped to the line and have the child match the letters that are there.

    Answer: This activity helps with letter identification. Using clothespins helps to increase finger strength, and helps to encourage an open thumb and web space, which is used in the tripod grasp. It also increases proprioceptive awareness to help with force during writing activities. Holding the card while working the clothespin helps with the concept of coordinating and stabilizing with one hand while working with the other hand.

Work Sheet 16-10. Feeding Scenario

Answers are bold.

1. Jacob is a 4-week-old infant born at 34 weeks gestational age. He has a diagnosis of bronchopulmonary dysplasia and is currently on oxygen via a nasal cannula. He was referred to occupational therapy for assistance with his nippling skills. The nurses report that he initiates sucking on the nipple but then quickly stops. He loses a lot of the formula from the oral cavity. What intervention strategies should be considered with Jacob?

   Answer: Consider changing to the Haberman nipple or thickening the formula to decrease the formula flow rate. If Jacob starts out sucking then stops, he is likely becoming disorganized by the formula entering the oral cavity. By slowing the formula down you can decrease the amount that is obtained per suck and can increase Jacob's ability to coordinate his suck/swallow/breathe pattern. Holding Jacob in a more upright position will also help to decrease the impact that gravity has on pulling the formula to the back of the mouth and increase the baby's time to coordinate his oral movements. You might also discuss with the physician increasing Jacob's oxygen slightly during the feeding process. This can help to increase coordination as well.

2. Jennifer is an 8-week-old infant born at 24 weeks gestational age. She has a cardiac abnormality and demonstrates hypotonia throughout her body. She spends much of her day sleeping in a side lying position. When supported in an upright position she tends to demonstrate an open mouth position. When presented with the bottle she demonstrates weak mouth closure and initiates a suck but doesn't seem to obtain much from the bottle. After about 5 minutes of working on the bottle, she tends to become drowsy and wants to fall back to sleep. What intervention strategies should you consider when working with Jennifer?

   Answer: Jennifer has low tone that is impacting her proximal stability and the strength of her mouth movements, resulting in poor nippling skills. Several things should be considered with Jennifer. Bundling could be tried to help improve her stability. Holding her in a semiupright side-lying position will also provide her with more stability and decrease the impact of gravity pulling her mouth open. Using a soft nipple will help decrease the strength of suck required. Providing firm, steady jaw support will help to increase the stability of her oral musculature. Chilling the nipple and/or formula will also help to increase alertness and the swallowing reflex.

3. Antoine is a 6-year-old male with a history of cerebral palsy who has been referred to you for treatment for his feeding difficulties. You observe his parents feeding him and note that they hold him in their lap during feedings. Antoine is noted to push into extensor patterns with his trunk, and his arms go into a high guard position (arms abducted to about 90° with elbows flexed) and his neck goes into extension. He almost lies in his parent's lap during feeding. You worry about aspiration in this position due to the neck extension. How would you instruct his parents to position him?

   Answer: Antoine needs to be positioned with more hip and knee flexion to help break up his extensor patterning. Although his parents might be able to hold him in their lap in more hip/knee flexion, it is unlikely that they will be able to feed him and manage his tone at the same time. It is also not age appropriate for Antoine to be held in his parent's lap for feeding. Antoine should be positioned in his wheelchair or a specialized feeding chair to facilitate hip and knee flexion and help break up his extensor patterning.

4. Jessica is a 2-month-old female who is on gastric tube (g-tube) feedings due to aspiration noted on her modified barium swallow. Her parents hope to be able to feed her orally in the future. You are working on a program with the family to help Jessica be able to progress from tube feedings to oral feedings. What might you recommend to the family to help Jessica maintain a suck pattern in preparation for later oral feedings?

   Answer: It is a good idea to recommend that the family provides Jessica with a pacifier each time she is receiving a tube feeding. This helps to keep her sucking pattern strong (albeit nonnutritive) and helps her associate the sucking process with becoming full. You might also recommend that they wipe Jessica's face before and after each tube feeding. Children with oral feedings receive much input to the facial area, with food getting on their face during the feeding process and having their faces wiped during and after the feeding process. Children with tube feedings do not have the problem of food getting on their face during meals and therefore often have a decrease of sensory input to the facial area.

(continues)

Work Sheet 16-10. Feeding Scenario *(continued)*

5. Angelica is a 4-year-old female with low tone of unknown etiology. She demonstrates low tone throughout her trunk, extremities, and facial area. During feeding she tends to demonstrate an open mouth posture and often loses the bolus from the oral cavity. What things might you do in treatment to help decrease her open mouth posture during spoon feedings?

Answer: Jessica demonstrates poor jaw control. It would be a good idea to use a three-point jaw support technique or support with your index or middle finger under her jaw and your thumb resting under her lower lip to provide improved lip closure (illustrated in Case-Smith, 2005, p. 501, Figure 14-6). You should also be sure that Angelica is positioned well with good support being provided. You might try reclining her slightly so that there isn't as much of a pull of gravity downward on her jaw. Be sure to keep her head in alignment with her body and her chin tucked.

6. John is a 3-year-old male who is having problems transitioning to drinking from a regular cup. When he attempts to drink from the cup, the liquid spills between the cup and his lips. What enters the oral cavity makes him cough and sputter. What can you do to help John learn to transition to a regular cup?

Answer: Have John's parents use a thickening agent to thicken the liquid they are presenting him in the cup. The slower movement of the liquid will give him more time to coordinate his arm movements and lip and tongue movements in presenting the liquid to the oral cavity. The thickened liquid will move more slowly, allowing John to prepare for the entrance of the liquid into his mouth. The thickened liquid is heavier and provides more input to the lips and tongue during movement. It also is more adhesive and maintains more of a bolus formation, rather than the thin liquid that flows quickly and easily.

7. Elijah is a 5-year-old male who demonstrates poor motor control. With UE reaching activities he often demonstrates over- or underreaching of his target. He frequently uses too much force in activities. His parents report that their major concern for him at this time is his inability to scoop food off of his plate. What could you do to help Elijah improve his ability to complete this task?

Answer: Try using Dycem or another nonslip product under Elijah's dish to keep it from moving during his attempts to get the food off the plate. Use a scoop bowl to provide a good edge to scoop the food against and to give Elijah a clue as to when to try to change the force used in the task. You might try placing some light cuff weights on Elijah's wrists to give him more input and help dampen his excess movement patterns and/or try using a weighted utensil.

8. Tiffany is a 4-year-old female who demonstrates a weak gross grasp and poor grip reflex. She attempts to self-feed with a spoon but often ends up dropping the spoon when attempting to scoop the food onto the spoon, bringing the spoon to her mouth, or both. She is becoming very frustrated with the task overall and often refuses to eat unless her parents feed her. What can you do to help Tiffany complete this task more independently?

Answer: Try presenting Tiffany with a spoon that has a built-up handle. There are also many commercially available plastic molded children's spoons that are lighter and have adaptive handles where the child can slide his or her hand through, so a portion of the handle is in the palm and a portion goes around the dorsum of the hand. If needed, the bottom portion of this handle can also be built up to accommodate decreased grasping skills.

Work Sheet 16-11. ADL

1. You are working with a child and having him place pennies into a penny bank. What ADL skill could you be addressing with this activity?

   A. Tying shoes
   B. Donning shirt
   C. Buttoning
   D. Zipping

   Correct Answer: C. This activity works on the in-hand manipulation skills needed to manage the button through shifting and translating it in the hand and then on placing the button (penny) into the buttonhole (slot of the penny bank).

2. You are working with a child and are completing an activity where you have the child sitting on a bench and you have placed five hoops around the child's waist. You are having the child take the hoop from around the waist, up over the head, and then trying to throw the hoop onto a post a few feet in front of him or her. What ADL skill could you be addressing with this activity?

   A. Zipping
   B. Donning a shirt
   C. Doffing a shirt
   D. Buttoning

   Correct Answer: C. Because of going from the child's waist to overhead, you are working on taking the shirt off, but you could also address donning if, after completing the preceding task, you have the child put the hoops back over the head and around the waist after you take them off the post.

3. You are working with a child and are having the child play tug-of-war with you to help strengthen his or her grasp. What ADL skill could you be addressing with this activity?

   A. Buttoning
   B. Pulling up pants
   C. Zipping
   D. Brushing hair

   Correct Answer: B. Zipping and buttoning require more pinch strength than gross grasp strength, which is truly what is addressed in tug-of-war. Brushing hair requires sustained grasp on the brush but not as much active grasp against resistance as is required in pulling up your pants.

4. You are working with a child and are having the child grasp a beanbag animal then put his or her arm through a tube (such as an empty oatmeal container with both ends cut off) and then drop the animal into a basket. What ADL skill could you be addressing with this activity?

   A. Buttoning
   B. Donning a shirt
   C. Zipping
   D. Pulling up pants

   Correct Answer: B. This activity simulates putting an arm through a sleeve.

5. You are working with a child in treatment and begin by having the child pinch and pull theraputty. You then use a pair of plastic, child-size tweezers to pick up small plastic animals placed at arm's length and then sustain the grasp to place them in a small container near the child's body. What ADL skill could you be addressing with this activity?

   A. Zipping
   B. Donning pants
   C. Buttoning
   D. Tying

   Correct Answer: A. This activity addresses sustained pinch strength and mimics arm moving during sustained pinch.

(continues)

Work Sheet 16-11. ADL *(continued)*

6. You are working with Tony, a 7-year-old little boy. In treatment, you are having him play Connect Four, a game where you place checkers in slots and see who is the first to get four in a row of a particular color. What ADL skill could you be addressing with this activity?

 A. Feeding skills
 B. Gross grasp skills
 C. Buttoning skills
 D. Bathing skills

 Correct Answer: C. This works on a portion of buttoning, which is placing an object (button) into a slot (buttonhole).

7. You are working with a child with mental retardation, and his parents are concerned because he is not yet toilet trained at 4 years of age. What do you tell his parents?

 A. There are larger diapers available and they should call their durable medical equipment (DME) company to get some because it is not likely that he will be toilet trained.
 B. Many children with mental retardation just take longer to potty train and you can help them with some strategies to progress him along.
 C. They should begin to remodel their bathroom because it is likely that he will not be independent with toileting.
 D. Children with mental retardation have difficulty with sequencing activities, and because toileting requires the appropriate sequencing of several tasks, it is unlikely that the child will be able to be toilet trained.

 Correct Answer: B. Although the other statements might be true to a point and/or could be used appropriately during some point of treatment, the first place to start is evaluating the child and helping the parents address strategies to address the issues the child is having with developing independence in toileting.

8. The child you are trying to dress continues to go into an asymmetric tonic neck reflex (ATNR) pattern. What would be the *best* thing to tell the parents to do to help make dressing the child easier?

 A. Gently roll the baby toward you so that the baby's head comes into midline and his or her arms relax, making dressing easier.
 B. It will be easier to get the shirt on if you dress the extended arm first and then the flexed arm.
 C. It will be easier if you dress the flexed arm first and then the extended arm because the flexed arm is closer to the head and easier to get in.
 D. It would be best to dress the child in a sitting position because this is how a child at that age would be dressing.

 Correct Answer: A. Although B is true, it would be better to help inhibit the ATNR pattern by bringing the baby's head into midline through rolling him or her into side lying.

9. Your 5-year-old patient, Luke, has decreased upper extremity strength and decreased hand strength. He is having problems with pulling up his pants after they are put on. Your goal is for him to be independent in donning his pants. What would be the *best* activity to use during treatment?

 A. Placing his leg through a ring
 B. Placing rings over his feet
 C. Playing tug of war
 D. Stepping into a box

 Correct Answer: C. You are specifically addressing Luke pulling up his pants after they are on. The other activities help in getting his legs in the pants.

10. Jennifer is an 8-year-old female with a history of developmental delay. She has difficulty with putting her clothes on in the appropriate order. Which activity would be the *best* to do with her during treatment?

 A. Play games or sing songs that help to identify body parts.
 B. Use a set of sequencing cards that depict a child completing the different stages of dressing.
 C. Change Jennifer's positioning during dressing, such as having her sit supported in the corner to dress.
 D. Provide wrist loops to make it easier for Jennifer to pull up her clothing.

 Correct Answer: B. Although the other activities can be used to help with dressing, using sequencing cards is the best activity to help Jennifer put her clothes on in order.

Family-Centered Pediatrics in Occupational Therapy

CHAPTER 17

Susan Ann Talley

OBJECTIVES

1. Describe how the types of clinical reasoning affect the role of the occupational therapist when working with families of children with disabilities.
2. Apply the International Classification of Functioning, Disability and Health (ICF) to the role of the occupational therapist with families of children with disabilities.
3. Explain how families are affected when raising a child with a disability.
4. Apply educational strategies to assist families to make environmental modifications and promote activities to improve participation of children with disabilities and their families in appropriate occupational roles.
5. Describe how cross-cultural competence can facilitate interactions and implementation of interventions for families of children with disabilities.
6. Compare and contrast the response of families when a child is born with, or acquires an impairment of, body structure and function leading to a disability.
7. Describe and apply the roles of an occupational therapist when working with families of children with disabilities.
8. Identify and apply strategies useful to facilitate family-therapist collaboration in the implementation of treatment interventions for a child.

KEY TERMS

International Classification of Functioning, Disability and Health, http://www.who.int/classifications/icf/en/

Table 17-1 Key Terms

Case-Smith, 2005, pp. 7–8	Crepeau, Cohn, & Schell, 2009
Clinical reasoning	Caregiver occupations, pp. 15–21
Cultural competence	Clinical reasoning, p. 314
Cultural contexts	Cultural competence, pp. 55–57, 580–581
Family adaptation	Cultural contexts, pp. 55–67

(continues)

Table 17-1 Key Terms *(continued)*

Case-Smith, 2005, pp. 7–8	Crepeau, Cohn, & Schell, 2009
Family occupations	Family occupations, pp. 580–581
Family-centered care/family-centered service	Family-centered care, p. 35
Family–therapist collaboration	Participation, p. 182
Occupation	Therapeutic relationship, pp. 328–337
Participation	
Therapeutic relationship	

INTRODUCTION

Welcome to Day 25 of your study guide. You have just completed the chapters on providing examinations, evaluations, and interventions for children who have impairments of body structure and function that interfere with children's occupations. Families experience many changes when raising a child with a disability including, but not limited to, changes in interaction patterns, activities, social and community participation, demands on time and resources, expectations for the child and family, and educational and employment opportunities. This chapter focuses on the roles occupational therapists assume when working with families of children with disabilities and how to facilitate therapist–family collaboration to improve outcomes for the family and child.

Use the outline in this chapter to review the pertinent concepts, strategies, and evidence for working successfully with families of children with disabilities. Complete the corresponding work sheets to reinforce your understanding of the concepts, strategies, and other considerations.

OUTLINE

1. Theories of clinical reasoning

(Case-Smith, 2005, pp. 2–5, Table 1-1)
(Crepeau, et al., 2009, pp. 318–321)

These theories of clinical reasoning are important to provide a framework when developing a plan of care for a child and his or her family. These theories will provide you with different questions you will want to answer when developing therapist–family collaboration. The type (or types) of clinical reasoning you use will help you better understand and develop the most efficient and effective interventions to facilitate the occupational roles of children and their families as well as facilitating the therapist–parent relationship.

    a. These are the most common types of clinical reasoning used by pediatric occupational therapists:
        i. Scientific (Case-Smith, 2005, p. 3; Crepeau, et al., 2009, pp. 318)
        ii. Narrative (Case-Smith, 2005, p. 4; Crepeau, et al., 2009, p. 320)
        iii. Pragmatic (Case-Smith, 2005, p. 4; Crepeau, et al., 2009, pp. 320–321)
        iv. Interactive (Case-Smith, 2005, p. 4; Crepeau, et al., 2009, pp. 321)
        v. Ethical (Case-Smith, 2005, p. 4; Crepeau, et al., 2009, p. 319, 322)
        vi. Conditional (Case-Smith, 2005, pp. 4–5; Crepeau, et al., 2009, p. 319)
    b. Work Sheet 17-1: Using Clinical Reasoning to Make Family-Centered Clinical Decisions (Case-Smith, 2005, pp. 3–5; Crepeau, et al., 2009, pp. 314–327)

Use this chart to summarize the information you have learned about types of clinical reasoning. There are three columns for you to complete.

        i. In the first column describe the primary characteristics of the type of each type of clinical reasoning.

    ii. In the second column list questions you might ask of the family or information you will want to gather that will facilitate your use of each type of clinical reasoning to understand the occupational roles of the child and the parents or caregivers or both.

    iii. In the last column, for each type of clinical decision making, describe how the information gathered may impact your intervention with the parents or caregivers or both to facilitate the occupational roles of the child and family.

2. International Classification of Functioning, Disability and Health (ICF) http://www. who.int/classifications/icf/en/

(Case-Smith, 2005, pp. 7, 58)

(World Health Organization, 2002)

    This enablement model from the World Health Organization (WHO) provides a framework in which to organize a variety of information to understand all aspects of a child's functioning relative to any disability or health issue. This is useful in developing a plan of care. Each area can be of more significance at different times, depending on the response of the family to their child's particular needs. Activities and participation will provide you with a great deal of information about the occupational roles of the child and his or her family. The personal and environmental factors will help you understand the context in which these occupational roles occur and may provide you with insight when working with the parents or caregivers or both to provide a family-centered plan of care. The WHO Web site has a great deal of useful information about the ICF.

    a. Body functions and structures

(Case-Smith, 2005, p. 7)

        i. The occupational therapist assesses the physical structures and the physiological functioning of the child's body. These will include such factors as strength, power, range of motion, sensory processes and integration, postural tone, and eye–hand co-ordination, to name a few. The occupational therapist identifies both areas of strengths and impairments.

    b. Activities and participation

(Case-Smith, 2005, p. 8)

        i. These levels focus on the child's and the family's capacity to engage in occupations, both from an individual perspective and at the societal level. This involves both the ability to do a specific activity (e.g., handwriting) and to use those activities in appropriate environments (e.g., writing in school for an assignment).

    c. Personal and environmental factors

(Case-Smith, 2005, p. 8)

    d. The environment interacts with all levels of functioning, activities, and participation. Environmental considerations include the physical, and psychosocial, and cultural environments provided by the parents, caregivers, community, and society.

    e. Work Sheet 17-2: Using the International Classification of Functioning, Disability and Health with Families of Children with Disabilities

Use this chart to summarize the information you have learned about the ICF, paying particular attention to those areas that involve the family. There are four columns for you to complete.

        i. In the first column describe the types of examinations and evaluations you might perform to assess a child's body functions and structures.

        ii. In the second column list the questions you might ask the family, or information you might want to gather, about the child's and family's activities and participation.

        iii. In the third column, list the questions you might ask of the family or information you might want to gather about the environments that the child or family participates in or would like to participate in.

    iv. In the last column list the questions you might ask the family or information you might want to gather about the personal characteristics of the child or family.

3. Occupational roles of children

(Case-Smith, 2005, pp. 5, 92–113)

    The occupational roles of children develop by their participation in family activities and are impacted by the cultural and physical contexts. Play is the predominant occupation of children. It is important for the occupational therapist to evaluate the child's ability to engage in meaningful activities and assume appropriate roles and routines, as well as how this affects the family, as individuals and as a whole. The assessment includes finding out the concerns of the parents, other family members, and other adults who are part of the child's day-to-day lived experiences. The occupational roles of a child evolve over the course of his or her growth and development.

    a. Play (Case-Smith, 2005, pp. 96–99, 104–105, 110–111, Boxes 4-1 through 4-9)
    b. Activities of daily living (ADL) (Case-Smith, 2005, pp. 522–532)
    c. Instrumental activities of daily living (IADL) (Case-Smith, 2005, pp. 522–532)
    d. School (Case-Smith, 2005, pp. 157–158, 800–826)

4. Occupational roles of families

(Case-Smith, 2005, pp. 118–121)

    Families are a key component when working with children. It is in the context of the family and its daily, weekly, and annual routines and activities that children learn and practice their occupational roles. It is the contexts of a family's beliefs, values, and culture that shape the occupational activities of the child and family members. Consequently, the occupational therapist evaluates not only the occupations of the child but also the occupations of the family and how the child's special needs affect those family occupations. The occupational therapist is then better prepared to support the family and child by selecting interventions that complement the family's values, resources, and culture.

    a. Home management
    b. Caregiving
    c. Employed work
    d. Education
    e. Play
    f. Leisure
    g. Outcomes (Case-Smith, 2005, pp. 118–119, Box 5-1)
        i. Cultural identity (Case-Smith, 2005, p. 8)
        ii. Emotional well-being
        iii. Routines and habits
        iv. Readiness for child's occupations

5. Family responses to a child with impairments or disabilities

(Case-Smith, 2005, pp. 121–138)

    A family is a dynamic system that strives to adapt and respond to changes or stressors introduced to the system. When a child in a family has a significant developmental or health problem, the family attempts to cope and adapt to the changes in routines, behaviors, and activities. The ability of a family to respond is influenced by many contextual factors such as available resources, values, beliefs, and cultural traditions, to name a few. The occupational therapist attempts to facilitate positive and adaptive responses within the family when planning and implementing an intervention plan. To do so requires familiarity with how families respond to a child with impairments or disabilities.

    a. Initial responses (Case-Smith, 2005, pp. 127–128)
    b. Ongoing responses (Case-Smith, 2005, pp. 133–135)
        i. Early childhood
        ii. School age

    iii. Adolescence

    iv. Adulthood

  c. Family resources

    i. Financial (Case-Smith, 2005, pp. 19, 145–146, 128, 482–483)

    ii. Human (Case-Smith, 2005, p. 128)

    iii. Time (Case-Smith, 2005, p. 129)

    iv. Emotional (Case-Smith, 2005, pp. 129–130)

  d. Family structure and systems (Case-Smith, 2005, pp. 119–121, 124–127, 135–138)

6. Developing a family–therapist partnership

(Case-Smith, 2005, pp. 15, 25–26, 138–144, 394–396, 851, 872–873)

(Crepeau, et al., 2009, pp. 33–42, 183)

    Families are the primary social context for children. As stated earlier in this chapter, it is in the context of the family, in the daily, weekly, and annual routines and activities, that children learn and practice their occupational roles. The context of family beliefs, values, and cultures shapes the occupational activities of the child and other family members. It is vital that the occupational therapist form a collaborative partnership with the parents and other family members. Family-centered care uses the values and priorities of the family as the central theme in providing occupational therapy services.

  a. Family-centered services

(Case-Smith, 2005, pp. 25–26, 57–58, 703, Box 21-2, 870)

(Crepeau, et al., 2009, pp. 33–42, 183)

  b. Activities and participation

    i. ADL (Case-Smith, 2005, p. 130)

    ii. Recreation and leisure (Case-Smith, 2005, pp. 130–131)

    iii. Socialization (Case-Smith, 2005, p. 132)

    iv. Community (Case-Smith, 2005, pp. 132–133)

  c. Interpersonal relationships (Crepeau, et al., 2009, pp. 328–337)

    i. Therapeutic use of self

    ii. Partnering (Case-Smith, 2005, pp. 139–140, 620, 895)

    iii. Information (Case-Smith, 2005, pp. 139–140)

    iv. Cultural competence (Case-Smith, 2005, pp. 18–21, 93–94, 103–104, 108–109, 112, 123–124, 140–141, 269–270, 524; Crepeau, et al., 2009, pp. 55–65, 580–581)

    v. Service provision (Case-Smith, 2005, pp. 141–142)

    vi. Autonomy (Case-Smith, 2005, p. 142)

  d. Methods of communication (Case-Smith, 2005, pp. 142–144, 703)

    i. Formal and informal meetings (Case-Smith, 2005, pp. 142–143)

    ii. Written and electronic communication (Case-Smith, 2005, pp. 143–144)

  e. A parent's perspective

(Case-Smith, 2005, pp. 154–159)

    In the appendix to Chapter 5 in Case-Smith (2005), Beth Ball, an occupational therapist and a mother of three children with disabilities, writes about her experience as a parent. This is a good illustration of the lived experiences of a parent of a child with impairments of body structures and functions that impact activities and participation.

  f. Work Sheet 17-3: Case Studies: Implementing Family-Centered Care

Use the following case studies to complete the work sheet to describe the impact on occupational roles of the child and family, how the family is responding, and how to facilitate the family-therapist partnership.

Case Study 1. Jenny was born 6 months ago at 32 weeks gestation with a birth weight of 4 lbs 5 oz. She is the first child of Maria, a 22-year-old single mother. Maria lives alone with Jenny in a one-bedroom, fifth-floor apartment. There is an elevator in the building. Maria is employed as a computer consultant and is able to work from home a majority of the time. Maria's mother lives approximately 1 hour away and is able to assist with taking care of Jenny when Maria must go to a client's location for her job. Jenny's father is not involved in her care and lives in another state.

Jenny has been referred for occupational therapy services by her pediatrician. Jenny has not been gaining weight as expected and is at the 10th percentile for weight, 20th percentile for length, and 50th percentile for head circumference. She has been diagnosed with hydrocephalus and has a shunt that is draining well. Maria reports that Jenny cries frequently, has difficulty with feedings, sleeps irregularly, and doesn't like to be held. Consequently, Jenny spends most of her time in her crib or on a blanket on the floor, usually on her back. Maria reports that Jenny does not yet roll over or hold her head up well and seems stiff sometimes. Maria states that she feels stressed; for example, she is concerned that Jenny cries unexpectedly while being held and rocked.

Case Study 2. David is 7 years old and lives with both of his parents, his sister Janie, and his baby sister Isabelle, who is 18 months old, in a two-story home on several acres. He is in the first grade in a rural public elementary school. He rides to and from school on a bus with his older sister Janie, who is 10 years old.

David's parents state that he has always been a wild child and is always getting in trouble. He has difficulty behaving around the house, never seeming to sit still or get his chores done—unlike Janie, who is "a very easy child" in their opinion. David didn't sleep through the night until he was 2 years old and still resists going to bed. He is a very picky eater and is unwilling to try new foods. He also is a very cautious child when it comes to climbing, jumping, and other similar physical activities. David's father is concerned that David is not very athletic and will be shunned by other boys his age.

Yesterday David's teacher phoned to ask to meet with David's parents. She is concerned about his behavior in the classroom and that he is not making progress as expected after 3 months into the school year. The teacher feels he is distractible, fidgety, and doesn't pay attention for very long. David also seems to be picking fights with some of his classmates, especially when he is standing in line or is in situations that require close contact with the other children. During recess he avoids climbing on the playground equipment or engaging in other physical activities. The teacher is also concerned that it is difficult for him to engage in fine motor activities.

Case Study 3. Allison is 14 years old and has a diagnosis of spastic diplegic cerebral palsy. She lives with her mother and father and three siblings (Jaime, 16 years old; Kayla, 15 years old; and Michael, 8 years old). Allison's family has recently moved to a new Midwestern suburban city because her mother had a job transfer. All of the children were very involved in extracurricular activities, including sports and music, in their previous town and hope to be involved here as well. Both sets of grandparents lived near their previous home; there are no relatives located in this new city.

Allison will be starting at the public high school in 6 weeks and will be mainstreamed into most classes. Allison is able to use loftstrand crutches and bilateral ankle-foot orthoses (AFOs) for shorter distances, and she uses a motorized scooter for community mobility. Handwriting is slow and tedious for Allison. She has tested at or above grade level for most of her classes.

Allison's mother reports that her daughter tends to be shy and slow to warm up. She expresses concern about obtaining services in the new town and how Allison will fit in at the new school and in the community. They have had mixed experiences with therapy providers in the past and are leery about finding occupational and physical therapists that they feel they can work with. Allison's parents are wondering what will happen later this year when Allison becomes eligible for driver's education because Jaime recently earned her driver's license. Allison is concerned about what classes she will be taking, what her teachers will be like, if she'll make any friends, or if anyone will make fun of her.

WORK SHEETS

Work Sheet 17-1. Using Clinical Reasoning to Make Family-Centered Clinical Decisions

Table 17-2 Using Clinical Reasoning to Make Family-Centered Clinical Decisions

Type of Clinical Reasoning	Describe the main characteristics of this type of clinical reasoning.	What questions might you ask the parents or family based on this type of clinical reasoning?	How will this information influence your intervention plan for the parents or family?
Scientific			
Narrative			

Work Sheet 17-2. Using the International Classification of Functioning, Disability and Health with Families of Children with Disabilities

Table 17-3 Using the International Classification of Functioning, Disability and Health with Families of Children with Disabilities

Body Function and Structure	Activities and Participation	Environmental Context	Personal Characteristics or Attributes
Describe the types of examinations and evaluations you might perform to assess body function and structure.	List questions you might ask of the family, or information you might want to gather, about the child's and family's activities and participation.	List questions you might ask of the family, or information you might want to gather, about the environments that the child or family participates in or would like to participate in.	List questions you might ask of the family, or information you might want to gather, about the personal characteristics of the child or family.

SUGGESTED RESPONSES

Suggested responses may include, but are not limited to, the following:

Table 17-4 Suggested Responses Work Sheet

Body Function and Structure	Activities and Participation	Environmental Context	Personal Characteristics or Attributes

Work Sheet 17-3. Case Studies: Implementing Family-Centered Care

Table 17-5 Case Studies: Implementing Family-Centered Care

	Case Study 1: Jenny	Case Study 2: David	Case Study 3: Allison
	6 months old *Premature birth:* *32 weeks gestation*	*7 years old* *No diagnosis*	*14 years old* *Diagnosis: spastic diplegia*
Occupation of the child: Indicate the known information that impacts the child's occupational role within the context of the family for each case study.			
What concerns do you have, or what other information would you want to know, to facilitate the child's occupational role within the context of the family?			

REFERENCES

Case-Smith, J. (Ed.). (2005). *Occupational therapy for children* (5th ed.). St. Louis, MO: Mosby.

Crepeau, E. B., Cohn, E. S., & Schell, B. A. B. (Eds.). (2009). *Willard and Spackman's occupational therapy* (11th ed.). Philadelphia: Lippincott Williams & Wilkins.

World Health Organization. (2002). International classification of functioning, disability and health. Retrieved July 2, 2008, from http://www.who.int/classifications/icf/en/

Exhibit 1-1 Stress Vulnerability Scale

In modern society, most of us can't avoid stress. But we can learn to behave in ways that lessen its effects. Researchers have identified a number of factors that affect one's vulnerability to stress—among them are eating and sleeping habits, caffeine and alcohol intake, and how we express our emotions. The following questionnaire is designed to help you discover your vulnerability quotient and to pinpoint trouble spots. Rate each item from 1 (always) to 5 (never), according to how much of the time the statement is true of you. Be sure to mark each item, even if it does not apply to you—for example, if you don't smoke, circle 1 next to item six.

		Always	Sometimes			Never
1.	I eat at least one hot, balanced meal a day.	1	2	3	4	5
2.	I get 7–8 hours of sleep at least four nights a week.	1	2	3	4	5
3.	I give and receive affection regularly.	1	2	3	4	5
4.	I have at least one relative within 50 miles on whom I can rely.	1	2	3	4	5
5.	I exercise to the point of perspiration at least twice a week.	1	2	3	4	5
6.	I limit myself to less than half a pack of cigarettes a day.	1	2	3	4	5
7.	I take fewer than five alcohol drinks a week.	1	2	3	4	5
8.	I am the appropriate weight for my height.	1	2	3	4	5
9.	I have an income adequate to meet basic expenses.	1	2	3	4	5
10.	I get strength from my religious beliefs.	1	2	3	4	5
11.	I regularly attend club or social activities.	1	2	3	4	5
12.	I have a network of friends and acquaintances.	1	2	3	4	5
13.	I have one or more friends to confide in about personal matters.	1	2	3	4	5
14.	I am in good health (including eyesight, hearing, and teeth).	1	2	3	4	5
15.	I am able to speak openly about my feelings when angry or worried.	1	2	3	4	5
16.	I have regular conversations with the people I live with about domestic problems—for example, chores and money.	1	2	3	4	5
17.	I do something for fun at least once a week.	1	2	3	4	5
18.	I am able to organize my time effectively.	1	2	3	4	5
19.	I drink fewer than three cups of coffee (or other caffeine-rich drinks) a day.	1	2	3	4	5
20.	I take some quiet time for myself during the day.	1	2	3	4	5

(continues)

Exhibit 1-1 Stress Vulnerability Scale *(continued)*

Scoring Instructions: To calculate your score, add up the figures and subtract 20.

Score Interpretation:
A score below 10 indicates excellent resistance to stress.
A score over 30 indicates some vulnerability to stress.
A score over 50 indicates serious vulnerability to stress.

Self-Care Plan: Notice that nearly all the items describe situations and behaviors over which you have a great deal of control. Review the items on which you scored three or higher. List those items in your self-care plan. Concentrate first on those that are easiest to change—for example, eating a hot, balanced meal daily and having fun at least once a week—before tackling those that seem difficult.

Source: Exhibit courtesy Copyright 2009 Stress Directions, Inc., Lyle H. Miller and Alma Dell Smith, Boston, MA www.stressdirections.com

Exhibit 5-1 Reflection Question Journal

1. What? (What have I accomplished? What have I learned?)

2. So what? (What difference did it make? Why should I do it? How is it important? How do I feel about it?)

3. Now what? (What's next? Where do we go from here?)

Source: Exhibit courtesy of Live Wire Media.

Occupational Functioning Special Practice Settings (Days 26–31)

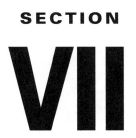

Occupational Rehabilitation/ Return to Work Programming: Functional Capacity Evaluation, Ergonomic Assessment, Job Site Evaluation, Work Hardening, and Work Conditioning

CHAPTER 18

Jon Nettie

OBJECTIVES

1. Define functional capacity evaluation, ergonomic assessment, job site evaluation, work hardening, work conditioning, job coaching, light duty programming, and work tolerance screening.
2. Choose the most appropriate discipline for the patient based on previous rehabilitation outcomes.
3. Understand the purpose for functional capacity evaluation, ergonomic assessment, job site evaluation, work hardening, job coaching, work tolerance screening, and light duty programming.
4. Understand the components of a functional capacity evaluation, ergonomic assessment, job site evaluation, work hardening, work conditioning, job coaching, work tolerance screening, and light duty programming.
5. Recognize what makes up a difficult patient.
6. Demonstrate proper documentation.
7. Understand the use of lumbar supports.
8. Recognize the levels of education needed to promote proper health and awareness of occupational therapists' roles in decreasing the patient's days away from work, which translates to less worker compensation costs to the employer and allows the supervisor and/or upper management to meet budgetary goals.
9. Apply knowledge to clinical and work-related settings.

KEY TERMS

Table 18-1 Key Terms

Chaffin & Andersson, 1996, pp. 1–2 Isernhagen, 1995, pp. 3–37, 70–85, 410–444, 443–462, 480
Activity restriction
Carrying
Climbing
Disability
Dysfunction
Ergonomic assessment
Function
Functional capacity evaluation
Impairment
Job coaching
Job site evaluation
Lifting
Light duty programming
Physical demands (never, rare, occasionally, frequently, and continuously)
Pulling
Pushing
Work categories (sedentary, light, medium, heavy, very heavy)
Work conditioning
Work hardening
Work tolerance screening

INTRODUCTION

Welcome to Days 26 and 27 of your study guide. This chapter will provide you with information that will allow you to choose the appropriate medium(s) to assist you in getting patients and returning them back to work. It will allow you to properly document outcomes for work, clinical, insurance, and legal systems. It will also allow you to choose the right level of education given to the patient's supervisors, upper management, and union when placing the injured or ill worker back into the workplace.

OUTLINE

1. **History of occupational medicine programs**

   (Chaffin & Andersson, 1996 pp. 1–2; Isernhagen, 1995, pp. 634–636)

   a. *Founding father of occupational medicine or ergonomics, Bernardino Ramazzini* (Diseases in Occupations, 1713)
   b. *Little association between work and injury until industrial resolution (17th century)*
   Source: Courtesy of Susan Isernhagen, PT, DSI Solutions, Duluth, MN

   c. *Movement into workers' compensation laws in the 20th century plus development of the Americans with Disabilities Act (ADA) and Equal Employment Opportunity Act (EEO)*

   d. *Big move was in 1970 in the development of Occupational Safety and Health Act (OSHA)*

Source: Copied with permission from D. Chaffin, G. B. J. Andersson, and B. J. Martin, *Occupational Biomechanics*, 4th ed., J. Wiley and Sons, New York, NY, 2006.

     i. *Community care concept*
     ii. *Delivery network*
     iii. *On-site miniclinics*
     iv. *Broad-based services*

2. Employer wants

   a. *Centralized services*
   b. *Closer relationships*
   c. *On-site education*
   d. *Before the employer can get what it wants, we (PT/OT/PTA/OTA) need to offer something*

     i. *To whom: Physicians, patients, insurers, case managers, employers*
     ii. *What: Work hardening/work conditioning (WH/WC), functional capacity evaluations (FCE), job site analysis (JSA), job coaching (JC), ergonomic evaluations (EE), light duty programming (LDP)*

Source: Courtesy of Lauren Hebert, DPT, OCS, Smart Care Physical Therapy, Dixfield, ME. The following sources are used throughout this chapter:

Source: Susan Isernhagen, PT, DSI Solutions, Duluth, MN (Isernhagen, 1995, pp. 410–418); *Source*: Courtesy of Leonard Matheson, PhD, EPIC Rehab, Chesterfield, MO (Matheson, 1999); *Source*: Robin Saunders, MSPT, Empi, Inc. (Saunders, 1996).

3. Functional capacity evaluations (see Appendix A)

   a. *Layman's definition: A functional capacity evaluation (FCE) is a 2- to 4-hour evaluation that will look at one's current physical abilities. There will be an evaluation period where the therapist will assess ROM, strength, and subjective pain complaints. There will also be a self-perception evaluation where you as the patient will give the therapist an idea of where you feel you are functionally. When the subjective portion and the screening portion are completed, you will then move into the functional part of the evaluation. Here the therapist will run through several tests to look at sitting, standing, walking, squatting, lifting (floor to waist, waist to waist, waist to shoulder [curl], and waist to overhead [press]), pushing and pulling, carrying bilaterally and unilaterally, kneeling, crawling, and fine motor tasks [gripping, pinching]. The therapist will take your safety into account. If you feel the need to stop a subtest you have the right to do so. The therapist will ask, however, why you needed to stop, and this will be documented. Furthermore, if the therapist sees poor body mechanics being used, he or she will stop you, reeducate you on how to correct the body mechanics, and then resume. If your body does not allow you to resume then you will be told that this subtest is completed. Do expect to have some residual and next-day soreness following this aggressive evaluation. You can combat the symptoms through medication prescribed by your doctor or by using ice.*

Source: Robin Saunders, MSPT, Empi, Inc.

   b. Purpose
     i. Appropriateness
     ii. Allows goals to be developed for returning to work
     iii. Gives baseline
     iv. Helps to identify various limiting factors and restrictions for returning to work
     v. Identifies prognosis, frequency, and duration
     vi. Identifies necessity for other services (vocational rehab, specialized PT/OT, job site evaluation)

   c. Components
     i. Interview (medical history, job history, etc.)

      ii. Neuromuscular evaluation (done short/sweet, quickly/efficiently)

          I. Get a baseline of manual muscle testing to compare to the functional evaluation

          II. Do not want the client to feel like a patient but more of an employee/worker

      iii. Functional baseline evaluation

          I. Baseline evaluation will include standing, walking, sitting, squatting, crawling, lifting (waist to waist, floor lift, shoulder lift, overhead lift), carrying, push/pull, climbing (stairs and ladder), forward bending (repetitive and sustained), reaching (repetitive and sustained), hand functioning (grip, grasp, and pinch), and activity.

          II. *Client "sorts" (patient's perception of his or her function as it relates to the injury); this will also help identify any possible inconsistencies.*

      Source: Courtesy of Leonard Matheson, PhD, EPIC Rehab, Chesterfield, MO (see Appendix B)

      iv. Goal setting and recommendations

      v. Documentation

          I. Inconsistencies

          II. Symptom magnification *Source*: Susan Isernhagen, PT, DSI Solutions, Duluth, MN

          III. Nontest behavior *Source*: Susan Isernhagen, PT, DSI Solutions, Duluth, MN

          IV. Goals

          V. Recommendations

          VI. Work categories (see Appendix C)

4. Work hardening/work conditioning

    a. *Layman's definition: Work hardening occurs at least 3 days a week, if not daily. It will last from 2 to 8 hours per day. The average time in the clinic is 4 hours. You will initially start out with an evaluation by the therapist to get a baseline level of history of your injury, your current rehabilitation status, and goals for returning to the same type of occupation. While in the work hardening program you will be total-body reconditioned, which means you will work on all parts of the body, not just the injured area. There will also be aerobics work to get your endurance up as well as generalized strengthening and work simulation. You will be allotted breaks every couple of hours, and a lunch hour will be provided if needed. You need to dress casually and comfortably. If there is specific attire that you wear at work, you may be required to wear that attire in the program, especially if it requires that you wear heavy boots or specific equipment. You will be reevaluated every 2 to 4 weeks to assist the therapist and physician in the progression of your rehabilitation program.*

    Source: Robin Saunders, MSPT, Empi, Inc.

    b. Justify work hardening/work conditioning

      i. *Should be different from general PT/OT*

      ii. *It must be more than just exercise*

      iii. *Must communicate with more than just the physician*

      iv. *Need to have careful tracking of outcomes*

      v. *Need to have specific and focused work goals*

      vi. *Very specific and focused evaluation*

    c. *Work hardening versus work conditioning*

      i. *Interdisciplinary versus unidisciplinary*

      ii. *Physical, behavioral, vocational versus physical and functional*

      iii. *Daily 3 to 4 hours versus daily 2 to 4 hours*

      iv. *Work-simulated activities versus work-related activities*

    d. *Entrance criteria: Work hardening versus work conditioning*

      i. *Work hardening*

          I. *Unable to return to previous job capacity because of pain, dysfunction, postinjury, or illness*

          II. *Good prognosis*

      III. *Job-oriented goals*
      IV. *Client understands he or she will return to work following the program*
      V. *Work hardening not contraindicated and the physician agrees with the plan*
      VI. *No psychological issues, chemical dependency, symptom magnification, or other areas that will interfere with progress toward the goal*
      VII. *Goal obtainable within 6 to 8 weeks*

    ii. *Work conditioning*
      I. *Unable to return to previous job capacity because of pain, dysfunction, post-injury, or illness*
      II. *Good prognosis*
      III. *Good job-oriented goals*
      IV. *Client understands he or she will improve function to return to work following the program*
      V. *Work conditioning not contraindicated and the physician agrees with the plan*
      VI. *No psychological issues, chemical dependency, symptom magnification, or other areas that indicate the need for work hardening or other services*
      VII. *Goal reachable within 2 to 8 weeks*

e. *Work hardening/work conditioning trial*
    i. *Client who has not met entrance criteria*
    ii. *Must meet entrance criteria within 2 weeks or be discharged*
    iii. *All symptom magnifiers automatically receive a 2-week trial.*
    iv. *Almost all clients of a clinical trial will participate in work hardening programs, not work conditioning.*
    v. *Make sure documentation states that this is only a trial.*

f. *Estimation of frequency and duration*
    i. *You may be wrong about the initial setting of your frequency and duration, so progress reports are important to let appropriate parties know that an extension may be needed (e.g., In week two or five the patient is falling behind in goal acts because of [specify] factors and may require an additional 2 weeks).*

g. *Goal problems*
    i. *Goal set too high*
    ii. *Goal set too low (game playing by the client)*
    iii. *Stated goals are different than actual goals.*
    iv. *No functional goals or no goal set at all*
    v. *Goals incongruent with insurance goals*
    vi. *Goals incongruent with employer's goals*

h. *Work hardening/conditioning exit criteria*
    i. *Client meets goal.*
    ii. *Client stops progressing toward goal.*
    iii. *Program becomes medically contraindicated.*
    iv. *Client wishes to discontinue.*
    v. *Client is noncompliant.*
    Source: Courtesy of Leonard Matheson, PhD, EPIC Rehab, Chesterfield, MO

5. Client types: Easy versus difficult
Source: Courtesy of Lauren Hebert, DPT, OCS, Smart Care Physical Therapy, Dixfield, ME (Hebert, 1999, pp. 3–5)

a. *Easy client*
    i. *Client is willing to work hard (motivated).*
    ii. *Client wants to be involved in his or her goal setting and progression.*
    iii. *Steady weekly progress*

b. *Difficult client*
    i. *Has predetermined mind-set of being disabled*
    ii. *Shows improvement of reinjury during the last week of the program*

      iii. *Shows improvement of reinjury during the first week after returning to work*

      iv. *Shows improvement in all areas except job-pertinent activities*

      v. *Malingerer: Uses illness or other incapacity to avoid duty or work*

          I. *Assigns motivation to the behavior*

      vi. *Magnifier: Causes symptoms to appear greater to gain more importance*

          I. *Describes behavior but not motivation*

          II. *Magnification also present when the client has a true pathology*

  c. *Specific types of difficult patients*

      i. *Refugee: Symptoms provide an escape from an apparently unresolved conflict of life situation.*

      ii. *Game player: Symptoms provide an opportunity for positive gain.*

      iii. *Identified patient: Patient's role eclipses and contains all of the other possible roles that he or she might have.*

          I. *You may confront the malingerer or magnifier but must phrase appropriately (e.g., I know you may be having symptoms, but I will not put you into any harm. If I see that you are approaching harm or using faulty body mechanics, I will make the appropriate changes so that you may continue).*

6. Documentation

(Hebert, 1999, pp. 1–5)

  a. *What to avoid*

      i. *Incomplete and inaccurate work sheets*

      ii. *Statement and notes related to attitude rather than behavior*

          I. *Don't: Client did not appear to understand body mechanic instruction.*

          II. *Do: Client demonstrated poor techniques despite 30 minutes of one-on-one instruction.*

      iii. *Conclusions about functional abilities without supporting facts*

          I. *Don't: Client is unable to lift 40 pounds from the floor.*

          II. *Do: Client exhibits shakiness or change in technique when lifting 40 pounds from the floor level.*

      iv. *Poor handwriting*

      v. *Excessive detail to unrelated activities or conclusions*

      vi. *Failure to document important conversations with related parties*

  b. *Difficult documentation*

      i. *Direct and to the point*

          I. *Activity was discontinued by the client due to complaints of pain; however, no change in technique or signs of increased effort, such as (specify), were noted.*

          II. *Client reports that he or she cannot perform (specific work activities) because of pain, however, there is no objective basis to limit the client from performing the activity. Returning to work that involves performance of that activity would be unsuccessful because of the client's subjective limitations. Return to work that involves (specify) would be more successful.*

          III. *Due to the inconsistencies noted, it is impossible to determine objective capabilities of the patient; however, there are some reasonable suggestions for rehabilitation management.*

7. Work simulation

  a. *Be creative*

      i. *Break the job down into specific parts and work them in order to achieve total job duty.*

8. Back to school

(Continuing Education Course Notes, 1996a)

(Continuing Education Course Notes, 1996b)

a. *Basics*

    i. *Basic information given over a short period of time to allow the client to be functional and independent*

    ii. *Correct the patient's goal of pain reduction (because pain reduction may not always be possible); help set up appropriate priorities*

    iii. *Basic information*

        I. *Basic spinal anatomy*

        II. *Basic body lifting mechanics instruction*

        III. *Home exercise program*

        IV. *Posture reeducation*

        V. *Pain management techniques*

    iv. *Advanced information*

        I. *Neutral spine concept*

        II. *Emphasize critical need for spinal stabilization*

        III. *Home exercise program for spinal stabilization and total body reconditioning*
        Source: Courtesy of Lauren Hebert, DPT, OCS, Smart Care Physical Therapy, Dixfield, ME

b. Lumbar back braces and belts

    i. *Why are low back muscles highly stretched when lifting?*

c. *Paraspinal muscles are relatively close to spinal motion segments.*

        I. *When lifting, carrying, pushing, and pulling loads, external load movements can become quite high depending on the position of the object and if it is in motion.*

d. *Why does the low back become highly stretched when lifting?*

e. *Paraspinal muscles are close to the motion segment of the rotational axis (centered at the disc); increased compression force is on the disc.*

f. *Is asymmetric lifting a special risk?*

g. *During twisting, lifting studies confirm that many different torso muscles are used to increase contractions in antagonism; therefore, the compression force is increased by 20 to 50%.*

h. *Does dynamic lifting cause high spinal forces?*

i. *Although people adjust downward toward their lifting capabilities, the paraspinal muscles will cause very high spinal compression force to be the same level as static positioning.*

j. *Static analysis may underestimate capabilities for highly dynamic jobs by 15 to 50%.*

k. *Do you know when the back is overstressed?*

l. *No. It may be 24 to 48 hours after the trauma has occurred before symptoms become evident.*

m. *The National Institute for Occupational Safety and Health (NIOSH) is part of the Centers for Disease Control and Prevention (CDC) within the U.S. Department of Health and Human Services. NIOSH is the federal institute responsible for conducting research and making recommendations for the prevention of work-related injuries and illnesses. NIOSH publication No. 94-127 (October 1996, updated June 10, 1997), Back Belts: Do They Prevent Injury?, states that the decision to use back belts should be a voluntary decision by both the employer and employee. Back belt use should not be mandatory.*

NIOSH noted the following points:

n. *There is a lack of scientific evidence that back belts work.*

o. *Workers who wear belts may attempt to lift more weight than they would without a belt. A false sense of security may subject workers to greater risk of injury.*

p. *Workers and employers should redesign the work environment and work tasks to reduce lifting hazards rather than rely solely on back belts to prevent injury.*

q. *The research needed to adequately assess the effectiveness of back belts will take several years to complete. In the interim, workers should not assume that back belts are protective.*

r. *The psychological theories for the need of lumbar supports*

s. *The decision to wear a belt is a personal choice; however, NIOSH believes that workers and employers should have information available to make the decision.*

t. *Individual perception = biomechanical stress + no self-control over risk factors*

u. *If one is properly educated in the use of correct body and lifting mechanics, one does not need a belt; however, if one cannot obtain proper self-control to relieve fears and anxiety, a belt may be used to give the person control; then the person takes into his or her own hands the need to use or not use a belt in threatening situations.*

Source: Copied with permission from D. Chaffin, G. B. J. Andersson, and B. J. Martin, *Occupational Biomechanics*, 4th ed., J. Wiley and Sons, New York, NY, 2006.

v. Overall conclusion

   i. Lumbar muscles produce greater than 1000 pounds of force. How can the use of proper body and lifting biomechanics help prevent low back pain?

   I. Keep the load close.

   II. Keep the load off the floor.

   III. Keep torso as vertical as possible with proper lumbar curvature.

   IV. Do not jerk or move quickly with loads.

   V. Avoid side lifting and twisting, especially with heavy loads.

   VI. Ergonomic programs reduce the risks of lifting tasks.

   VII. Employers that rely on back belts to prevent injury should be aware of the lack of scientific evidence supporting their use. NIOSH does not recommend the use of back belts to prevent injuries among workers who have never been injured.

9. Neck school

(Continuing Education Course Notes, 1996a)

(Continuing Education Course Notes, 1996b)

   a. *The focus is the same as the back-to-school concept, except the emphasis is on scapular stabilization, upper extremity strengthening versus lumbar stabilization, and lower extremity strengthening*

   Source: Lauren Hebert, DPT, OCS, Smart Care Physical Therapy, Dixfield, ME

10. Job site analysis (see Appendix D)

Source: Lauren Hebert, DPT, OCS, Smart Care Physical Therapy, Dixfield, ME (Hebert, 1999, pp. 1–6)

   a. *Layman's definition: A job site analysis (JSA) is when the therapist comes out to the job site. There, the occupation will be evaluated for risk factors that may cause and/or aggravate symptoms. When these risk factors are determined, recommendations for minimizing and/or eliminating them will be given. Additionally, any equipment that may be needed to help minimize and reduce the symptoms will be recommended.*

   b. *Job coaching may also be included in this evaluation to work on proper body and lifting mechanics while trying to minimize risk factors.*

   c. *The job site evaluation may last anywhere from 1 to 4 hours based on the complexity of the job.*

   d. *Purpose: The procedure is based on system analysis techniques, which utilize proactive approaches to develop a detailed, open-ended evaluation of facilities, equipment, tools, prostheses, and work methods to recognize and evaluate specific work activities associated with potential and harmful exposures to generic risk factors.*

   e. *Team: PT/OT/PTA/OTA/ATC*

   i. *Workers*

   ii. *Work supervisors*

   iii. *Safety and health professionals*

   f. *Equipment*

   i. *Video recorder*

   ii. *Camera*

      iii. *Force measuring equipment*
      iv. *Basic measuring tools*
      v. *Stopwatch*

  g. *Ergonomic risk factors*
      i. *Forceful exertions*
      ii. *Awkward postures*
      iii. *Local contact stressors*
      iv. *Vibration*
      v. *Temperature extremes*
      vi. *Repetitive or prolonged activities*

  h. *Report background*
      i. *Background history (medical and work history)*
      ii. *List of associated observable risk factors*
      iii. *List of corrective measures*
      iv. *List of job-specific stretching exercises*
      v. *Plan (include further worker and management training on low back and neck pain and disorders of the upper extremities)*

  i. *Education plan*
      i. *Neck and arm program*
         I. *Train management and the union on all the things that create injuries and claims. Discuss costs (biomechanics, medical signs and symptoms, ergonomics, worker behaviors and attitudes, policies). All management must attend or the program may fail.*
         II. *Train employees more on fatigue avoidance and getting rid of work discomfort and pain rather than the disease process. Do not discuss politics.*
      ii. *Low back program*
         I. *Same as neck and arm program, but teach employees the signs and symptoms and outcomes of low back injuries, and provide more motivational education to become and stay healthy.*

      Source: Courtesy of Lauren Hebert, DPT, OCS, Smart Care Physical Therapy, Dixfield, ME

11. **Workstation facts (ergonomic desk analysis) (see Appendices E and F)**

Source: Courtesy of Back Designs Incorporated, Novato, CA (Back Designs, Inc., 2007, p. 1)

  a. *According to the U.S. Bureau of Labor Statistics, nearly 2 million workers become injured simply by sitting at their desks. Postures, repetitive motions, and office equipment positioning are among the factors that cause these accumulative trauma disorders. Workplace injuries are not inevitable, and workers can be safe if the appropriate measures are taken.*

  b. *Most individuals who work in an office setting are provided with a desk and the equipment needed to perform the job. This does not necessarily have to limit an individual into a locked position based on the amount of space, technology, or funds available. Changing some of the placements of the items that are used in an individual's daily occupation can help decrease tension, chronic pain complaints, and daily aches and pains.*

  c. *Because different individuals have different types of body styles and sitting postures, a chair must be designed appropriately for the individual and his or her functional needs. Optimally, the chair should have adjustable armrests, lumbar support, and some type of control to lock the back into place for better posture during prolonged computer or desk work. Furthermore, one should be positioned in a 90-90-90 position. This is when the feet are flat on the floor and the knees and hips are at 90° angles. This puts the body into the comfort position for work. If a person is then too low to do desk or computer work, the chair seat should be raised so the person can work comfortably. If the person's feet then dangle, a footrest is needed.*

  d. *The body enjoys change, so the sitting position (posture) should be altered throughout the day. Change the settings of the chair. Change the placement of paperwork. However,* *one thing that must not change is the placement of the computer monitor. It should always be in front to prevent neck, shoulder, and upper back strain from continuously looking to one side.*

e. *By being aware of a person's body and surroundings, work can be a lot less stressful. Please see Appendix G for an ergonomic on-site job assessment sample report.*

Source: Courtesy of Back Designs Incorporated, Novato, CA

12. Job coaching* (see Appendix H)

Source: Lauren Hebert, DPT, OCS, Smart Care Physical Therapy, Dixfield, ME (Hebert, 1999, pp. 1–2)

a. *On-site job coaching with an employee or employer or both, upon the employee returning to work provides documentation of compliance or noncompliance with recommendations to return to work safely with or without restrictions. The therapist will also assist with implementation of proper body and lifting mechanics, with emphasis on correct utilization of work techniques.*

13. Work tolerance screening*

(Hebert, 1999, pp. 3–4)

a. *Work tolerance screening is an intensive 1-day evaluation during which the physical demand of work is simulated in a controlled setting. This helps to determine an individual's ability to return to his or her previous job or perform critical demands of a new job prior to the development of a formal vocational plan.*

14. Light/modified duty programming*

(Hebert, 1999, pp. 5–6)

a. *The development of a light/modified duty program helps to prevent lost work days and reduce workers' compensation claims and payouts. This is done through education recognition and commitment of all employees, supervisors, upper management, medical staff, and the safety department.*

*Job coaching, work tolerance screening, and light/modified duty programming are areas in occupational rehabilitation that require continuing education and training

Source: Lauren Hebert, DPT, OCS, Smart Care Physical Therapy, Dixfield, ME.

CASE STUDIES

Case Study 18-1.   Match the following:

A   **1.** A female patient is injured and is off work. Her husband is glad she is not working and can care for their children at home.

C   **2.** A male patient has a lawyer and is suing for negligence.

B   **3.** A single mom is injured and now has attendant care for laundry and housekeeping chores.
   A. Refugee
   B. Identified patient
   C. Game player

Case Study 18-2.   A 42-year-old male with a rotator cuff tear and repair is a tool and dye maker. He loads parts from a pallet on the floor and places them into a machine. He reaches into the machine. The reach is approximately 16 inches, and the weights vary from 2 to 20 pounds. He also has to close the sliding door (that sticks from time to time) and push a lever up and to the right to start the machine. What exercises and/or education can you come up with to help him with his job?

Case Study 18-3.   Which of the following are examples of proper documentation?
   A. Patient cannot lift 20 pounds.
   B. Patient complains of pain constantly and is therefore magnifying.
   C. Patient has not demonstrated proper body and lifting mechanics during a 30-pound unilateral carrying test over a distance of 20 feet. The patient exhibits trunk stiffening and cannot

control appropriate faulty body and postural mechanics. Patient had been instructed on proper maintenance of body mechanics over a 50-minute period and still did not demonstrate proper control.

D. Patient dropped the box and could not explain his inability to hold it; therefore, he is malingering.

Case Study 18-4.   The physician asks you to dispense a lumbar support to his patient. The patient is returning to work in a week. His job is in the heavy category as defined by the U.S. Department of Labor. This is defined as lifting on an occasional basis with weight up to and exceeding 100 pounds independently. The doctor says the lumbar support will help protect his back. What do you say to the doctor?

Case Study 18-5.   You are asked to educate an employer on minimizing work injury claims and possible lost workdays. Please list some suggestions that you would discuss with management and supervisors versus employees themselves.

REFERENCES

Back Designs, Inc. (2007). *Ergonomic design for the home and work office.* Novato, CA: Author.

Chaffin, D., & Andersson, G. B. (1996). *Occupational biomechanics-course lecture notes* (5th ed.). Ann Arbor: University of Michigan.

Continuing Education Course Notes. (1996a). *Ergonomics: Job analysis and field studies.* Ann Arbor: University of Michigan.

Continuing Education Course Notes. (1996b). *Occupational ergonomics.* Ann Arbor: University of Michigan.

Hebert, L. (1999). *Development of claims prevention and ergonomic consulting practice-course lecture notes.* Dixfield, ME: Smart Care.

Isernhagen, S. J. (Ed.). (1995). *Comprehensive guide to work injury management.* Duluth, MN: Aspen.

Matheson, L. (1999). *Functional capacity evaluation: Getting started.* Keene, NH: Roy Matheson & Associates.

Saunders, R. (1996). *Industrial rehabilitation: Techniques for success.* St. Paul, MN: Empi, Inc.

CASE STUDY RATIONALE

Case Study 18-1
1. **A.** The patient's husband is happy and less stress is in the household.
2. **C.** Monetary gain.
3. **B.** High stress as a single parent. She now has help.

Case Study 18-2
1. Perform body mechanic instruction.
2. Teach patient appropriate abdominal bracing, hip hinging, joint protection, and trunk posture.
3. Perform lifting tasks from the floor with weight ranging from 2 to 20 pounds with good body mechanics.
4. Perform outward reaching over distances of 6 to 16 inches with weight ranging from 2 to 20 pounds focusing on proper body and lifting mechanics.
5. Use a Thera-Band to simulate the motions needed to push the lever to start the machine and/or use a BTE isokinetic machine to help simulate numerous work-related activities.

Case Study 18-3.   **Correct Answer: C.** This describes the most objective findings to explain why things are occurring. Choices A, B, and D have no significant objective measures to back up the documentation.

Case Study 18-4.   You should state that you want to educate the patient on the use of the brace. Include education and discussion that the brace is a psychological aide and is to be used as an adjunct to proper body and lifting mechanics. The patient must realize that the brace will not prevent low back injury. You should also discuss proper problem-solving skills with regards to testing weight and to achieve assistance when needed.

Case Study 18-5.   With management and supervisors, you need to make sure you discuss the need to allow individuals to report claims so one may identify potential risks. Start education on proper body and lifting mechanics, pain management techniques, and additional ergonomic intervention. You should also discuss workplace politics and attitudes as they relate to how the employees/supervisors may react to injuries.

With regard to the employees, you should talk about fatigue avoidance, stretching, and exercise rather than disease processes. Do not discuss politics.

APPENDIX A

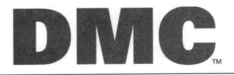

DMC™
Rehabilitation Institute
of Michigan

Source: Courtesy of Rehabilitation Institute of Michigan/The Detroit Medical Center.

Rehabilitation Institute of Michigan
Occupational Rehabilitation Services
Functional Capacity Evaluation
Generic

Client Name: C., J.
Insurance: Workers' Compensation
Diagnosis: Closed head injury and thoracic fracture
Physician: Dr. L. H.
Case Manager: R. Y., RN

Date: December 11, 2008
Injury Date: July 26, 2007
Mechanism of Injury: Fall from scaffold

Summary/Conclusions

A functional capacity evaluation was completed on Mr. C. to achieve a baseline of his current capacity.

General objectives of his performance have demonstrated to be within the heavy to very heavy category as defined by the US Department of Labor. Based on maximal effort testing, the reliability of Mr. C is considered acceptable. There were no inconsistencies noted.

Mr. C performed the functional subtests at a generally steady pace. Endurance to the tasks performed was generally fair to good. Flexibility was noted to be good for the upper extremities and good for the lower extremities. Instruction of proper body mechanics was required. Subjective pain complaints were not verbalized. No pain behaviors were observed.

He reports his pain generally being a 0/10.

Reason for Referral:

To set general functional baseline level to determine capabilities of returning to work full duty for entrance into work hardening program prior to returning to work.

Major Limiting Factors:

1. Some minor biomechanical issues with regards to lifting. Patient needs to work on control of items in front of him versus twisting.
2. Mild endurance/deconditioning for heavy work.

Recommendations:

Based on maximal effort testing, the patient demonstrated the ability to perform the following:

1. Unlimited sitting.
2. Unlimited standing.
3. Sit-to-stand as needed.
4. Unlimited community distance walking.
5. Ability to squat lift with weight up to 85 pounds on an occasional basis.
6. Ability to level lift to a height of 48 inches from the floor with weight up to 50 pounds on an occasional basis.
7. Ability to lift to the height of shoulder at 54 inches from the floor with weight up to 50 pounds on an occasional basis.
8. Ability to lift overhead to a height of 76 inches from the floor with weight up to 50 pounds on an occasional basis.
9. Ability to bilateral carry with weight up to 50 pounds over a distance of 500 feet on an occasional basis.
10. Ability to unilaterally carry right and/or left with weight up to 33 pounds on an occasional basis.
11. Ability to generate a static pull force on average of 104 pounds and a static push force on average of 108 pounds.
12. Ability to load a standard cart with weight totaling 280 pounds and then pushes and manipulated over surfaces of tile, carpet and ramps totaling approximately 5000 feet.
13. Ability to stair climb unlimited. Ability to carry 50 pounds up two flights of steps independent with no handrail.
14. Ability to climb a standard A-frame ladder with weight up to 50 pounds and then set the weight at a height of 76 inches from the floor on shelving units and then retrieve.
15. Ability to ascend a 12 foot ladder and perform manual manipulation of tools on the Bennett test (working with nuts, bolts, and screws and transferring from one side of the box to the other).
16. Ability to forward bend on an occasional basis with weight ranging from 15 pounds to 85 pounds.
17. Ability to reach from heights of 24 to 76 inches from the floor with weight ranging from 3 pounds to 50 pounds on an occasional basis.
18. Ability to perform sustained overhead reaching at the Valpar 9. He performed activities from panel 2 to panel 1 and panel 2 to panel 4, which required kneeling and blind manipulation.
19. Unlimited fine motor gripping and grasping.
20. Patient did extremely well during this evaluation. Patient should be able to return to work full duty unrestricted. It is, however, recommended if he chooses to return to work immediately following revisit with physician that he pace himself back into full duty over a month's time. He had worked very aggressively and diligently within the therapy clinic, but the activities there cannot simulate "real world activities." If he does not pace himself appropriately, he will fatigue very quickly and have the potential of burning himself out and therefore put him at risk of injury due to failure of proper body mechanics. If he feels he can pace himself appropriately, then he can enter back into the work force independently and without restrictions.

If he feels he cannot pace himself appropriately, then it is recommended that he enter into a work hardening program on a daily basis for 1 month to advance to more aggressive ballistic activity, lifting and carrying, body mechanics and endurance retraining.

Dr. H., thank you for this referral. If you have any questions or comments, please contact me at (313) 555-5555. My office hours are M, T, Th 7:00 a.m. to 4.00 p.m. Wednesday and Friday from 7:00 a.m. to 2.00 p.m.

Sincerely,

Jon Nettie, PT   cc: R. Y., RN

I. Background Information (provided by participant)

History of Injury:

    a) Injury date: July 26, 2007

    b) Incident resulting in injury: Patient fell off a scaffold at work and landed on his back and head.

    c) Primary region of injury: Thoracic vertebrae fractures with closed head injury. Closed head injury created significant amount of swelling requiring cranial surgery, afterwards an infection set in and a skull prosthetic was then inserted with a regime of antibiotics and the infection was then cleared.

    d) Last date worked: July 26, 2007

    e) Previous treatments: Physical therapy, occupational therapy, and speech therapy

    f) Past medical history: Patient did experience one seizure on October 23, 2008 while in physical therapy. He has not had one since.

    g) Test results: Not applicable

    h) Surgeries: July 27, 2007, November 2007, and August 2008

    i) Medications: OTC meds prn

    j) Next medical follow-up: January 23, 2009

Major Physical Complaints:

None

II. Vocational

    a) Employer: O.S. Construction

    b) Job Title: Construction foreman

    c) Workstation Setup: Commercial

    d) Length of Employment: 17 years

    e) Job Status: Workers' compensation

    f) Vocational Plans: Return to work full duty

Critical Demands:

Oversee all aspects of projects, lifting and carrying with weight up to 50 pounds, lifting overhead with weight up to 25 pounds. Ladder and scaffold work, prolonged standing, walking, kneeling, crawling, and occasional stair climbing.

III. Educational:

Associates degree in architecture.

IV. Social History:

    a) Age: 50 years old

    b) Marital status: Married

V. Musculoskeletal Assessment:

Upper Extremity Status:

Table 18-2 Upper Extremity Status

	R-AROM	R-MMT	L-AROM	L-MMT
Shoulder Flexion	WNL	WNL	WNL	WNL
Extension	WNL	WNL	WNL	WNL
Abduction	WNL	WNL	WNL	WNL
Adduction	WNL	WNL	WNL	WNL
Internal Rotation	WNL	WNL	WNL	WNL
External Rotation	WNL	WNL	WNL	WNL
Horizontal Abduction	WNL	WNL	WNL	WNL
Horizontal Adduction	WNL	WNL	WNL	WNL
Elbow Flexion	WNL	WNL	WNL	WNL
Extension	WNL	WNL	WNL	WNL
Forearm Supination	WNL	WNL	WNL	WNL
Pronation	WNL	WNL	WNL	WNL
Wrist Flexion	WNL	WNL	WNL	WNL
Extension	WNL	WNL	WNL	WNL
Scapular Stabilizers	WNL	WNL	WNL	WNL

UE Sensation: WNL
Edema: None noted

AROM: Cervical spine: Forward bending: WNL
Backward bending: WNL
Rotation (R): WNL
Rotation (L): WNL
Side bending (R): WNL
Side bending (L): WNL

Lower Extremity Status:

Table 18-3 Lower Extremity Status

	R-AROM	R-MMT	L-AROM	L-MMT
Hip Flexion	WNL	WNL	WNL	WNL
Extension	WNL	WNL	WNL	WNL
Adduction	WNL	WNL	WNL	WNL
Abduction	WNL	WNL	WNL	WNL
Internal Rotation	WNL	WNL	WNL	WNL
External Rotation	WNL	WNL	WNL	WNL
Knee Flexion	WNL	WNL	WNL	WNL
Knee Extension	WNL	WNL	WNL	WNL
Dorsiflexion	WNL	WNL	WNL	WNL
Plantarflexion	WNL	WNL	WNL	WNL
Inversion	WNL	WNL	WNL	WNL
Eversion	WNL	WNL	WNL	WNL

LE Sensation: WNL
Balance: Good
Edema: None noted

AROM: Lumbar spine   Forward bending: WNL
Backward bending: WNL
Rotation (R): WNL
Rotation (L): WNL
Side bending (R): WNL
Side bending (L): WNL

FUNCTIONAL CAPACITY EVALUATION SUB-TESTS

1. Spinal Sort: (Please see Table 18-6)

The Spinal Sort was used to assess Mr. C.'s current self-perception.

This is an activity sort using 50 pictures, each of which has a work activity picture and a description of a familiar utensil, tool, device, or implement.

The client sorts the pictures according to his perceived ability to use each item in the sort.

An analysis of Mr. C.'s sort indicates that he views himself as being able to use approximately 84% of the items at a regular rate of speed. See Table 18-6 for a list of functional activities.

He views himself as being able to use approximately 16% of the items in conjunction with a break. See Table 18-6 for a list of functional activities.

He views himself as unable to use approximately 0% of the items.

The display of Mr. C.'s sort indicates that he views his abilities to be within the heavy category as defined by the US Department of Labor. This puts him at the 99th percentile of injured individuals.

2. Sitting:

Test Performance:

Single duration demonstrated: 35 minutes

Pain Rating: (0–10 scale) 0/10
Resting Heart Rate: 68 bpm

Major Limiting Factors:

None

3. Standing:

Test Performance:
Longest duration observed: 75 minutes
Pain Rating: (0–10 scale) 0/10
Resting Heart Rate: 68 bpm

Major Limiting Factors:

None

4. Walking:

Test Performance:
½ mile in 8 minutes and 41 seconds
Pain Rating: (0–10 scale) 0/10
Heart Rate:

> Pre-test: 72 bpm
> Post-test: 98 bpm
> Recovery (one minute after): 81 bpm

Major Limiting Factors:

None

5. Squatting:

Test Performance:

> Repetitive Squat:
> Unloaded: 10/10 full squats completed

Loaded leg lift:

> Occasional: 85 lb.
> Frequent: 43 lb.

Pain Rating: (0–10 scale) 0/10
Heart Rate:

> Pre-test: 81 bpm
> Post-test: 136 bpm

Major Limiting Factors:

Repetitive unloaded: None.
Repetitive loaded: Failure of proper body mechanics with weight greater than 85 pounds. Patient demonstrated use of lifting through the back versus the legs with weight greater than 85 pounds.

6. Lifting:

Isoinertial Lift

      (a) Level Lift: To a height of 48 inches from the floor
           Occasional: 50 lb.
           Frequent: 25 lb.
      (b) Knuckle to shoulder: To a height of 54 inches from the floor
           Occasional: 50 lb.
           Frequent: 25 lb.
      (c) Shoulder to overhead: To a height of 76 inches from the floor
           Occasional: 50 lb.
           Frequent: 25 lb.

Pain Rating: (0–10 scale) 0/10
Heart Rate:

      Pre-test: 88 bpm
      Post-test: 120 bpm

Major Limiting Factors:

None.

7. Carrying:

Test Performance: Bilateral Carry Test

      Occasional: 50 pounds × 500 feet.
      Frequent: 25 pounds × 500 feet

Test Performance: Unilateral Carry Test

Right Hand:	Left Hand:
Occasional: 33 pounds × 20 feet	Occasional: 33 pounds × 20 feet
Frequent: 17 pounds × 20 feet	Frequent: 17 pounds × 20 feet

Pain Rating: (0–10 scale) 0/10
Heart Rate:

      Pre-test: 84 bpm
      Post-test: 128 bpm

Major Limiting Factors:

None

8. Pushing/Pulling:

Test Performance:

Chattilon Dynamometer

Table 18-4 Chattilon Dynamometer

Static Force	Trial 1	Trial 2	Trial 3	Average
Static pull force	102 lb	110 lb	108 lb	104 lb
Static push force	100 lb	110 lb	115 lb	108 lb

Pain Rating: (0–10 scale) 0/10
Transport:

> Type: Cart
> Load amount: 280 pounds
> Distance: 5000 feet

The patient had to load eight 35-pound cinderblocks and then push them over tile, carpet, and ramps.
Pain Rating: (0–10 scale) 0/10

Major Limiting Factors:

None for both

9. Climbing:

Test Performance:
Stairs:

> Client achieved 15 steps with no weight and client achieved 30 steps with 50 pounds.

Pain Rating: (0–10 scale) 0/10
Heart Rate:

> Pre-test: 68 bpm
> Post-test: 98 bpm
> Recovery (One minute after): 72 bpm

Ladder:

> Client achieved 3/3 rungs on an A-frame ladder with 50 pounds. Client achieved standing on the ladder for 10 minutes on a 12-foot A-frame ladder while performing the Bennett test.

Pain Rating: (0–10 scale) 0/10

Major Limiting Factors:

None

10. Forward Bending:

Based on maximal effort testing, patient demonstrated the ability to forward bend on an occasional basis with weight ranging from 15 pounds to 85 pounds on an occasional basis.
Pain Rating: (0–10 scale) 0/10

Major Limiting Factors:

None

11. Reaching:

Based on maximal effort testing, patient demonstrated ability to reach from heights of 24 inches to 76 inches from the floor with weight ranging from 3 pounds to 50 pounds on an occasional basis.
Pain Rating: (0–10 scale) 0/10

Major Limiting Factors:

Sustained overhead reaching at the Valpar 9 from panel 2 to panel 1 focusing on overhead work and then panel 2 to panel 4 focusing on kneeling blind "work." Patient completed this task in 5 minutes and 55 seconds.

12. Hand Function:

Hand Dominance: Right
Test Performance:

Jaymar Pinch Dynamometer - Gross Grasp

Grip Strength

Table 18-5 Grip Strength

Position	Hand Settings	Trial #1	Trial #2	Trial #3	Average	CVs
Narrowest	#1	R = 56 lb L = 75 lb	R = 54 lb L =65 lb	R = 57 lb L = 63 lb	R = 59 lb L = 68 lb	R = 6.0% L = 8.4%
	#2	R = 110 lb L = 103 lb	R = 97 lb L = 97 lb	R = 95 lb L = 97 lb	R =100 lb L = 99 lb	R = 6.6% L = 2.9%
Widest	#3	R = 98 lb L = 100 lb	R = 95 lb L = 98 lb	R = 99 lb L = 95 lb	R = 97 lb L = 98 lb	R = 1.8% L = 2.1%
	#4	R = 100 lb L = 91 lb	R = 97 lb L = 86 lb	R = 94 lb L = 85 lb	R = 97 lb L = 87 lb	R = 2.5% L = 3.0%
	#5	R = 86 lb L = 85 lb	R = 90 lb L = 82 lb	R = 85 lb L = 80 lb	R = 87 lb L = 82 lb	R = 2.5% L = 2.5%

*Pain Rating: (0–10 scale) 0/10; CVs = coefficients of variation

Major Limiting Factors:

None
Comments:

Average for patient's age at:
Position #2: Dominant 113.6 lb, nondominant 101.9 lb

APPENDIX B

Table 18-6 Performance Assessment and Capability Testing (PACT) Spinal Function Sort

#		Able (1)	Restricted (2, 3, 4)			Unable (5)	?
1	Place/Bottle/Floor	1	2	3	4	5	?
3	Push/Pull/Vacuum	1	2	3	4	5	?
5	Place or Retrieve 5# Waist to Eye-Level	1	2	3	4	5	?
7	Lower 10# Eye-Level to Floor	1	2	3	4	5	?
9	Lift 10# Floor to Eye-Level	1	2	3	4	5	?
11	Load 20# Trunk of Auto	1	2	3	4	5	?
13	Unload 20# Trunk of Auto	1	2	3	4	5	?
15	Unload 2 x 10# Trunk of Auto	1	2	3	4	5	?
17	Paint Brush Eye-Level	1	2	3	4	5	?
19	Wash Dishes Sink	1	2	3	4	5	?
21	Light Bulb Overhead	1	2	3	4	5	?
23	Cut Lumber	1	2	3	4	5	?
25	Pour Soap	1	2	3	4	5	?
27	Load/Unload Dish Washer	1	2	3	4	5	?
29	Push Heavy Door	1	2	3	4	5	?
31	Pull Heavy Door	1	2	3	4	5	?
33	Carry 10# Stool	1	2	3	4	5	?
35	Carry 20# Groceries	1	2	3	4	5	?
37	Climb Stepladder	1	2	3	4	5	?
39	Sweep Push Broom	1	2	3	4	5	?
41	Lower 50# Crate Eye-Level to Floor	1	2	3	4	5	?
43	Lift 50# Crate Eye-Level to Floor	1	2	3	4	5	?

#		Able (1)	Restricted (2, 3, 4)			Unable (5)	?
2	Retrieve/Tool/Floor	1	2	3	4	5	?
4	Push/Pull Shopping Cart	1	2	3	4	5	?
6	Place or Retrieve 5# Waist to Overhead	1	2	3	4	5	?
8	Lower 10# Crate Bench to Floor	1	2	3	4	5	?
10	Lift 10# Crate Floor to Bench	1	2	3	4	5	?
12	Lower 20# Crate Eye-Level to Floor	1	2	3	4	5	?
14	Lift 20# Crate Floor to Eye-Level	1	2	3	4	5	?
16	Lift 20# Box Floor to Bench	1	2	3	4	5	?
18	Hammer Nails	1	2	3	4	5	?
20	Trim Face-Place	1	2	3	4	5	?
22	Install Face-Plate	1	2	3	4	5	?
24	Pull Nail	1	2	3	4	5	?
26	Move Barrel with Dolly	1	2	3	4	5	?
28	Dig with Shovel	1	2	3	4	5	?
30	Get into Driver's Seat	1	2	3	4	5	?
32	Get out of Driver's Seat	1	2	3	4	5	?
34	Carry 30# Bucket	1	2	3	4	5	?
36	Carry 10# Groceries x 2	1	2	3	4	5	?
38	Carry 20# Bucket Up Stepladder	1	2	3	4	5	?
40	Sweep Kitchen Broom	1	2	3	4	5	?
42	Lower 50# Crate Bench to Floor	1	2	3	4	5	?
44	Lift 50# Tool Box Floor to Bench	1	2	3	4	5	?

(continues)

Table 18-6 Performance Assessment and Capability Testing (PACT) Spinal Function Sort *(continued)*

#		Able (1)	Restricted (2, 3, 4)			Unable (5)	?
45	Lower 100# Crate Eye-Level to Floor	1	2	3	4	5	?
46	Lower 100# Crate Bench to Floor	1	2	3	4	5	?
47	Lift 100# Crate Floor to Eye-Level	1	2	3	4	5	?
48	Lift 100# Crate Floor to Bench	1	2	3	4	5	?
49	Paintbrush Eye-Level	1	2	3	4	5	?
50	Place or Retrieve 5# Waist to Overhead	1	2	3	4	5	?

Section 1 Total

(4x)	(3x)	(2x)	(1x)	

Section 2 Total

(4x)	(3x)	(2x)	(1x)	RPC	% tile

Dis	Dk	Int
0 - 2	0 - 3	1
0 - 2	4+	2
3 - 4	na	3
5+	na	4

Name: _____
Date: _____   ER: _____

FCE at:	PDC Sedentary	PDC Light	PDC Medium	PDC Heavy	PDC Very Heavy
RPC Score:	100 - 110	125 - 135	165 - 175	180 - 190	196+

Source: Courtesy of Leonard Matheson, PhD, EPIC Rehab, Chesterfield, MO.

APPENDIX C

Physical Demand Characteristics of Work

Table 18-7 Physical Demand Characteristics of Work

Physical Demand Level	Occasional (0–33% of the Workday)	Frequent (34–66% of the Workday)	Constant (67–100% of the Workday)	Typical Energy Required
Sedentary	10 lbs	Negligible	Negligible	1.5–2.1 METS
Light	20 lbs	10 lbs and/or walk/stand/push/ pull of arm/leg controls	Negligible and/or push/pull of arm/ leg controls while seated	2.2–3.5 METS
Medium	20–50 lbs	10–25 lbs	10 lbs	3.6–6.3 METS
Heavy	50–100 lbs	25–50 lbs	10–20 lbs	6.4–7.5 METS
Very heavy	Over 100 lbs	Over 50 lbs	Over 20 lbs	Over 7.5 METS

Source: Courtesy of Leonard Matheson, PhD, EPIC Rehab, Chesterfield, MO.

APPENDIX D

Job Site Evaluation

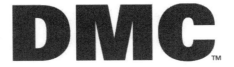

DMC™ Rehabilitation Institute of Michigan

Source: Courtesy of Rehabilitation Institute of Michigan/The Detroit Medical Center.

March 19, 2008

Job Site Evaluation   **A. B.**
Physician: Dr. J. B.
Diagnosis: Low back pain
Insurance: Workers' Compensation
Case Manager: B. B., RN
Railroad Safety Manager: D. C.

This evaluation was completed at American National Rail Road, Appalachian Railway.

The client is to carry his grip bag, weighing anywhere from 20–60 pounds over gravel and dirt surfaces. The surfaces may be extremely uneven and loose. Approaching the train engine, the client may put one bag up on the train while reaching up overhead and he will then carry the remainder of his bags up to the front of the engine and carry them up the stairs. He will climb up onto the engine and retrieve his grip along the engineer side of the engine.

He sits in a chair of good ergonomic design. It has lumbar support that provides the appropriate support for the low back. The large engine chair swivels to the left, which allows for better access to the controls.

He will have to access the engine and walk to the back and around to the conductor side of the train to work the hand brake. This will take anywhere between 30 to 50 rotations of the brake wheel. While doing so, he needs to brace his lower abdominals during this activity in order to maximize his stability and minimize his symptoms.

On the Grand Trunk Engine, chairs do not swivel excessively due to an arm pad located to the left of the seat, up under the window. This arm pad is along the side of the wall. The chair does not give sufficient support to the low back if the engineer needs to locate or swivel in the chair to operate the controls. The hand brake, however, is located at the front of the engine on the conductor side and is a ratchet style. The ratchet style hand brake can require between 30 and 50 pumps in order to lock the train into position. If there is room on the deck of the train, two hands can be used, as well as squatting. The employee could turn slightly and switch hands to prevent fatigue static positioning to one side.

While riding in the engine, the employee is responsible for hooking up train cars to the engine. As the trains connect, there is some "jarring." The engine idles at rest. The idling creates some vibratory bouncing in the chairs. The range of forces generated can vary based on the amount of cars to be hooked. Additionally, when the engine starts to initiate movement forward there will be varying degrees of force put on the engine and with the cab itself, creating some additional jarring forces.

The engineer primarily sits in the engine, but does not leave it unless he has to switch out his crew. However, if there is a major emergency, he will leave the engine and have to work on cranking down the hand brakes. The conductor is the employee who has to do the most manual duties with some help from stationmasters.

It would benefit the patient to receive a Saunders lumbar support. This will give him maximum support, as well as maintaining his flexibility to continue to perform his activities.

At this point, he has performed other activities independently and with good body and lifting mechanics. There are no significant complaints of discomfort. He should be able to perform all the above-mentioned duties unrestricted and full, acting only as an engineer (i.e., only driving the train and occasionally applying a hand brake). When he reaches a destination, it is beneficial if he stands up and stretches into backward bending and rotation to the right, since the majority of his positioning is in sitting and with rotation to the left.

Based on the patient's progression within the clinic, job site analysis and review of the doctor's evaluation, it is recommended that the client return back to full duty in conjunction with a lumbar support. He should be able to maintain the job based on the job description as discussed with the train yard desk manager. As long as he uses proper body mechanics, stretching, and the lumbar support, he should be able to return back to work position unrestricted.

PLAN: Continue the work hardening x1 week and plan for discharge with release back to work. Patient may benefit from continuation of work hardening for at least 2 to 4 weeks following the return back to work, to manage any symptoms that may occur while performing prolonged activities and getting reacclimated to the job.

Dr. B., thank you for this referral. If you have any questions or comments, please contact me at (313) 555-5555. My office hours are M, T, Th 7:00 a.m. to 4.00 p.m., Wednesday and Friday from 7:00 a.m. to 2.00 p.m.

Sincerely,
Jon Nettie, PT
Source: Courtesy of Rehabilitation Institute of Michigan/Detroit Medical Center

APPENDIX E

Ergonomic Design for the Work and Home Office
Source: Courtesy of Back Designs Inc., Novato, California. The ergonomic chair (see additional information at http://www.backdesigns.com/store/How-to-fit-an-ergonomic-chair-W9C230.aspx).

Recommended Use:

Since different individuals have different types of body styles and sitting postures, a chair must be designed appropriately for the individual and their functional needs.

A. Vision:
   An individual's vision during different activities may affect their sitting posture. Sometimes raising a computer screen or using a slant board or copy holder can help solve sitting problems better than a chair.

B. Seat height:
   The seat of a chair should support the individual's thighs evenly while their feet and legs rest comfortably on the floor, foot rest, or knee rest. In a traditional office chair, the seat's front edge height should match the length of the lower leg (popliteal height). Most office chairs have a height adjustment. If an individual is short in stature and is given a standard chair, using a foot rest, foot platform, or foot ring may be appropriate. This is only for upright and reclined tasks. Foot rests generally don't work for forward tasks since they may constrain postures and increase slumping.

C. Foot depth:
   An individual must allow 1–3 inches of space behind the knees to avoid excessive pressure. Use a deeper seat for reclining, and a shallower seat for activities that require forward sitting. Larger individuals will prefer a larger surface for weight distribution.

D. Seat width:
   The conventional seat should be at least two inches wider than the individual's thighs. Remember, the seat width can affect armrest width.

E. Seat tilt:
   Most people prefer a forward tilting seat for forward sitting, a nearly horizontal seat for upright sitting, and a backward tilting seat for reclining. Some chairs offer a "free float" seat tilting, which adjusts automatically with your body weight shifting.

F. Seat cushion:
   To help distribute one's weight better, a seat with a contour, extra padding, or variable density upholstery materials is an option. Less contoured or firmer seats will allow an individual to move easier in the seat.

G. Backrest height:
   A backrest will depend on the amount of activity that an individual is engaging in. For reclining, the backrest should reach the upper back or neck depending on how far the person reclines. For upright sitting, the backrest only needs to support the low back and perhaps the upper back. For forward activity, support for the low back is sufficient although some people prefer no back support at all.

H. Backrest height adjustment:
   Backrest contour should match the placement of the spinal curves. Women sometimes need higher lumbar backrest placement and lower upper back and neck rest placement than men. The backrests on most chairs are height adjustable.

I. Backrest pivot:
   The backrest may pivot forward and back on a central axis. This will allow for greater movement in the low back and the upper back. This, however, may be uncomfortable if spinal flexibility is limited. Most of today's office chairs do not have the backrest pivot.

J. Seat to backrest angle:
   An individual's thigh-torso angle will influence their spinal posture. One must match their neutral thigh torso posture to their chair. By having appropriate adjustments, the individual

will be able to maintain a neutral spine posture that will keep the low back comfortable. For example, the low back curve deepens into an arch as your thigh torso angle opens when you reach overhead. On the other hand, the low back flattens as your thigh torso angle closes (e.g., sitting on a low stool).

K. Adjustment controls:
   All adjustment controls should be within easy reach from a sitting position. This is important for seat and backrest tilt controls.

L. Armrest height:
   Armrests should be used to support the arms, not to support the body. Armrests are used for upright and reclined sitting neck and back fatigue, and ease back and leg loads when entering and exiting the chair. Some office chairs have adjustable armrests. Armrests are not always recommended for computer data entry. The more active the task (e.g., intense data entry), there is less necessity for the armrest. The less active the task (intermittent data entry), there is more necessity for the arm support.

M. Armrest depth:
   Armrest for reclined or non-desk activities should support the entire forearm. For desk work, the armrest should be recessed to allow for easy access to the work surface. Support of just the elbow may be sufficient.

N. Distance between armrest:
   A correctly placed armrest may take some of the stress of the neck and back and helps the individual get in and out of the chair more efficiently. An armrest that is narrow interferes with arm movement and an armrest that is too wide is not used for full rest or support. Some chairs have an adjustable armrest width.

O. Swivel:
   A chair that swivels will allow the individual to move efficiently at his work station. They will be able to change their reach and line of vision with less body twisting. If the individual does precise or fine motor work, a swivel chair may cause them to feel unstable.

P. Base:
   A large diameter base provides greater stability. If the individual prefers a chair that tilts far back or sits at high counter heights, a large base will be much more important.

Q. Gliders and casters:
   Carpet casters are standard on most chairs. They are useful for moving forward and away from the table or desk. Use hard casters for carpet, use soft casters for hard (e.g., wood or tile) floors. Glides and braking casters are used for special applications. See article on casters at http://www.backdesigns.com/store/Chair-casters-can-affect-your-health-W43C230.aspx.

R. Upholstery:
   Upholstery depends on the manufacturer. Most seats and back rests are made of high-density foam to give years of comfort under normal use. Most chairs are covered with nylon or a blended fabric. Upholstery costs increase as you move into leather or leather-based materials.

THE ERGONOMIC OFFICE

Source: Courtesy of Back Designs, Inc., Novato, CA (see updated information at http://www.backdesigns.com/store/The-homemade-ergonomic-office-W56C132.aspx).

Most individuals who work in an office setting are "given" a desk and the equipment needed to perform the job. This does not necessarily have to limit an individual into a locked position based on the amount of space technology, or funds available. Changing some of the placements of the items that are used in an individual's daily occupation can help decrease tension, chronic pain complaints, and daily aches and pain. The following suggestions on areas to pay attention to and their solutions may be helpful.

1. Computer Screen:

A. Screen too low?
   A low screen may force one's head into a forward and down position, thus straining the neck and upper back. **Easy solution:** Put the screen on top of a phone book, a sturdy box,

or on top of the CPU (the main computer). **Money solution:** A monitor valet allows for easy positioning of the screen, forward and back and up and down. It will help free up valuable desk space. Prices range from $25 to several hundred dollars.

B. Screen too high?

This forces the head to tilt back and the chin to move forward, thus straining the neck and possibly causing headaches.

Easy solution: Place the computer screen directly on the desk rather than on top of a phone book or CPU. **Money solution:** Extension cables to help relocate the CPU some distance from the screen may help. Floor CPU units will help free up desk space. Floor stands are priced $25 and up. Extension cables are priced at $10 and up.

C. Screen distance?

The best distance from which to read a computer screen is generally much greater than reading distances for papers and books. Typical distances for reading from a paper or book is from 15″ to 25″. Computer screens should be much farther away, sometimes 30″ or more.

Maximum viewing distance: First of all, there is no maximum viewing distance. As long as you can comfortably discern the information on the screen it's not too far away. Maximum viewing distance is limited only by the size and clarity of the characters on the screen. Guidelines that specify a viewing distance of, say, 24″ to 30″ have no basis for the 30″. The "arm's-length" recommendation has even less basis—there is no correlation between visual capability and arm length.

Minimum viewing distance: How close is too close depends on your Resting Point of Vergence (RPV). That's the distance at which your eyes converge with no stimulus for convergence, like in the dark. Studies show that people with far Resting Points of Vergence are less able to tolerate close viewing distances. People with short RPVs have no problem with farther viewing distances.

The RPV averages about 45″ looking straight ahead and about 35″ at a 30° downward gaze angle. Someone with an RPV of 15″ might not have a problem with a 15″ viewing distance which would cause eyestrain for someone with an RPV of 50″. We commonly see inadequate distance between a computer user and a CRT monitor, often between 18″–30″.

Get the monitor back as far as possible, depending on your visual abilities, the screen display characteristics and your software interface. If possible, you should also lower it and tip it back so the top of the screen is farther from your eyes than the bottom of the screen.

Most desktop surfaces are too shallow for proper placement of a conventional CRT monitor. CRT monitors require a deeper desk, or the monitor needs to extend over the back edge of the desk, or you'll need to place your monitor on a separate table placed behind your desk. In an office setting, two workers could place their desks back-to-back, with each worker's monitor placed on the other worker's desk.

Flat panel monitors allow more distant placement of the computer screen on shallow desks.

Don't overlook other factors, such as glare, luminance balance, screen contrast, mental stress, and refraction. Some people need corrective eyeglasses or a different prescription for more comfortable viewing.

See http://www.backdesigns.com/store/Monitor-Positioning-Guidelines-W22C132.aspx for updated information.

D. Screen glare problems?

Glare may make the screen difficult to see and fatigue the eyes. It may also lead to headaches. Glare from a window overhead can make it difficult to see the displays. If a window or light source is behind the screen, the screen contrast becomes too dark to see. **Easy solution:** Reorient the screen so that it is perpendicular to the light source. Fashion a screen shade or hood from cardboard and tape, being careful not to cover the screen ventilation holes. Vertical blinds can let in natural light while shading direct sunlight. **Money solution:** If one is unable to reorient the screen to avoid the glare or change the light source, a glare screen or hood is recommended. These are priced at $50 and up.

2. Wrist Rest:

If a desk has edges that irritate the wrists and forearms, a wrist rest is recommended. A wrist rest can also possibly relieve aches and fatigue in the hands, arms, shoulders, and neck by increasing the support of the wrists and hands. A wrist rest will also help maintain a neutral posture in the wrists and arms.

Wrist rests are not for everyone. Generally, they are best used to rest upon when you pause between keystrokes, not while you are actively keying. Also, be certain that the wrist rest does not force you to reach uncomfortably far to access your keyboard. You may need a wrist rest if the hard edges of your desk irritate your wrists and forearms. For some, wrist rests can also relieve aches and fatigue in your hands, arms, shoulders, and neck by increasing the support to your arms. Some people also use wrist rests to help maintain neutral postures in the wrist and arms. Be conscious of your overall function while in the chair. Fixating the arms or wrists may lead to increased strain in the small structures of the hands and in the neck and upper back.

Easy solution: Fold a hand towel to the same height as the keyboard. The towel may be taped to the desk so that it does not slip or fold. You may want to change the towel weekly because it will tend to compact and collect dirt and body oils. Additionally, most keyboards have legs in the back that can also change the angle of the wrist position. It is recommended that for one-third of the day, the legs be up, for another third of the day, the legs be down, and for another third of the day, a small increment of about 1/4 inch be placed at the front part of the keyboard to tilt the keypad up at the front. **Money solution:** Purchase a standard forearm support. These are priced at $15–$100.

3. Data Entry:

Reading and writing on a flat surface will tend to put a posture of forward head, rotation, and side bending to one side. The majority of the time this is done to the nondominant side. Prolonged use in this area may cause neck and upper back problems. **Easy solution:** Prop a clipboard at an angle against a thick book. The bottom edge of the clipboard may need to be taped so that it does not slide. **Money solution:** A copy holder that is upright or angled can be purchased in various sizes to hold from a single page up to a book. Copy holders are priced at $19–$200.

4. Desk:

A. Desk too high?
A desk that is too high will usually cause a person to raise their chair height, which allows their feet to dangle and not touch the ground. This may allow one to feel unbalanced and compromise circulation in the feet. Furthermore, a desk that is too high may allow one to shrug their shoulders to reach the desk, straining the neck and upper back. **Easy solution:** Cut down the legs on the desk if possible. If not, the chair needs to be raised and a footrest needs to be established. A small step stool, a sturdy box, or a number of old phone books all make a good footrest. A footrest with increased surface area is best because it allows for an ease in foot placement underneath the desk. **Money solution:** Most office chairs have a pneumatic lift that adjusts the chair's height. A commercial footrest that angles and has a height adjustment will range in price from $30–$200. Additionally, a keyboard valet that lowers the keyboard may help with input and prevent the need of getting a chair that adjusts up, thereby eliminating the footrest.

B. Desk too low?
A desk that is too low can force a person to slump or strain their entire back. The ideal desk is one that is just at or just above the elbow height. However, if much writing is done, the desk should be slightly higher than the elbow crease. For keyboard entry, the desk should be slightly lower than the elbow. Ideally, the person should fit their chair first before they fit the desk height. **Easy solution:** Place wood blocks under each of the desk legs. Stock lumber may already be at the correct height to maintain the proper height of the deck. Add layers as needed to adjust to the proper height. **Money solution:** Off-the-shelf desk raising devices are available. They are easy to install and fit most desks. They range in price at $30–$100.

5. Chair:

A. Chair too low?

Sitting on a seat that is too low forces one to move into a forward head posture or slump position. This may strain the neck and upper back. Having a seat at the correct height will allow the feet to rest comfortably on the floor with the thighs and buttocks evenly and fully supported. **Easy solution:** Put a folded beach towel or slab of foam underneath the seat and secure it with tape. **Money solution:** Fabric covered seat cushions and wedges range in price from $15–$200.

B. Uncomfortable backrest?

The backrest on a chair should naturally follow the body contours. If it does not, it may tend to force the individual into a forward head or slumped posture causing strain on the neck and upper back. **Easy solution:** Roll a hand towel into a comfortable diameter and tape it accordingly. Then secure it to the back of the chair at a height that fits the small of the back. A small pillow could also be used. **Money solution:** There are severe portable lumbar supports commercially available with special straps for attachment. These range in price from $20–$200.

C. Chair seat too long?

When the chair seat is too long the knees cannot be properly positioned at a 90 degree fashion to allow the feet to sit comfortable on the floor. This forces the individual to slouch and strain the low back unless they are sitting at the edge of the chair seat. Sitting at the edge of the chair seat may cause fatigue and strain into the low back. **Easy solution:** Place a filler between the back and the chair's backrest. This can be a seat cushion, pillow, or towel. It should be the same thickness as the seat is long and can be padded to match the contours of the low back. **Money solution:** There are portable back supports commercially available that combine both space filler and contours for the back. They range in price from $20–$200.

D. Ergonomic seating:

See "Staying Healthy at Work/Home" handout on the following page for specifics on what makes a good ergonomically designed chair.

6. Mouse:

A. Too much mouse movement?

Using a mouse requires repetitive shoulder and finger movements, which can irritate the shoulder, neck, and wrist areas. **Easy solution:** Switch to a trackball control. Using the trackball allows the individual to roll the fingers and the palm of the hand, allowing for easier and more fluid motions than the mouse. Additionally when using a trackball control, a wrist support is needed as when used in keyboard entry. The speed of the mouse may also be increased and there may be a loss of precision control with trackball use. This is useful if the individual works on a large or wide screen monitor. Some software packages help control the speed and some have a "ballistic gain" feature built in which causes the pointer to move farther when the mouse is moved faster.

B. Hard to reach mouse?

The shoulder and neck can be strained if the individual has to reach too far for the mouse. Frequent movement between the mouse and keyboard can also cause excessive strain. **Easy solution:** Switch to a trackball control. There is less shoulder movement and less reach is needed. Additionally, the mouse can be moved closer to the keyboard. This may be a problem if the keyboard sits in a tray, which has no room for a mouse. A small keyboard platform may also have accommodation for a mouse or a trackball.

C. Clicking difficulty?

Repeated button clicking can lead to arm and finger fatigue and pain. This is evident in high incidences of data entry. **Easy solution:** Switch to a mouse or trackball that requires less force to activate a button (example: Microsoft mouse). Additionally, the mouse can be set up so that the hands are alternated for use. Furthermore, a pointing device or software with a drag lock feature such as Mac Power Click software or Kensington Thinking Mouse can be used. These devices allow you to click on an object and the computer software holds the object for you without having to keep the button depressed.

D. Pointing device size?

The pointing device can be too big or too small depending on the size of one's hands. This can cause strain on the ring or pinkie fingers. For persons having small hands, a pointing device wider than 2–4 inches or a three-button pointing device may be too large. **Easy solution:** If a smaller pointing device is needed, try switching to a narrower profile mouse or a pointing pen. Additionally, one may switch to a trackball control. Furthermore, if a pointing device is used, try not to keep the hand on it when not in use.

E. Rest:

Repetitive extension of the fingers and hands or continuous holding of the fingers and hands suspended over the pointing device can lead to elbow, forearm, and shoulder fatigue and soreness, which may also lead to an exacerbation of neck pain. **Easy solution:** Rest the fingers gently on the pointing device to take the load off the hand and tendons. Additionally, use a forearm rest or wrist rest to take pressure off and put the hand in a more neutral position.

STAYING HEALTHY AT WORK/HOME

According to the U.S. Bureau of Labor statistics, nearly 2,000,000 workers become injured simply by sitting at their desks. Posture, repetitive motions, and office equipment positioning are among the factors that cause these accumulative trauma disorders. Workplace injuries are not inevitable and workers can be safe if these few easy guidelines are followed:

1. **Posture:**
   - When viewing the computer screen, make sure the head is upright and that the top of the screen is at eye level.
   - The shoulders should be in a relaxed position.
   - The arms should be close to the side and relaxed in a comfortable position, preferably resting on an armrest.
   - The elbows should be bent at a 100° angle and resting on an armrest when using a keyboard.
2. **Keyboard/Pointing Device:**
   - The home roll key should be positioned-directed in the center of the trunk of the body: The keyboard height and slope should adjust easily to allow the wrist to be in a slightly flexed position for 1/3 of the day, a neutral position for 1/3 of the day, and a slightly extended position for 1/3 of the day.
   - The pointing device should be within close reach and at the same level as the keyboard and may be alternated from right to left.
3. **Chair:**
   - The chair height should be adjusted so that the feet are flat on the floor.
   - Hips should be as far back in the chair as possible but not so as to compromise the back of the knee to induce circulation discomfort.
   - The chair back should support the lower back and upper back depending on the type of work being done at the desk.
   - The backrest height should be adjusted to provide maximum support.
   - The seat should be long enough and wide enough to support the hips and thighs to distribute the weight appropriately.
   - The chair should have armrests so that the arms can rest comfortably.
   - The chair height should be adjusted slightly at approximately 1/4–1/2 inch above the 90° hip position and below the 90° hip position to provide change throughout the day.
4. **Computer screen:**
   - The top of the screen should be slightly below eye level.

- The screen should be at the proper tilt and height so that it can be viewed without raising or lowering the chin.
- The screen should be approximately an arm's reach away.
- Documents should be placed on stands beside the monitor repositioned from right to left throughout the day.
- If there is a glare problem, move the monitor out of the path of the light source or get a glare screen.

5. Lighting:
- Sufficient light should be provided so that reading tasks can be done without straining the eyes.
- The screen should be glare-free from windows, lights, and services. Make appropriate changes as noted above under the computer screen.

In addition to changing the equipment into ergonomically designed positions to ease stress on the body, clients also need to stretch their joints and muscles that become shortened and tightened. Here are a few quick stretches that can be done at work. These exercises are to be repeated 1–3 times every 1–2 hours while working.

1. Neck stretch:
- Tilt the ear toward the shoulder and reach up while touching the top of the head with the palm of the hand. Hold for 10 seconds. Repeat 2–3 times on both sides.

2. Overhead reach:
- Take a deep breath and gently reach over your head with both arms. Hold for a few seconds, exhaling while lowering the arms slowly. Repeat 2–3 times.

3. Shoulder pinch:
- Place the arms behind the head. Relax the shoulders and squeeze the shoulder blades together. Keep the shoulders back and down, holding for 5 seconds. Repeat 2–3 times.

4. Chair rotation stretch:
- Sitting in the chair, wrap the feet around the chair legs. Reach behind the body, grab the back of the chair, and pull gently to increase a stretch into the midback. Hold for 5–10 seconds. Repeat 2–3 times.

5. Forearm stretch:
- Hold the arms straight at waist height and face the fingers up. Hold the fingers and stretch the wrist back. Make sure the fingers and thumbs are kept together. Hold for 5–10 seconds. Repeat 2–3 times.
- Repeat this by stretching into a downward motion of the wrist and hands as well.

6. Promote change:
- Every so often the client must stand up and move around and walk to allow change in the body from a prolonged sitting position. Purposely place the printer and other peripherals away from the desk to encourage the client to get up, move, and walk about.

APPENDIX F

Ten Tips for an Ergonomic Workstation
Source: Courtesy of Back Designs, Inc., Novato, California.

1. Place the monitor directly in front and center of the user.
2. Place the monitor at a distance of more than 16 inches from the user and no more than an arm's length away. The viewing angle should be between 0 and 18 degrees.
3. Keep the CPU within arm's reach, but off of the work surface.
4. Place the work surface at a height that allows legs to fit comfortably underneath with feet flat on the floor. Use a footrest if needed.
5. Keyboard should be located at a height that allows the worker to key with the upper arms hanging relaxed on the shoulders.

6. Elbows should be roughly at right angles to allow the wrist to be fairly straight.
7. Keyboard should be at a slightly negative tilt (bottom row is tilted up towards the ceiling).
8. Place the pointing device (mouse) at the same height as the keyboard and as close to the keyboard as possible.
9. Always maintain contact with the backrest of the chair to minimize back discomfort.
10. Take various 20-second to 2-minute rest periods between regularly scheduled breaks. This allows for improved circulation and nutrition waste exchange.

APPENDIX G

Ergonomic Assessment Report

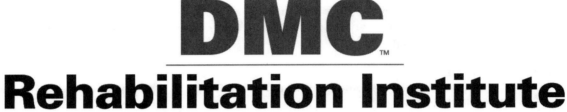

Source: Courtesy of Rehabilitation Institute of Michigan/The Detroit Medical Center.

December 5, 2008
Ergonomic Assessment Report   **H. I.**
Physician: Dr. F. M.
Diagnosis: Thoracolumbar strain
Insurance: PPOM

Subjective:

The patient stated that back on May 14, 2008, she was pulling a bag of landscaping rocks out of the front of her car. She set them down on the ground and started to drag them to the garage. Not wanting to leave scratch marks on the concrete, she lifted the bag and carried it into the garage in a hunched position. She stated that she began to feel pain the following morning. The early pain was manageable, however, by May 20, 2008, it went to the low back and right flank area. This pain was so bad that she had her husband take her to the emergency room. On May 22, 2008, the patient returned back to the emergency room secondary to her pain symptoms being much more intense than on May 20, 2008. She underwent occupational and physical therapy from the end of May through July, for treatment of low back pain. She stated that therapy helped moderately. She was discharged from occupational and physical therapy and then went to a chiropractor from August to November of 2005.

She underwent an MRI in September 2008, which was negative. She went back to her primary care physician and occupational and physical therapy was reinstated. She started this on October 10, 2008, and is currently attending therapy.

She is still moving considerably slower and continues to complain of significant weakness and pain while engaging in functional activities. The majority of her symptoms are currently on the side of her body. She notes an increase of symptoms while at home and in the work setting.

Objective:

Functional Assessment: A functional assessment was done to assess the functional activities that occur in her workplace. Assessing the functional workplace activities will allow for postural changes to ease symptoms and maximize productivity in the workplace. This will help by conserving energy and the ability to perform household activities once returning home following her workday. Minimizing her symptoms and maximizing her functional capacity will facilitate home- and work-related activities so that she is not sedentary and involved in a cyclic pain pattern.

The patient works while seated in a chair with a poor ergonomic design; for example the chair has no adjustable armrests or seat tilt and height adjustment. The seat back tension is on the lowest setting, which causes the chair to recline, giving minimal low and upper back support, as well as forcing the patient to move forward in her chair. In other words, she has no support while seated. Additionally, the seat depth is too long, which produces compressive forces along the popliteal area (back of the knee), and if she sits fully back into the chair, it causes an excessive posterior pelvic tilt and a forward head posture. The patient currently uses a towel for lumbar support.

When performing data entry, she does not have proper elbow support, which will cause shoulder elevation and shoulder and neck strain over time. She tends to move into a slouched position, increasing postural strain due to the seat depth (too deep) and use of a towel roll. In order to accommodate for her current injury (e.g., difficulty reaching on the right), she has moved the mouse to the left side. She has to reach out to manipulate the mouse on the tabletop. Once she switched the mouse to the left side it was still on a right-handed configuration. Through the control panel, the mouse function was switched to a left-handed configuration with a right click. She can practice using the new mouse setup under accessories and in the utility files. The current keyboard tray does not have a mouse attachment.

The monitor is a 12-inch monitor and is set approximately 12 inches away from her seated work position. The height is at an appropriate level as she works in her chair. The monitor is slightly too far away, which can cause forward head posturing due to eyestrain since she wears contacts.

The patient performs a significant amount of data input. She completes writing tasks on the left side of the computer. She has to perform writing activities, as well as data input while following items off of a worksheet. This puts her into an abnormal posture. She has to reach to the right and to the number keyboard, as well as rotate and laterally flex to read the computer screen. This is all in conjunction with mousing, as well as working on spreadsheets and other computer tasks.

She has a need to access binders from an overhead bin and from a tall file cabinet. This creates excessive pain, especially as she reaches for objects. Due to her pain, she reports weakness and difficulty reaching and pulling items overhead.

The patient does have a roller mat.

Risk Factors:

1. Poor ergonomically designed chair. No adjustable armrest, no significant back adjustments, seat depth too large, no seat tilt, no significant lumbar/thoracic support.
2. Computer monitor too far away.
3. Poor posture when performing data entry.
4. Overhead lifting and reaching to grasp for binders.
5. Poor position of the mouse requiring excessive reach.

Correct Recommendations:

Consult with an ergonomic office supply company. Here the patient can be properly fitted for a chair that fits all of the needs of the patient. The chair should include a proper seat depth, seat height adjustment, seat tilt, back adjustment (which can lock at varying degrees of angle), adjustable armrest (to move up and down and in and out), and casters to allow for rolling on the current floor mats. A proper chair will allow for better support during work-related activities while decreasing postural strain.

1. The monitor, which is too far away, has been drawn 6 inches closer to allow for less postural strain; especially as the day wears on and her contacts may be difficult to use due to

the dryness of her office. She requires wetting drops intermittently to prevent tackiness and haziness of her eyes by the end of her work shift. If the wetting drops do not help, then an antiglare screen is recommended since the workstation is directly underneath fluorescent lights.

2. When performing data entry, she must switch desk work from the right to the left side of the computer every couple of hours. Additionally, she needs to turn the monitor to approximately a 45-degree angle to reduce strain on her neck while performing data entry. She also needs to bring the mouse over to the side that she is working. With the highly repetitive nature of shifting from side to side, a cordless mouse may be purchased. This will allow for an ease in transfer ability of the mouse from position to position. Also, the cordless mouse can put her in the most optimal posture needed to perform mousing activities. The computer is a bit older and therefore may need to be upgraded to accommodate a standard cordless mouse. Additionally, with the data input, it is recommended that she use a paper stand. This could be moved from side to side when she switches the mouse positions as well. A view stand also may be needed where it can be set up in front of her cube and not allow for any rotational motion as she views documents versus spreadsheets.

3. Binders should be moved from off the high file cabinet and brought over to the overhead bin. There is less of a reach with the overhead bin and she should be able to manage them at her desktop easier than worrying about reaching overhead and carrying them to her workstation. She would need to move the "blank checks" binder to the file cabinet located to the right of her overhead bin and notify appropriate personnel of the new location.

Since the patient has a significant amount of pain complaints and weakness, it is difficult for her to turn the monitor herself. Therefore, she is going to use a device 15 inches or longer (e.g., ruler) and her body weight as leverage to turn the screen from right to left; for example, cutting a dowel rod or broom handle at least 24 inches in length will facilitate this activity and minimize her symptoms while grasping, pushing, and pulling the monitor.

Assessment:

With the patient's continued pain complaints it is recommended that she continue with occupational and physical therapy. Additional scapular progressive resistive exercises (PREs) and continuation of Feldenkrais and stretching may be continued.

Plan:

Continue occupational and physical therapy, progressing as tolerated. Recommend implementation of the corrective recommendations to help minimize symptoms within the workplace. By minimizing work symptoms it will allow for conservation of energy and improved performance of functional activities at work and at home.

Dr. F. M., thank you for this referral. If you have any questions or comments, please contact me at (313) 555-5555. My office hours are M, T, Th 7:00 a.m. to 4.00 p.m., Wednesday and Friday from 7:00 a.m. to 2.00 p.m.

Sincerely,

Jon Nettie, PT

APPENDIX H

Job Coaching Report

DMC™
Rehabilitation Institute of Michigan

Source: Courtesy of Rehabilitation Institute of Michigan/The Detroit Medical Center.

December 13, 2008

Job Coaching Report	**G.S.**
Physician:	Dr. M. U.
Diagnosis:	Rhabdomyolitis
Insurance:	DMC Care
Supervisor:	Ms. M.

Background Information:

The patient is a 46-year-old female who works at Harper Hospital as a lactation nurse. Several months ago she started noticing symptoms of increasing fatigue, muscle weakness, and muscle pain, as well as an antalgic gait pattern. She went to her family doctor regarding these symptoms. Her primary care physician thought it might be due to the new anti-seizure medication that she was on. The primary care physician sent her to a neurologist who was unsure of her symptoms, but definitely said that it was not the seizure medication Topamax. She was then sent to a rheumatologist who thought it might be lupus. After the test came back negative for lupus, she went to a second rheumatologist who felt that it was from the new cholesterol medication that she was on. The cholesterol medication was stopped and her symptoms ceased to progress.

The patient has undergone occupational and physical therapy in the past. She was attending therapy at the Rehabilitation Institute of Michigan (RIM) for approximately eight weeks until her medical insurance was exhausted. She is now under the care of her primary care physician and is attending outpatient occupational and physical therapy.

She states that she is about 75% better on good days and as much as 50–60% better on poor days.

She states that she is scheduled to undergo an MRI of the left hip.

The patient does have a history of seizures and was exposed to meningitis as a teen. The seizures have been controlled for several months and she has clearance from the neurologist regarding the seizures for all activities.

Brief Job Description:

As a lactation nurse she educates mothers on breast-feeding their babies. She needs to enter into the room, pick up the baby, and bring him or her over to the mother in the bed. Once there, she stands for 5–10 minutes while assisting the mother and baby in appropriate breast-feeding techniques. The job requires her to stand and walk almost continuously. The shortest distance that she is required to walk is between patient rooms, on the floor of 2-Weber North of Harper Hospital.

At times, she has to walk as far as the Brush wing, which is approximately a block away. Additionally, she helps coordinate education classes for outpatient parents regarding birthing and breast-feeding techniques. For the education classes, she has to take packets of information to a designated classroom. She has to carry 2–3 "bundles" of information to the classroom per class session. Once there she will then lay the items down and begin to make packets for each of the students.

She also gives tours of the hospital for prospective patients.

Objective:

Strength: Left shoulder flexion 4/5, abduction 4/5, right hip flexion 4–/5, right hip abduction 4–/5

Heart Rate: Resting heart rate 120 beats per minute. The patient states that she has a documented history (several years) of a high resting heart rate.

AROM: Within functional limits for both upper and lower extremities

Balance: Fair with wide base of support and eyes open

Gait: Uncontrolled gait pattern, almost ataxic. She tends to have little control of her left knee, moving at times into hyperextension. Occasionally, the left lower extremity will internally rotate and create a valgus stress of the left knee. She also has a decrease in hip extension with circumductive patterns. This gait pattern is non-efficient for prolonged ambulation.

She was evaluated on a standard cane, as well as Lofstrand crutches. The Lofstrand crutches have provided the most efficient gait pattern with the greatest control of the left lower extremity.

The patient has developed the habit to walk very quickly. By walking quickly, she feels that she has better control of her left lower extremity and this creates less pain. When she is told to slow down and concentrate on heel strike, stance phase, follow through, and toe off, more pain is generated into the hip and a lot less weightbearing is noted on the left lower extremity. Therefore, she relies a lot on momentum with a quick gait pattern.

She has demonstrated the simulation of walking into a room, picking up a child, and then walking to and standing at the edge of the bed. Although she presented with a gait deviation (limp), she should be able to perform this activity without any difficulties. Her seizures are controlled and should not be an issue in this matter.

Risk Factors:

1. Poor gait pattern
2. Decreased strength
3. Pain

Recommendations:

The patient should be able to return to work starting at a 4-hour workday. She should use the Lofstrand crutches if she is working only on the floor, going from room to room. She should not use a standard cane nor ambulate without any assistive devices until she approaches the patient's room. Once at the patient's room, she may leave the crutches outside the door or just inside the door. She has demonstrated the ability to walk while performing her work duties without incident. She can carry any and all materials needed for educational purposes in a backpack.

For walking longer distances (e.g., to the Brush floor of Harper Hospital), she would be best suited with some type of transportation device. An electric three- or four-wheeled scooter would be the most efficient. She could keep the scooter in her office or in a certain designated area on the floor. If she is paged, she can walk to the scooter with her Lofstrand crutches and transport them to her designated work area. Otherwise, ambulating this distance may cause increased fatigue and pain. As for tours of the hospital, the scooter would be the most appropriate mobility solution.

The patient needs to continue to work diligently with her supervisors to let them know of her capabilities and her current fatigue levels. She will start off returning to work at a 4-hour shift and then every 2 to 3 days, based on fatigue levels, she may increase her time by 1–2 hours. If there are any specific activities that cannot be resolved (i.e., through corrective recommendations designed to minimize symptoms and maximize productivity), the patient and/or supervisors need to page me at 54321 for consultation. Additionally, I could be consulted to follow up in one month's time to see how the patient is doing and to make any further comments or recommendations to the patient's supervisors and attending physicians.

Dr. M. U., thank you for this referral. If you have any questions or comments, please contact me at (313) 555-5555. My office hours are M, T, Th 7:00 a.m. to 4.00 p.m., Wednesday and Friday from 7:00 a.m. to 2.00 p.m.

Sincerely,

Jon Nettie, PT

Wheelchair Seating and Mobility

CHAPTER 19

Diane Thomson and Kimberlee Bond

OBJECTIVES

1. Demonstrate ability to determine an appropriate mobility device for each client.
2. Demonstrate components of and competence in performing a seating and positioning evaluation.
3. Describe the four types of postural deformities.
4. Demonstrate ability to apply knowledge of assessments into practical clinical scenarios.
5. Describe the occupational therapist's role within seating and positioning.
6. Demonstrate the ability to determine function versus fit when determining appropriateness of a wheelchair.
7. Describe the core concepts of the Human Activity Assistive Technology Model (HAAT).

KEY TERMS

Table 19-1 Key Terms

Cook & Polgar, 2008, pp. 545–555
Arm rest
Cognition
Context
Extrinsic enablers
Fixed deformity
Flexible deformity
Human Activity Assistive Technology Model
Intrinsic enablers
Lightweight wheelchair
Medicaid
Medicare

(continues)

Table 19-1 Key Terms (continued)

Cook & Polgar, 2008, pp. 545–555
Paralysis
Pelvic obliquity
Pelvic rotation
Planar
Power assist
Pressure ulcer
Psychosocial function
Rigid ultralightweight wheelchair
Scoliosis
Shearing
Tilt
Ultralightweight wheelchair
Windswept hip deformity

INTRODUCTION

Welcome to Days 28 and 29 of your study guide. Hopefully you are well on your way to completing your journey. This chapter will provide you with the process for assessing a client for the appropriate wheelchair by looking at the physical, environmental, social, cognitive, and psychological issues involved. Use the outline along with the references provided to gather information toward this goal. Case studies have been provided to allow for a better understanding of the concepts presented. These will provide an opportunity to reinforce the learning of the preceding concepts as well as applying the knowledge acquired.

OUTLINE

1. **Etiology of Human Performance Frame of Reference (also listed as Human Performance Model and Human Activity Assistive Technology Model)**

(Cook & Polgar, 2008, pp. 34–51)
(Pendleton & Schultz-Krohn, 2006, p. 38)

   a. Basic principles
      i. Studying human performance versus behavior within a context while completing an activity gives useful conclusions to address how technology is working for the subject.
      ii. Assistive technology can be useful in facilitation of performance in an activity.
   b. Human
      i. Who is completing the activity?
      ii. What intrinsic enablers are being used?

(Christiansen & Baum, 2005, pp. 373–385)

      I. Sensory input (i.e., visual or auditory input)
      II. Central processing (perception, motor control, cognition, psychological function)

        III. Effectors or motor output
      iii. Ability: Basic trait of person brought to task
      iv. Skill level: Level of proficiency
  c. Activity: Task needing to be completed
  d. Assistive technology: Object required to complete task (i.e., wheelchair for mobility)
  e. Context
      i. Setting
      ii. Social context
      iii. Cultural context
      iv. Physical context

2. History and physical, including environmental considerations

(Cook & Polgar, 2008, pp. 54–88, 91–142)

  a. Medical history
      i. Primary diagnosis, including date occurred/diagnosed
      ii. Secondary diagnoses, including limitations
      iii. History and progression of medical issues, including secondary issues
      iv. Recent and/or planned surgeries with limitations or need to wait until procedure completed noted
      v. Cardiorespiratory status, including effect on endurance
  b. Current seating/mobility (if applicable)
      i. Current wheelchair type, manufacturer, model, serial number (if available), seat dimension and overall width, age of device
      ii. Current wheelchair cushion type, manufacturer, serial number, age of device, seat dimension
      iii. Current style of back type, manufacturer, serial number, seat dimension, age of device
      iv. Parts that need to be replaced or repaired
      v. Reason for replacement
  c. Home environment
      i. Type of home
          I. Multilevel, ranch, condo, apartment, senior apartment, assisted living, long-term care
          II. Rented or owned
      ii. Ability to enter home: Ramp, lift, stairs (number of stairs), width of doorways
      iii. Ability to access rooms within home, including the bathroom as well as accessing upper and lower (i.e., basement) levels if needed
      iv. Amount of assistance at home
          I. How many hours?
          II. Who provides?
          III. What do they do?
  d. Transportation and community involvement

(Cook & Polgar, 2008, pp. 443–459)

      i. Type of transport vehicle (car, van, bus, ambulance)
      ii. Adaptation to vehicle (ramp, lift, tie-down system, locking system, hand controls)
      iii. Employment/education: If the consumer is currently employed and/or attending school; future plans
      iv. Community activities (e.g., travel, hobbies, and interests)
  e. Cognitive/visual status

(Cook & Polgar, 2008, pp. 54–88)

      i. Memory (single-step versus multiple-step commands)
      ii. Problem solving (cause and effect, topographical orientation)

       iii. Judgment: Safety issues (e.g., community mobility)

       iv. Attention/concentration

       v. Visual deficits (neglect, field cuts, partial or complete blindness, glasses or contacts, depth perception)

  f. Basic and instrumental activities of daily living status: How each of the following are addressed or affected by the use of a mobility device:

       i. Feeding

       ii. Grooming

       iii. Bathing

       iv. Dressing

       v. Toileting

       vi. Bowel (incontinent or continent)

       vii. Bladder (incontinent or continent)

       viii. Meal preparation

       ix. Household management

  g. Mobility skills and balance (sitting and standing if applicable)

       i. Transfers (type of transfer, all surfaces completed, assistance required)

       ii. Ambulation (distance, device, history of falls, safety issues and concerns)

       iii. Manual wheelchair propulsion (type of wheelchair trialed, distance, and time)

       iv. Power wheelchair operation (standard joystick versus specialty controls)

       v. Pressure relief (type performed)

       vi. Hours spent in wheelchair

       vii. Sitting balance (static versus dynamic, supported versus unsupported)

       viii. Standing balance (static versus dynamic, supported versus unsupported)

  h. Sensation

       i. Intact/impaired/absent

       ii. Areas affected

       iii. Presence/history of pressure ulcers (location and stage)

  i. Clinical criteria

       I. Mobility limitations causing inability to participate in mobility related activities of daily living (MRADL)

       II. Cognitive or sensory deficits that can be accommodated/compensated to allow for safe use of mobility device to participate in MRADL

       III. The ability or potential ability to safely use the mobility device

       IV. Environmental support for the use of the mobility device

       V. Sufficient function or ability to use the recommended equipment and find the least restricting device

3. Mat evaluation

(Cook & Polgar, 2008, pp. 179–212)

  a. Head and neck position

       i. Posture (functional, flexed, extended, rotated, laterally flexed, cervical hyperextension)

       ii. Ability to control head

  b. Upper extremity function

       i. Passive and active range of motion

       ii. Manual muscle test

       iii. Dexterity

  c. Trunk position

       i. Kyphosis

       ii. Lordosis

       iii. Scoliosis

       iv. Trunk rotation

  d. Pelvis position

       i. Pelvic tilt (anterior or posterior)

    ii. Pelvic obliquity (described by the low side)

    iii. Pelvic rotation

  e. Hip position

    i. Femur abducted or adducted at hip joint

    ii. Windswept deformity (check for dislocation)

    iii. Range of motion—client supine on mat—hip flexion with knee flexed to determine functional seating position

  f. Lower extremity function, including foot position

    i. Passive and active range of motion

    ii. Manual muscle test

    iii. Hamstring limitation

    iv. Foot positioning (neutral, dorsi flexed, plantar flexed, inverted, everted)

  g. Spasticity/tone

    i. Location

    ii. Effect on function

  h. Measurements

    i. Hip width (used to assist in determining width of wheelchair)

    ii. Hip to popliteal fossa (used to assist in determining depth of wheelchair)

    iii. Shoulder width

    iv. Chest width (used to assist in determining width of back)

    v. Chest depth (used to assist in determining length of lateral supports)

    vi. Knee to heel (used to assist in determining seat to floor height, length of leg rests)

    vii. Inferior angle of scapula (used to assist in determining height of back)

    viii. Top of shoulder (used to assist in determining height of back)

    ix. Top of head (used to assist in determining head rest placement)

    x. Elbow to mat (used to assist in determining arm rest height)

    xi. Elbow to wrist and finger tip (used to assist in determining arm rest length)

    xii. Foot length and width (used to assist in determining size of foot plates)

  i. Hierarchy of positioning

(Cook & Polgar, 2008, pp. 189–196)

    i. Pelvis and lower extremities: "The pelvis is the key point of control and its position affects the posture of the rest of the body" (p. 190).

    ii. Trunk: "Once the desired position in the pelvis and lower extremities has been obtained, the trunk is considered" (p. 192).

    iii. Head and neck: "With the pelvis, lower extremities, and trunk positioned, the head and neck positions are considered" (p. 195).

    iv. Upper extremities: "Support of the upper extremities is an essential component of the seating system" (p. 195).

4. Determination of wheelchair

(Cook & Polgar, 2008, pp. 408–442)

  a. Manual

    i. Folding frame

    ii. Rigid frame

    iii. Tilt in space

    iv. Recline

    v. Tilt and recline

  b. Power

    i. Front-wheel drive

      I. Stationary seat

      II. Tilt in space

      III. Recline

      IV. Seat elevator

    V. Power elevating leg rests and elevating foot platform
    VI. Combination of power seating devices
  ii. Midwheel drive
    I. Stationary seat
    II. Tilt-in-space
    III. Recline
    IV. Seat elevator
    V. Power elevating leg rests and elevating foot platform
    VI. Combination of power seating devices
  iii. Rear-wheel drive
    I. Stationary seat
    II. Tilt-in-space
    III. Recline
    IV. Seat elevator
    V. Power elevating leg rests and elevating foot platform
    VI. Combination of power seating devices

5. **Positioning considerations**

(Cook & Polgar, 2008, pp. 175–204)

  a. Cushions
    i. Foam
    ii. Gel
    iii. Fluid
    iv. Air
  b. Backs
    i. Planar
    ii. Curved
  c. Ancillary positioning devices (e.g., head rest, lateral thoracic support, arm support, hip and thigh guides, knee adductors, abductors, anterior chest support, pelvic positioning belt, foot positioning devices)
  d. Custom-molded seating

6. **Funding issues**

(Cook & Polgar, 2008, p. 143–161)

  a. Medicare
  b. Medicaid
  c. Private insurance
  d. Other sources

7. **Psychosocial issues**

(Cook & Polgar, 2008, pp. 75–78)

  a. Rejection of equipment
  b. Depression secondary to loss of independence

CASE STUDIES

Case Study 19-1. A 20-year-old male presents to the clinic with a diagnoses of T4 paraplegia and a history of ischial pressure ulcers that are currently closed.

  A. Would you recommend a manual or power wheelchair and why?
  B. What are the advantages and disadvantages of a folding wheelchair versus a rigid-frame manual wheelchair?
  C. List three cushion types that may be appropriate for this client.

Case Study 19-2. A 65-year-old male with C6 tetraplegia (also known as quadriplegia), who has used a manual wheelchair for 15 years, presents to the clinic with complaints of bilateral shoulder pain as well as increased fatigue due to being recently diagnosed with congestive heart failure. What type of wheelchair would you recommend and why?

Case Study 19-3. A 41-year-old woman with multiple sclerosis (MS) is able to ambulate with a walker; however, she reports multiple falls and shortness of breath during and immediately following walking short distances. She lives alone in a house with two steps to enter. She has had two exacerbations in the last 6 months with significant progression and weakness in bilateral upper and lower extremities.

    A. What factors are important to address within her environment before providing a wheelchair?
    B. What cognitive considerations should be made before providing a wheelchair?
    C. What are the psychological considerations (e.g., willing to accept transition of manual wheelchair versus scooter or power wheelchair)?
    D. Using principles of the Human Activity Assistive Technology Model, what are the major issues surrounding the client that affect her use of a wheelchair?

Case Study 19-4. An 8-year-old with cerebral palsy (CP) presents to the clinic with his parents for a wheelchair evaluation. He is unable to ambulate and has only used a stroller with his parents pushing him prior to this evaluation.

    A. What environments should be considered?
    B. What developmental issues should be considered?
    C. What type of wheelchair will increase his function and activity during his life roles?
    D. From whom is the information for the evaluation gathered?

REFERENCES

Christiansen, C. H., & Baum, C. M. (Eds.). (2005). *Occupational therapy: Performance, participation, and well-being* (3rd ed.). Thorofare, NJ: Slack.

Cook, A. M., & Polgar, J. M. (2008). *Cook & Hussey's assistive technologies: Principles and practice* (3rd ed.). St. Louis, MO: Mosby.

Pendleton, H. M., & Schultz-Krohn, W. (Eds.). (2006). *Pedretti's occupational therapy: Practice skills for physical dysfunction* (6th ed.). St. Louis, MO: Mosby.

CASE STUDY RATIONALE

Case Study 19-1

    A. Recommend a manual wheelchair secondary to a young male with no upper extremity issues. The manual wheelchair will allow for increased accessibility. At this level, he should be able to adequately perform pressure relief and position changes as well as higher-level wheelchair skills, such as wheelies, fall recovery, and stair bumping.

    B. An advantage of the folding-frame wheelchair is that it will fold for easy transport. A disadvantage is that it is heavier than a rigid-frame wheelchair and it has more movable parts, which cause increased maintenance issues. An advantage of the rigid-frame wheelchair is that it is lighter weight than a folding-frame wheelchair, requires less maintenance, is easier to transport, and has fewer movable parts, which decrease the shock to the shoulder joint and spine. A disadvantage is that it does not have removal parts, such as foot rests, which may make it more difficult for some clients to perform transfers because it limits the ability to place the feet on the ground.

    C. Three cushion types that may be appropriate for this client are air filled, dense foam with fluid overlay, and viscoelastic foam.

Case Study 19-2. A power wheelchair is required secondary to cardiac issues and shoulder overuse issues. A manual wheelchair will exacerbate these issues, and a power wheelchair will provide independent mobility while preserving upper extremity function for transfers.

Case Study 19-3

    A. Accessibility into and throughout the home (i.e., ramp and doorways), life roles (work, family, leisure interests, activities of daily living (ADL), instrumental activities of daily living (IADL), mobility related activities of daily living (MRADL)), and transportation needs

    B. Problem solving, memory, safety/judgment, topographical orientation

    C. Mood/coping skills, accepting progressive nature of disease. The therapist will need to address issues of mobility with the client's present and future needs as well as a discussion with the client to develop an understanding and acceptance of the recommended device.

    D. Human: Lives alone; cognitive status?
        Activity: Life roles (mother, employee, supervisor)
        AT: What device will be used (manual wheelchair versus scooter or power wheelchair)?
        Context: Where will the device be utilized (home, work, community)?

Case Study 19-4

    A. Home, school, playground/community

    B. Piaget's stages of human development (concrete operations). Children begin logical thinking surrounding concrete objects and activities. Can complete complex tasks with several steps forward and backward (e.g., using a dial in one direction to turn speed up and opposite direction to turn speed down). Can classify and sort objects by characteristics. Realizes multiple solutions for problem solving.

    C. Power wheelchair with power seat elevator will allow increased interactions with peers and increased mobility throughout all environments. Limitations may be transportation of a power wheelchair by the parents, ability to install ramps at home for access, and child's ability to safely maneuver the wheelchair.

    D. Child, parents, teacher, school-based clinicians, vendor

Exhibit 19-1

Seating/Mobility Evaluation

Name: _____	Date Referred: _____	Date of Eval: _____
Address: _____	Phone: _____	Physician: _____
_____	Age: ____ Sex: ____	OT: _____
Funding: _____	Height: _____	PT: _____
Referred By: _____	Weight: _____	Soc. Sec. No: _____

Reason for Referral:
Patient Goals:
Caregiver Goals:

MEDICAL HISTORY:

	ICD-9: ___ ICD-9: ___
Dx:	ICD-9: ___ ICD-9: ___
Hx / Progression:	
(Symptoms)	
Recent / Planned Surgeries:	

Cardio-Respiratory Status:	Comments:
☐Intact: ☐Impaired:	

CURRENT SEATING / MOBILITY: (Type – Manufacturer – Model)

Chair:	Age:
w/c Cushion : Age:	w/c Back : Age:
Reason for ☐Replacement / ☐Repair / ☐Update:	
Funding Source:	

HOME ENVIRONMENT:

☐House ☐Apt ☐Asst Living ☐LTCF ☐Alone ☐w/ Family-Caregivers:
Entrance: ☐Level ☐Ramp ☐Lift ☐Stairs   Entrance Width:
w/c Accessible Rooms: ☐Yes ☐No   Narrowest Doorway Required to Access:
Comments:

COMMUNITY ADL:

TRANSPORTATION: ☐Car ☐Van ☐Bus ☐Adapted w/c Lift ☐Ramp ☐Ambulance ☐Other:
Driving Requirements:
Employment / Education\al Requirements:
Other

COGNITIVE / VISUAL STATUS:

Memory Skills	☐Intact:	☐Impaired:	Comments:
Problem Solving	☐Intact:	☐Impaired:	Comments:
Judgment	☐Intact:	☐Impaired:	Comments:
Attn / Concentration	☐Intact:	☐Impaired:	Comments:
Vision:	☐Intact:	☐Impaired:	Comments:
Hearing:	☐Intact:	☐Impaired:	Comments:
Other:	☐Intact:	☐Impaired:	Comments:

(continues)

Exhibit 19-1 *(continued)*

Seating/Mobility Evaluation   Continued

ADL STATUS:	Indep.	Assist	Unable	Comments / Other AT Equipment Required
Dressing	☐	☐	☐	
Bathing:	☐	☐	☐	
Feeding:	☐	☐	☐	
Grooming/Hygiene:	☐	☐	☐	
Toileting	☐	☐	☐	
Meal Prep	☐	☐	☐	
Home Management	☐	☐	☐	
Bowel Management:	☐Continent	☐Incontinent		
Bladder Management:	☐Continent	☐Incontinent		

MOBILITY SKILLS:	Indep	Assist	Unable	N/A	Comments / History of Past Use
Bed ↔ w/c Transfers	☐	☐	☐	☐	
w/c ↔ Commode Transfers	☐	☐	☐	☐	
Ambulation:	☐	☐	☐	☐	Device:
Manual w/c Propulsion:	☐	☐	☐	☐	
Operate Power w/c w/ Std. Joystick	☐	☐	☐	☐	
Operate Power w/c w/ Alternative Controls	☐	☐	☐	☐	
Able to Perform Weight Shifts	☐	☐	☐	☐	Type:
Hours Spent Sitting in w/c Each Day:			Comments:		

SENSATION:

☐Intact ☐Impaired ☐Absent	Hx of Pressure Sores ☐Yes ☐No	Current Pressure Sores ☐Yes ☐No
Comments:		

CLINICAL CRITERIA / ALGORITHM SUMMARY

Is there a mobility limitation causing an inability to safely participate in one or more Mobility Related Activities of Daily Living in a reasonable time frame? Explain:	☐Yes ☐No
Are there cognitive or sensory deficits (awareness / judgment / vision / etc) that limit the users ability to safely participate in one or more MRADL's	☐Yes ☐No
If yes, can they be accommodated / compensated for to allow use of a mobility assistive device to participate in MRADL's? Explain:	☐Yes ☐No
Does the user demonstrate the ability or potential ability and willingness to safely use the mobility assistive device? Explain:	☐Yes ☐No
Can the mobility deficit be sufficiently resolved with only the use of a cane or walker? Explain:	☐Yes ☐No
Does the user's environment support the use of a ☐ Manual Wheelchair ☐ POV ☐Power Wheelchair: Explain:	☐Yes ☐No
If a manual wheelchair is recommended, does the user have sufficient function/abilities to use the recommended equipment? Explain:	☐Yes ☐No ☐N/A
If a POV is recommended, does the user have sufficient stability and upper extremity function to operate it? Explain:	☐Yes ☐No ☐N/A
If a power wheelchair is recommended, does the user have sufficient function/abilities to use the recommended equipment? Explain:	☐Yes ☐No ☐N/A

RECOMMENDATION / GOALS:

☐ Manual Wheelchair ☐ POV ☐Power Wheelchair: ☐Positioning System(Tilt/Recline/Elev/Standing) ☐Seating

Physical / Occupational Therapist: _____   Date: _____   Phone: _____

Physician: I have read & concur
with the above assessment   _____   Date: _____   Phone: _____

The information contained in this document was prepared solely to assist in preparing accurate, legitimate claims for reimbursement under Medicare, Medicaid and other insurance plans. Every attempt has been made to insure the information is accurate at the time of writing but payment policies, coverage guidelines and fee schedules change frequently. Nothing in these materials is intended to, or should be construed as a guarantee a claim will be paid and if paid, the amount. Questions on payment policy and coverage guidelines are best directed to the payor's ombudsperson or professional services department. Copyright Michael Babinec 2008. All rights reserved.

Exhibit 19-1 *(continued)*

Mat Evaluation: (NOTE IF ASSESSED SITTING OR SUPINE)

		POSTURE:	FUNCTION:	COMMENTS:	SUPPORT NEEDED
HEAD & NECK		❑ Functional ❑ Flexed ❑ Extended ❑ Rotated ❑ Laterally Flexed ❑ Cervical Hyperextension	❑ Good Head Control ❑ Adequate Head Control ❑ Limited Head Control ❑ Absent Head Control		
UPPER EXTREMITY		**SHOULDERS** Left Right ❑WFL ❑WFL ❑elev / dep ❑elev / dep ❑pro / retract ❑pro / retract ❑subluxed ❑subluxed	R.O.M. Strength:		
		ELBOWS Left Right ❑Impaired ❑Impaired ❑WFL ❑ WFL	R.O.M. Strength:		
WRIST & HAND		Left Right ❑Impaired ❑Impaired ❑WFL ❑WFL	Strength / Dexterity:		

	TRUNK	Anterior / Posterior	Left Right	Rotation

TRUNK

Anterior / Posterior			Left Right			Rotation
❑ WFL	❑ ↑ Thoracic Kyphosis	❑ ↑ Lumbar Lordosis	❑ WFL	❑ Convex Left	❑ Convex Right	❑ Neutral ❑ Left Forward ❑ Right Forward
❑ Fixed	❑ Flexible		❑ Fixed	❑ Flexible		❑ Fixed ❑ Flexible
❑ Partly Flexible	❑ Other		❑ Partly Flexible	❑ Other		❑ Partly Flexible ❑ Other

PELVIS

Anterior / Posterior			Obliquity			Rotation		
❑ Neutral	❑ Posterior	❑ Anterior	❑ WFL	❑ Left Lower	❑ Rt. Lower	❑ WFL	❑ Right	❑ Left
❑ Fixed	❑ Other		❑ Fixed	❑ Other		❑ Fixed	❑ Other	
❑ Partly Flexible			❑ Partly Flexible			❑ Partly Flexible		
❑ Flexible			❑ Flexible			❑ Flexible		

HIPS

Position			Windswept			Range of Motion	
❑ Neutral	❑ ABduct	❑ ADduct	❑ Neutral	❑ Right	❑ Left	Left Right	
						Flex: ____° ____°	
						Ext: ____° ____°	
❑ Fixed	❑ Subluxed		❑ Fixed	❑ Other		Int R: ____° ____°	
❑ Partly Flexible	❑ Dislocated		❑ Partly Flexible			Ext R: ____° ____°	
❑ Flexible			❑ Flexible				

(continues)

Exhibit 19-1 *(continued)*

Mat Evaluation: Cont'd

	Knee R.O.M.		Strength:	Foot Positioning		Foot Positioning Needs:
	Left	**Right**		☐ WFL ☐L ☐R		
KNEES & FEET	☐ WFL	☐ WFL	Hamstring ROM Limitations: (Measured at ___° Hip Flex) Left_____ Right_____	☐ Dorsi-Flexed ☐L ☐R ☐ Plantar Flexed ☐L ☐R ☐ Inversion ☐L ☐R ☐ Eversion ☐L ☐R		
	☐ Flex_____°	☐ Flex_____°				
	☐ Ext _____°	☐ Ext _____°				

	Balance		Transfers	Ambulation	
MOBILITY	Sitting Balance:	Standing Balance	☐ Independent	☐ Unable to Ambulate	
	☐ WFL	☐ WFL	☐ Min Assist	☐ Ambulates with Assistance	
	☐ Min Support	☐ Min Support	☐ Max Asst	☐ Ambulates with Device	
	☐ Mod Support	☐ Mod Support	☐ Sliding Board	☐ Independent without Device	
	☐ Unable	☐ Unable	☐ Lift / Sling Required	☐ Indep. Short Distance Only	

Neuro-Muscular Status:

Tone:

Reflexive Responses:

Effect on Function:

	Measurements in Sitting:	Left	Right		
	A: Shoulder Width				Degree of Hip Flexion
	B: Chest Width			H:	Top of Shoulder
	C: Chest Depth (Front – Back)			I:	Acromium Process (Tip of Shoulder)
	D: Hip Width			J:	Inferior Angle of Scapula
	** Asymmetrical Width			K:	Elbow
	D: Hip Width			L:	Iliac Crest
	E: Between Knees			M:	Sacrum to Popliteal Fossa
	F: Top of Head			N:	Knee to Heel
	G: Occiput			O:	Foot Length

** Asymmetrical Width: i.e., windswept hips or scoliotic posture; measure widest point to widest point

Additional Comments :
_____
_____

Summary of Postural Asymmetries :
_____

Physical / Occupational Therapist: _____ Date: _____ Phone: _____

Assistive Technology Supplier _____ Date: _____ Phone: _____

Physician: I have read & concur with the above assessment _____ Date: _____ Phone: _____

The information contained in this document was prepared solely to assist providers in preparing accurate, legitimate claims for reimbursement under Medicare, Medicaid and other insurance plans. Every attempt has been made to insure the information is accurate at the time of writing but payment policies, coverage guidelines and fee schedules change frequently. Nothing in these materials is intended to, or should be construed as a guarantee a claim will be paid and if paid, the amount. Questions on payment policy and coverage guidelines are best directed to the payor's ombudsperson or professional services department. Copyright Michael Babinec 2008. All rights reserved.

Source: Courtesy Invacare Corporation

Promoting Meaningful Occupations Through Assistive Technology, Home Accessibility, Driver Rehabilitation, and Community Mobility

Joseph M. Pellerito Jr., Rosanne DiZazzo-Miller, and Fredrick D. Pociask

OBJECTIVES FOR ASSISTIVE TECHNOLOGY

1. Be able to define assistive technology (AT).
2. Be able to define universal design.
3. Recognize the role of AT in facilitating participation in meaningful occupations.
4. Understand the Human Interface Assessment (HIA).
5. Recognize basic AT solutions for optimal safety and independence in activities of daily living (ADL) and instrumental activities of daily living (IADL).
6. Be familiar with the Americans with Disabilities Act (ADA) and guidelines for home and community accessibility.

KEY TERMS

Table 20-1 Key Terms 20a

Pendleton & Schultz-Krohn, 2006, p. 349 Radomski & Latham, 2008, p. 511
Augmentative and alternative communication (AAC)
Computer-aided design (CAD)
Electronic aids to daily living (EADL)
Infrared (IR)
Personal digital assistants (PDA)
Pneumatic
Power switching
QWERTY layout
Radio frequency (RF)
Rehabilitation technology
Speech synthesizer
Universal design
Word prediction

INTRODUCTION

Welcome to Days 30 and 31 of your study guide. This chapter is divided into the following two sections: (1) an overview of assistive technology (AT) and home accessibility and how they promote occupation; and (2) driver rehabilitation and community mobility, parts one and two. The latter is presented in sequence because driving and community mobility can logically be organized into a type of subcategory under the broader topic of AT. Irrespective of how these content areas are organized or presented, they are key areas that entry-level practitioners should understand.

OUTLINE

1. **Assistive technology (AT)**
   a. Human Activity Assistive Technology Model (HAAT)

   (Radomski & Latham, 2008, p. 512)

   - i. Four subsections
     - I. Human–technology interface
     - II. Processor
     - III. Activity output
     - IV. Environmental interface
   - ii. Ultimately, the HAAT model assists the AT professional with determining the best features for the equipment and furthermore allows the professional to adapt and modify it to the context of the client.

   b. Human Interface Assessment (HIA) Model

   (Pendleton & Schultz-Krohn, 2006, p. 351)

   - i. This model reviews client skills and abilities in four main areas
     - I. Motor
     - II. Process
     - III. Communication
     - IV. Activity demands

2. **Assessment**

   (Radomski & Latham, 2008, p. 516)

   a. The goals of the client serve as the forefront of all AT assessment and intervention practice.

   b. Structured interviews and questionnaires serve as important assessment tools when trying to identify a client's occupational performance within his or her daily roles.

   c. A seating evaluation is required in all AT assessments to promote proper alignment stability.

   d. An assessment of motor control is also required for the therapist to understand the strengths and challenges of the client. This will provide invaluable information on what types of AT devices and equipment are appropriate. This includes, but is not limited to, sensation, ROM, strength, endurance, and coordination to determine the most efficient and available AT devices for each client.

   e. Assess the appropriate switch type as well as the best area to mount it. Here the OT will address reliability of response, ability to perform timed responses, and ability to activate and deactivate the switch (Radomski & Latham, 2008, pp. 518–519).

   f. Basic orientation and cognitive skills are evaluated throughout the AT assessment.

   g. Visual impairments are a common cause of AT assessment and intervention. The OT's recommendation of AT devices will depend greatly on the client's visual abilities. "Visual acuity, eye ROM, visual field cuts, tracking, and figure–ground discrimination are assessed" (Radomski & Latham, 2008, p. 519).

3. Team members

(Radomski & Latham, 2008, pp. 515–516)

   a. OT
   b. SLP
   c. MSW (social worker)
   d. Seating and mobility specialist (may be an OT or PT)
   e. Teacher or vocational counselor
   f. Rehabilitation engineer
   g. Suppliers

4. Intervention

(Pendleton & Schultz-Krohn, 2006, pp. 352–366)
(Radomski & Latham, 2008, pp. 520–530)

   a. In terms of intervention, it is always important to note that for each high technology aid or device that is recommended, a low technology backup should also be available to the client.

      i. Computer access

         I. Input is how the client will enter information into the computer, most commonly through the use of a keyboard or mouse.

            a. Intellikeys
            b. Key guards
            c. Overlays
            d. Minikeyboard
            e. QWERTY layout
            f. Trackballs
            g. Touch screens
            h. Mouse emulation
            i. On-screen keyboards
            j. Speech recognition
            k. Optical character recognition
            l. Eye gaze
            m. Morse code
            n. Tongue-touch keypad
            o. Scanning

         II. Output (the computer's response to input from the client) is most commonly seen on the computer screen.

            a. Screen enlargement
            b. Text to speech
            c. Braille (display and embossing)
            d. Large print
            e. Auditory signals

   b. Augmentative and alternative communication (AAC) devices

      i. AAC devices range from paper and pencil (nonelectronic) to computerized speaking devices (electronic). The OT will need to determine which of the following are most appropriate after weighing the client's abilities in conjunction with the pros and cons of each of the following AAC options.

      ii. Synthesized or digitized
      iii. Static or dynamic
      iv. Vocal or nonvocal
      v. Dedicated or nondedicated
      vi. Orthography or representation

   c. Environmental access

       i. Electronic aids to daily living (EADL) promote client independence in a variety of areas including, but certainly not limited to, answering the telephone, operating the television and radio, and turning the lights on and off.

       ii. This area of AT is recommended for clients who require maximal or total physical assistance.

       iii. Working with a rehab engineer is important because the engineer will assist with providing input on electrical wiring, infrared (IR), and radio frequency (RF) transmissions.

          I. Simple EADL

             a. These usually consist of adapting access to a device by modifying the way the client can use it either by a type of switch, interface, or modified buttons.

          II. Complex EADL

             a. These are used primarily by clients who require maximal to total physical assistance.

             b. Complex EADL are oftentimes used in collaboration with an AAC or computerized system. A sip and puff device that interfaces with a computerized screen and is hooked up to the client's phone and home entertainment system is a good example of a complex EADL.

          III. Closed captioning

             a. This is oftentimes used for clients with auditory impairments. Watching television with the speech as text at the bottom of the screen is an example of closed captioning. This is often available through simply selecting that option on the user's television remote or television menu.

          IV. Closed-circuit television (CCTV)

             a. This is most appropriate for clients with visual impairments; it acts as a magnifier that uses a mounted camera to project magnification of a piece of paper onto a television screen.

          V. Braille note takers

             a. New technologies have made it possible for clients with low vision to take notes and either download them or print them from a Braille printer.

   d. Mobility and locomotion (as discussed in Chapter 19)

5. Specialized training

(Radomski & Latham, 2008, p. 532)

   a. Assistive technology provider (ATP)

   b. Certification through Rehabilitation Engineering and Assistive Technology Society of North America (RESNA)

       i. The aforementioned credential and certification are voluntary and provide a level of expertise and commitment to the assistive technology area of practice.

   c. Continuing education is a must for all OTs who practice in the area of AT.

6. Funding

(Radomski & Latham, 2008, p. 531)

   a. The Assistive Technology Act of 2004

       i. Provides grants to states that support AT needs of individuals

   b. The American with Disabilities Act of 1990

       i. Prohibits discrimination of, and requires access for, individuals with special needs in all areas of work and government

   c. Reimbursement

       i. Medical insurance

          I. Must show medical necessity

   d. Letter of medical necessity/justification

       i. The following information should be included in a letter of medical necessity:

    I. Client's roles and occupational performance

    II. Results from client/family interview

    III. Trial results of the recommended device

    IV. Cost analysis of alternative devices with a list of pros and cons

    V. How this device will enhance the client's occupational performance

7. Home and community accessibility

  a. The Americans with Disabilities Act (ADA) Standards for Accessible Design can be found at http://www.ada.gov/stdspdf.htm.

    i. This provides an OT with mandated guidelines for accessibility into buildings and facilities.

  b. Home evaluation and modification

    i. There are a number of online tools that can assist you with evaluating home environments and making appropriate recommendations for optimal safety and independence.

      I. Creating Accessible Homes http://www.ksre.ksu.edu/library/HOUS2/MF2213.pdf provides a quick checklist on accessible home features.

      II. The Comprehensive Home Evaluation Report (CHER) http://www.shdesigns.net/comptool.html is available for purchase and assists therapists with developing a comprehensive report that includes recommendations for home modifications and equipment.

      III. Tox Town http://toxtown.nlm.nih.gov/ is an interactive website that enables users to identify potential toxic hazards within their homes and communities.

    ii. Home evaluations and recommendations for modifications and equipment (e.g., durable medical equipment and assistive devices) complement AT consultation and recommendations; for example, OTs can recommend an environmental control unit through AT consultation. AT services can help identify the need for home evaluations.

      I. Review and learn home accessibility specifications including the following:
Pendleton & Schultz-Krohn, 2006, pp. 151–163
Radomski & Latham, 2008, pp. 310-388, 955–973
http://www.ksre.ksu.edu/library/HOUS2/MF2213.pdf

        a. Entrances

          i. Doorway openings

          ii. Locks and door handle types

          iii. Ramp specifications including rise and run ratios, turning platforms, handrails, surface types, and portable versus permanent

          iv. Thresholds

        b. Kitchens

          i. Cabinets (e.g., height, depth, width, locations, shapes, handle types)

          ii. Cook tops (e.g., gas or electric, control knob location, adaptive devices)

          iii. Counter spaces (e.g., height, depth, width, location, shape, types)

          iv. Fire extinguishers (e.g., types and locations)

          v. Ovens/microwaves (e.g., types and locations)

          vi. Refrigerator (e.g., types, storage variations, locations)

          vii. Sinks (e.g., height, depth, width, location, shape, types, disposal location, insulated pipes, faucet handle types)

        c. Bathroom

          i. Water heater temperature

          ii. Center floor drain

          iii. Faucet types

          iv. Floor spaces (e.g., turning radii)

          v. Grab bars

      vi.   Heating lamps
      vii. Non-slip flooring
      viii. Shower head types
      ix.   Shower types (e.g., roll-in shower and step-in shower)
      x.   Toilets and bidets (e.g., height and types)
      xi.   Tub types (e.g., old-fashioned-style tubs, standard tubs, specialty walk-in tubs)

  d. Bedrooms
      i.   Beds (sizes, types, locations, transfer aids)
      ii.   Bedroom locations
      iii.   Closets (e.g., types, sizes, locations, rod types)
      iv.   Furniture placement
      v.   Light switches (e.g., locations and types)

  e. Hallways

  f. Laundry rooms
      i.   Washers and dryers (e.g., styles and types)
      ii.   Sorting and folding tables (e.g., types, sizes, locations, permanent or portable)

  g. Indoor and outdoor stairways
      i.   Handrails
      ii.   Safety strips
      iii.   Color contrast
      iv.   Light switches (e.g., locations and types)
      v.   Step specifications

  h. General features
      i.   Alarm systems
      ii.   Call for help systems
      iii.   Door knobs
      iv.   Doors (e.g., types and sizes)
      v.   Electrical outlets (e.g., types and locations)
      vi.   Evacuation plans
      vii. Extension cords
      viii. Fire extinguishers (e.g., types and locations)
      ix.   Flooring (e.g., surface types and color contrast)
      x.   Light switches (e.g., locations and types)
      xi.   Indoor and outdoor maintenance plans
      xii. Phones (e.g., type and location)
      xiii. Smoke and carbon monoxide detectors (e.g., types and locations)
      xiv. Thermostats (e.g., types, height, locations)
      xv. Water temperature
      xvi. Windows (e.g., sizes, types, locations)

OBJECTIVES FOR DRIVER REHABILITATION AND COMMUNITY MOBILITY: PART ONE

1. Describe the different conceptual framework models that driver rehabilitation specialists use.
2. Explain the importance of the International Classification of Functioning, Disability and Health on the field of driver rehabilitation.
3. Explain the role that driver strategies and driving tactics may play in optimizing driver, passenger, and pedestrian safety.

KEY TERMS

Table 20-2 Key Terms 20b

Pellerito, 2006, pp. 3–22
Community mobility
Competencies
Driver rehabilitation specialist (DRS)
Instrumental activities of daily living (IADL)
International Classification of Functioning, Disability and Health (ICF)
Risk management

OUTLINE

1. Driver rehabilitation

(Pellerito, 2006, pp. 3–22)

- **a.** Driving is an important symbol of adult autonomy and independence.
- **b.** The independent community mobility afforded by driving has a major influence on an individual's quality of life.
- **c.** Most drivers with functional impairments have similar needs to drive and to maintain their community mobility as those of the general population.
- **d.** The professional services of driver rehabilitation specialists (DRS) can be invaluable in helping people with physical and/or cognitive limitations to maintain their community mobility and in protecting the safety of the individual driver and the public at large.
    - **i.** Driving provides a sense of personal competence and enables access to essential services and meaningful social interactions, and for older people it can support their ability to "age in place" in familiar surroundings.
    - **ii.** Independent community mobility influences the roles people assume, the formation and maintenance of primary and secondary group ties, the daily operation of households and businesses, the pursuit of meaningful activities in a variety of social settings, and the construction of positive self-concepts and high self-esteem more generally.
    - **iii.** The Association for Driver Rehabilitation Specialists (ADED) was formed in 1977 by a small group of professionals interested in sharing ideas about best practices and in developing formal and informal channels of communication.
    - **iv.** Professionals who successfully pass ADED's rigorous examination are granted the credential of Certified Driver Rehabilitation Specialist (CDRS).
    - **v.** Becoming a CDRS requires a DRS to pass an examination and to submit a series of reflective reports on their professional practice experiences.
        - **I.** This is still a voluntary process that DRSs may or may not undertake.
        - **II.** Most CDRSs have a background in OT; however, CDRSs may also be driver educators, physical therapists, pharmacists, and/or owners of commercial driving schools. Occupational therapists have expertise in assessing the individual's holistic status (i.e., mind, body, and spirit), including an understanding of how medical conditions and impairments can impede driver readiness. The occupational therapist working as a driver rehabilitation specialist is therefore often recognized as possessing an ideal professional background to perform predriving or clinical driver rehabilitation evaluations.

2. Clinical evaluations

(Pellerito, 2006, pp. 103–139)

    a. Programs offering clinical evaluations provide only key information that can be used by the driver rehabilitation team members. They also help to identify clients who are at risk and provide concrete data to support decisions to discontinue the evaluation process before the client has received an on-road evaluation.

    b. Programs offering clinical evaluations and simulator assessments

        i. Driving simulators offer many advantages

            I. The capability to assess clients' responses to challenging stimuli, including animate and inanimate obstacles; how they cope during variable inclement and clement weather conditions; their topographic orientation in familiar and unfamiliar environments; and night driving performance.

            II. Simulators may also bridge the gap between clinical and on-road evaluations by providing a tangible way for clients to practice driving skills after narrowly failing a clinical or on-road evaluation.

    c. Programs offering comprehensive driver rehabilitation evaluations and more

        i. These programs ensure that the client is provided with a comprehensive driver evaluation.

        ii. After the comprehensive evaluation has been completed, additional services should include driver training and/or addressing alternative community mobility as a critical IADL.

        iii. Alternative community mobility may include assisting clients and their caregivers with identifying viable and safe alternatives to driving, or riding as a passenger in, motor vehicles.

    d. Conceptual frameworks that are used by rehabilitation professionals play a key role in underpinning their evaluation procedures and guiding their observations, decisions, and intervention processes.

        i. The following models are the most relevant for driver rehabilitation and community mobility services:

            I. The Model of Human Occupation

            II. The Person–Environment–Occupation Model

            III. Canadian Model of Occupational Performance

            IV. The Occupational Adaptation Model

3. Models that identify driving as one of the most important IADL can be instructive in guiding DRSs in providing driver rehabilitation, evaluation, and training services.

(Pellerito, 2006, pp. 6–8)

    a. The Model of Human Occupation (MOHO)

        i. Key components of the MOHO framework include the following constructs:

            I. Volition: The thoughts, feelings, and motivations related to particular activities

            II. Habituation: Behavioral routines and patterns

            III. Performance capacity: Influenced by physical and mental abilities and by subjective experiences

            IV. Environmental influences, physical and social, that affect performance

    b. The Person–Environment–Occupation Model

        i. Highlights transactional interrelationships between the person, environment, and occupation (i.e., elements that influence human performance)

    c. Canadian Model of Occupational Performance (CMOP)

        i. The CMOP emphasizes interactional issues and performance factors relevant to a person's age and lifestyle.

    d. The Occupational Adaptation Model

        i. Central to this model is the notion that humans learn to adapt to the demands of their activities within a particular environment.

The process of evaluating drivers with functional impairments should reliably screen (i.e., filter out) those individuals whose driving performance would present an unacceptable risk to themselves, other drivers, prospective passengers, pedestrians, and public and private property.

  e. World Health Organization International Classification of Functioning, Disability and Health (ICF)

     i. The ICF provides a standard lexicon (i.e., universal vocabulary) for describing interrelationships among health, disability, functioning, and other related issues such as driving.

     ii. The full version of the ICF has two parts: Part 1: Functioning and Disability and Part 2: Contextual Factors.

     iii. Part 1 is subdivided into Body Functions and Structures and Activities and Participation.

     iv. Part 2 is subdivided into Environmental Factors and Personal Factors.

     v. The ICF classification system may help DRSs to describe more consistently the nature and extent of client problems and related factors.

  f. Risk management frameworks

     i. Driving is a hazardous activity.

       I. Driving a vehicle in ordinary traffic is an inherently hazardous activity for drivers, passengers, and pedestrians alike.

     ii. Crash risk varies according to the age and/or medical condition of the driver.

       I. Crash risk increases with increasing age beyond approximately 75 to 80 years of age.

       II. The review by Charlton et al. (2004) found that people who are diagnosed with dementia, epilepsy, multiple sclerosis, psychiatric disorders, schizophrenia, sleep apnea, alcohol abuse, or cataracts had a relative risk at least double that of people in control groups.

     iii. Balance injury risk and a client's desire to drive.

       I. The process of evaluating functionally impaired drivers should reliably screen (i.e., filter out) those individuals whose driving performance would present an unacceptable risk to themselves, other drivers, prospective passengers, pedestrians, and public and private property.

OBJECTIVES FOR DRIVER REHABILITATION AND COMMUNITY MOBILITY: PART TWO

1. Describe the different conceptual framework models that driver rehabilitation specialists use.
2. Explain the importance of the International Classification of Functioning, Disability and Health on the field of driver rehabilitation.
3. Explain the role that driver strategies and driving tactics may play in optimizing driver, passenger, and pedestrian safety.
4. Realize that the client is at the center of the driver rehabilitation team.
5. Be familiar with the five service delivery models.
6. Understand the National Mobility Equipment Dealers Association's role in the adaptive mobility industry.

KEY TERMS

Table 20-3 Key Terms 20c

Pellerito, 2006, pp. 53–74
Ancillary team members
Certified Driver Rehabilitation Specialist (CDRS)
Clinical driving screen
Clinical reasoning
Community mobility
Comprehensive driver rehabilitation evaluations
Driver remediation plan
Driving cessation or retirement plan
Employment plan
Evidence-based practice
Key driver rehabilitation services
National Mobility Equipment Dealers Association (NMEDA)
Occupational therapist specializing in driver rehabilitation
Occupational therapy (driving) generalist
Primary team members
Vehicle modifier

OUTLINE

1. Primary team members

(Pellerito, 2006, pp. 53–57)

    a. The driver rehabilitation specialist (DRS) plays the central role in providing efficacious driver rehabilitation and, more recently, community mobility services to clients and their caregivers.

        i. DRSs work with ancillary team members to help ensure that clients achieve their driver rehabilitation goals, community mobility goals, or both.

        ii. There is a distinction between the DRS and CDRS credentials.

        iii. Professionals who provide driver rehabilitation services may or may not have completed the requirements set forth by the Association for Driver Rehabilitation Specialists (ADED).

        iv. DRSs may hold occupational therapy credentials, they may be OTs who are also certified driver educators, and they may be other health professionals (e.g., pharmacists, physical therapists, recreation therapists) or certified driver educators.

    b. Clients and their caregivers

        i. The client is at the center of the driver rehabilitation team.

        ii. It is mutually beneficial for the client, DRS, and other team members when a client's full participation in the decision-making process is encouraged and expected.

        iii. The caregiver often fills in the blanks and provides valuable insight that the client may be lacking or unwilling to provide.

    c. Vehicle modifier

        i. The vehicle modifier is also known as the mobility equipment dealer or vendor.

    ii.   The vehicle modifier plays a primary role in the provision of driver rehabilitation and community mobility services.

    iii.   Vehicle modifiers do much more than their name implies; for example, they often help the client and DRS identify the optimal vehicle type and vehicle modifications that maximize the client's safety as a driver or passenger after accessing or exiting a vehicle with efficiency.

    iv.   Reputable mobility equipment dealers are members of the National Mobility Equipment Dealers Association (NMEDA).

d. Case manager

    i.   A case manager is a professional who represents the funding entity.

    ii.   Case managers often have a professional background in social work, nursing, or some other allied health profession.

    iii.   The case manager provides a communication link between the other driver rehabilitation team members and the third-party payer's professional who has the authority to authorize payment for services, vehicle modifications, and equipment (e.g., the insurance company's claims adjuster).

2. Driving retirement or cessation

(Pellerito, 2006, pp. 425–454)

a. When it is determined that a client is no longer able to drive safely with or without restrictions, the DRS should be compelled to assist his or her client with identifying and using community mobility resources for dependable alternative transportation.

b. Access to dependable alternative transportation is an essential IADL and is necessary to fully empower clients who no longer drive.

    i.   Alternative transportation options are often unfamiliar to clients and caregivers who have relied on driving a motor vehicle as their primary (and more often their sole) method of transportation.

c. Most driver rehabilitation programs in the United States are primarily set up to help clients safely drive a car, van, or truck with or without modifications.

d. Only a few driver rehabilitation programs have adopted the notion that community mobility must be addressed by exploring alternative transportation options as an integral part of the comprehensive driver rehabilitation evaluation.

3. Service delivery models

(Pellerito, 2006, pp. 58–67)

a. Service delivery models provide the contexts or environments in which key driver rehabilitation and community mobility services are offered and delivered.

b. The most common models currently in existence in the United States include:

    i.   Traditional medical model

    ii.   Community-based model

    iii.   Vocational rehabilitation model

    iv.   University model

    v.   Veterans Affairs model

c. The traditional medical model

    i.   The medical model features programs that are housed within a hospital, rehabilitation center, and/or a freestanding outpatient clinic.

    ii.   Occupational therapy generalists may perform a predriving screen and then refer their clients to an occupational therapist specializing in driver rehabilitation.

    iii.   A DRS is the only professional prepared to perform a comprehensive driver rehabilitation evaluation that includes the clinical and on-road evaluations.

    iv.   Some facilities employ driver educators to perform some of or the entire on-road portion of the comprehensive driver rehabilitation evaluation after the occupational therapist specializing in driver rehabilitation has completed a clinical evaluation.

    v.   Technology can be used at any point during the evaluation–training–follow-up continuum of care. For example, DRSs may use driving simulators, virtual reality technology, or off-street areas set up as closed circuit courses; each of these tools afford clients opportunities to participate in training programs more fully because they can practice remedial skills in a protected environment.

    vi. If the medical model includes an occupational therapist and a driver educator who provides driver rehabilitation services, they should maintain an ongoing dialogue face to face, over the telephone, and on the Internet before, during, and after the on-road driving evaluation.

    vii. The interpretation of the clinical evaluation and the on-road evaluation are typically presented to the client by the occupational therapist with the driver educator present to answer questions that may be raised by the client, his or her caregiver, or both.

    viii. Some clients may need a driving evaluation only for clearance to drive after completing their rehabilitation program.

    ix. A client may need additional on-road training to learn compensatory techniques, how to use unfamiliar adapted driving aids, and/or to improve his or her defensive driving techniques.

    x. Some clients may not successfully pass the on-road driver evaluation and should be assisted with developing either a driver remediation plan or driver cessation plan.

    xi. If remedial steps are not appropriate or prove to be ineffective and the client is no longer a candidate for driving, the DRS can do much more than simply provide a list of alternative transportation resources (e.g., city bus services, dial a ride, taxis, senior volunteer services, and mass transit) for the client and his or her caregivers to peruse.

    xii. Actively helping clients and their caregivers identify and use alternative transportation is an essential service that every DRS should be prepared to provide.

    xiii. If a vehicle modification is required, a vehicle prescription is completed.

    xiv. It is the vehicle modifier's responsibility to educate the client about vehicle maintenance, equipment warranties, and emergency procedures.

    xv. On completion of the vehicle modification and the on-road training program, the DRS fills out a medical examination report that lists the client's restrictions.

    xvi. In most cases the client is contacted for a special road test. If the client passes the road test with the Department of Transportation Motor Vehicle Division (DOT MVD) road tester, he or she is issued a restricted driver's license.

    xvii. Collaboration between the specialists, client, caregivers, and vehicle modifier is the key to making certain that any concerns are addressed before the prescription is finalized and costly mistakes are made.

    xviii. Client restrictions may include driving only when using hand controls, driving during the daytime, and/or driving within a specified area.

  d. The community-based model

    i. Services within the community-based model are typically offered by driving schools that are state licensed and employ driver educators and/or driving instructors.

    ii. Community driving programs usually do not require a physician's referral to see a client for driver rehabilitation services.

    iii. The clients seen by driver educators, and especially driving instructors, usually do not present the kinds of complex medical diagnoses that occupational therapists address on a routine basis.

    iv. If the DRS notes any further problem areas, he or she should refer the client to the appropriate healthcare specialist for a consultation.

    v. Very few of these programs address alternatives to driving because community mobility and driving cessation is, in all likelihood, never formally addressed.

    vi. Referrals received by DRSs working in community-based programs can originate with vocational rehabilitation counselors, family physicians, allied health therapists working as generalists or specialists, physiatrists, vehicle modifiers, ophthalmologists, and case managers, among others.

e. The independent entrepreneur community-based model

  i. This model features a professional, such as an occupational therapist, who has opened a for-profit driving program.

  ii. Private practices are state-licensed driving schools and require a physician's referral to work with clients and caregivers.

  iii. These programs follow the same format as the medical model.

  iv. Many private practices employ DRSs who travel to a client's neighborhood to conduct the clinical and on-road evaluations and on-road training.

  v. This type of program features an occupational therapist who conducts the clinical and on-road evaluations, plans and implements driver training regimens, and generates prescriptions for vehicle modifications and adapted driving aids.

f. The vocational rehabilitation (VR) model

  i. The VR model is a state-funded model that, like other service delivery models, employs DRSs credentialed in diverse professional fields of study.

  ii. Clients work with VR counselors to develop an employment plan, which may or may not include driver rehabilitation services.

  iii. After a prescription is submitted, a bidding process will determine which vendor will perform the necessary vehicle modifications and conduct the client–vehicle fitting session(s).

    I. VR programs generally require that there must be at least three bids received from qualified vendors.

    II. If driving can assist a client in securing gainful employment, the VR counselor often refers the client to a DRS for a comprehensive driving evaluation.

g. The university model

  i. The university model is often state and/or federally funded and located either on a university campus or within a university-affiliated teaching hospital setting.

    I. This model usually employs occupational therapists who specialize in driver rehabilitation. Some programs also employ a driver educator.

    II. A doctor's referral is required for a client to enroll in the program.

  ii. Universities place importance on research, education, and service; therefore, driver rehabilitation programs can potentially assist faculty members and DRSs in these endeavors.

  iii. University-based programs are generally provided on a fee-for-service basis and may be supported in part by grant funding.

  iv. Programs may also offer some kind of pro bono services to clients living in the respective communities that are underserved and would otherwise be unable to receive driver rehabilitation services.

h. The Veterans Affairs (VA) model

  i. The VA model features federally funded driver rehabilitation programs for American veterans who are either service connected or nonservice connected.

  ii. After the veteran's legal eligibility has been determined, he or she is referred for a physical and/or psychological examination to determine whether the veteran is able to undergo special driver training.

    I. If the client is service connected, then he or she can apply for a vehicle grant for approximately $11,000 (one-time grant).

    II. Vehicle modifications will be provided to enable the client to drive independently or ride as a passenger in a vehicle with optimal comfort and safety.

  iii. The service-connected veteran is generally viewed as a higher priority than nonservice-connected veterans.

  iv. For a veteran to be considered service connected, his or her disability (e.g., health condition, traumatic injury, disease) must have occurred or be traceable to the time period when he or she was enlisted in the military.

4. National Mobility Equipment Dealers Association (NMEDA)

(Pellerito, 2006, pp. 68–74)

    a. NMEDA is primarily composed of Dealer Members.

        i. The association also has manufacturers as a secondary membership (Associate Members).

        ii. A third component of the membership is known as the Professional Members.

    b. Many of the advances in this industry can be attributed to the association.

        i. NMEDA has developed a comprehensive set of guidelines to "direct the mobility equipment industry toward consistency, quality and compliance," as it states in its preamble.

    c. NMEDA created a Quality Assurance Program (QAP) for its dealers.

        i. Under this program a dealer's shop can be accredited in any or all of three categories, depending on the types of work being done at that shop.

        ii. The Professional Members include DRSs, rehabilitation engineers, vehicle modification inspectors, state and federal government employees with a role in the industry, and others.

        iii. The types of accreditation are Mobility Equipment Installer, Structural Vehicle Modifier, and High-Tech Driving System Installer.

5. Roles of the vehicle modifier

(Pellerito, 2006, pp. 68–74)

    a. Primary role: Structural Vehicle Modifier and High-Tech Driving System Installer

        i. The categories of work responsibilities correspond to the types of QAP accreditation: Mobility Equipment Installer, Structural Vehicle Modifier, and High-Tech Driving System Installer.

    b. Ancillary role: Client–Vehicle Fitting, Vehicle Selection, and Equipment Trials

    c. Client–Vehicle Fitting: As part of the driver rehabilitation team, the dealer/technician works closely with the DRS and consumer during the client–vehicle fitting. This is to ensure that all equipment is positioned to optimize the functional recommendations of the DRS, consumer choice, and technical feasibility.

WORK SHEET

Work Sheet 20-1. Assistive Technology Worksheet

Match the following legislation with its impact on the provision of assistive technology equipment and services (Cook & Polgar, 2008):

C

e

1. _e_ Rehabilitation Act of 1973, as amended

2. _c_ Assistive Technology Act of 1998

3. _d_ Americans with Disabilities Act of 1990

4. _a_ The Developmental Disabilities Assistance and Bill of Rights Act

5. _b_ Individuals with Disabilities Education Act Amendments of 1997

a. Provides grants to states for developmental disabilities councils, university affiliated programs, and protection and advocacy activities for people with developmental disabilities.

b. Every child, under this law, has a right to free and appropriate education. Includes children with disabilities to be educated with their peers. Allows assistive technology devices and services for students 3 to 21 years old.

c. Section 508 mandates equal access to electronic office equipment for all federal employees; mandates rehabilitation technology as a primary benefit to be included in an individual written rehabilitation plan (IWRP).

d. Prohibits discrimination on the basis of disability in employment, state and local government, public accommodations, commercial facilities, transportation, and telecommunications, all of which affect the application of assistive technology.

e. Addressed for the first time in legislation, the expansion of assistive technology devices and services, and mandates consumer-driven assistive technology services.

Match the following accessibility features with its appropriate option (Cook & Polgar, 2008):

C

e

6. _d_ Display & Readability

7. _e_ Sounds & Speech

8. _a_ Keyboard Options

9. _b_ Mouse Options

10. _c_ Accessibility Utility

a. Dvorak Layout

b. SnapTo

c. Text-to-Speech

d. Screen Resolution

e. Narrator

(continues)

Work Sheet 20-1. Assistive Technology Worksheet *(continued)*

Match each device with appropriate consumer requirements (Cook & Polgar, 2008):

11. _D_ Standard Keyboards	A. The consumer must be able to read text, decipher graphics or icons, locate and follow a small mouse cursor, have good figure-ground perception, and distinguish color.
12. _A_ Standard Computer Displays	
13. _B_ Standard Mouse Control	B. The consumer must be able to demonstrate range of motion, strength, coordination, and timing.
_C_	C. The consumer must be able to hold or make controlled contact, move and stop the mouse cursor at a desired location, and activate a button at the appropriate time.

Place in order the correct steps in the service delivery process, beginning with the first (1) and ending with the last (6) (Cook & Polgar, 2008):

14. _2_ Initial evaluation

15. _4_ Recommendations and Report   *3*

16. _3_ Follow-along   *6*

17. _5_ Implementation   *4*

18. _1_ Referral and Intake

19. _6_ Follow-up   *5*

REFERENCES

Charlton, J. L., Koppel, S., O'Hare, M., Andrea, D., Smith, G., Khodr, B., et al. (2004). *Influence of chronic illness on crash involvement of motor vehicle drivers* (Literature Review No. 213). Melbourne, Australia: Monash University Accident Research Centre.

Cook, A. M., & Polgar, J. M. (2008). *Cook and Hussey's assistive technologies: Principles and practice* (3rd ed.). St. Louis, MO: Mosby.

Pellerito, Jr. J. M. (Ed.). (2006). *Driver rehabilitation and community mobility: Principles and practice*. St. Louis, MO: Mosby.

Pendleton, H. M., & Schultz-Krohn, W. (Eds.). (2006). *Pedretti's occupational therapy: Practice skills for physical dysfunction* (6th ed.). St. Louis, MO: Mosby.

Radomski, M. V., & Latham, C. A. T. (Eds.). (2008). *Occupational therapy for physical dysfunction* (6th ed.). Philadelphia: Lippincott Williams & Wilkins.

Exhibit 1-1 Stress Vulnerability Scale

In modern society, most of us can't avoid stress. But we can learn to behave in ways that lessen its effects. Researchers have identified a number of factors that affect one's vulnerability to stress—among them are eating and sleeping habits, caffeine and alcohol intake, and how we express our emotions. The following questionnaire is designed to help you discover your vulnerability quotient and to pinpoint trouble spots. Rate each item from 1 (always) to 5 (never), according to how much of the time the statement is true of you. Be sure to mark each item, even if it does not apply to you—for example, if you don't smoke, circle 1 next to item six.

	Always	Sometimes			Never
1. I eat at least one hot, balanced meal a day.	1	2	3	4	5
2. I get 7–8 hours of sleep at least four nights a week.	1	2	3	4	5
3. I give and receive affection regularly.	1	2	3	4	5
4. I have at least one relative within 50 miles on whom I can rely.	1	2	3	4	5
5. I exercise to the point of perspiration at least twice a week.	1	2	3	4	5
6. I limit myself to less than half a pack of cigarettes a day.	1	2	3	4	5
7. I take fewer than five alcohol drinks a week.	1	2	3	4	5
8. I am the appropriate weight for my height.	1	2	3	4	5
9. I have an income adequate to meet basic expenses.	1	2	3	4	5
10. I get strength from my religious beliefs.	1	2	3	4	5
11. I regularly attend club or social activities.	1	2	3	4	5
12. I have a network of friends and acquaintances.	1	2	3	4	5
13. I have one or more friends to confide in about personal matters.	1	2	3	4	5
14. I am in good health (including eyesight, hearing, and teeth).	1	2	3	4	5
15. I am able to speak openly about my feelings when angry or worried.	1	2	3	4	5
16. I have regular conversations with the people I live with about domestic problems—for example, chores and money.	1	2	3	4	5
17. I do something for fun at least once a week.	1	2	3	4	5
18. I am able to organize my time effectively.	1	2	3	4	5
19. I drink fewer than three cups of coffee (or other caffeine-rich drinks) a day.	1	2	3	4	5
20. I take some quiet time for myself during the day.	1	2	3	4	5

(continues)

Exhibit 1-1 Stress Vulnerability Scale *(continued)*

Scoring Instructions: To calculate your score, add up the figures and subtract 20.

Score Interpretation:
A score below 10 indicates excellent resistance to stress.
A score over 30 indicates some vulnerability to stress.
A score over 50 indicates serious vulnerability to stress.

Self-Care Plan: Notice that nearly all the items describe situations and behaviors over which you have a great deal of control. Review the items on which you scored three or higher. List those items in your self-care plan. Concentrate first on those that are easiest to change—for example, eating a hot, balanced meal daily and having fun at least once a week—before tackling those that seem difficult.

Source: Exhibit courtesy Copyright 2009 Stress Directions, Inc., Lyle H. Miller and Alma Dell Smith, Boston, MA
www.stressdirections.com

Exhibit 5-1 Reflection Question Journal

1. What? (What have I accomplished? What have I learned?)

2. So what? (What difference did it make? Why should I do it? How is it important? How do I feel about it?)

3. Now what? (What's next? Where do we go from here?)

Source: Exhibit courtesy of Live Wire Media.

WORK SHEET ANSWERS

Assistive Technology Worksheet Answers

1. __C__ Rehabilitation Act of 1973, as amended

2. __E__ Assistive Technology Act of 1998

3. __D__ Americans with Disabilities Act of 1990

4. __A__ The Developmental Disabilities Assistance and Bill of Rights Act

5. __B__ Individuals with Disabilities Education Act Amendments of 1997

a. Provides grants to states for developmental disabilities councils, university affiliated programs, and protection and advocacy activities for people with developmental disabilities.

b. Every child, under this law, has a right to free and appropriate education. Includes children with disabilities to be educated with their peers. Allows assistive technology devices and services for students 3 to 21 years old.

c. Section 508 mandates equal access to electronic office equipment for all federal employees; mandates rehabilitation technology as a primary benefit to be included in an individual written rehabilitation plan (IWRP).

d. Prohibits discrimination on the basis of disability in employment, state and local government, public accommodations, commercial facilities, transportation, and telecommunications, all of which affect the application of assistive technology.

e. Addressed for the first time in legislation, the expansion of assistive technology devices and services, and mandates consumer driven assistive technology services.

---

6. __D__ Display & Readability

7. __C__ Sounds & Speech

8. __A__ Keyboard Options

9. __B__ Mouse Options

10. __E__ Accessibility Utility

a. Dvorak Layout

b. SnapTo

c. Text-to-Speech

d. Screen Resolution

e. Narrator

---

11. __B__ Standard Keyboards

12. __A__ Standard Computer Displays

13. __C__ Standard Mouse Control

A. The consumer must be able to read text, decipher graphics or icons, locate and follow a small mouse cursor, have good figure-ground perception, and distinguish color.

B. The consumer must be able to demonstrate range of motion, strength, coordination, and timing.

C. The consumer must be able to hold or make controlled contact, move and stop the mouse cursor at a desired location, and activate a button at the appropriate time.

(continues)

Assistive Technology Worksheet Answers *(continued)*

14. __2__ Initial evaluation

15. __3__ Recommendations and Report

16. __6__ Follow-along

17. __4__ Implementation

18. __1__ Referral and Intake

19. __5__ Follow-up

Documentation, Management, Insurance, and Working with a Certified Occupational Therapy Assistant (COTA) (Days 32–35)

Documentation of Occupational Therapy Practice

Deborah Loftus

OBJECTIVES

1. Explain the purpose and methods for correct occupational therapy documentation.
2. Understand and implement the Occupational Therapy Practice Framework terminology as it relates to documentation.
3. Demonstrate the ability to write appropriate measurable, client-centered, short- and long-term goals.
4. Apply knowledge of applicable regulations, guidelines, and reimbursement systems, such as Medicare and supplemental insurances, as it relates to the documentation of occupational therapy practice.
5. Demonstrate competence in the following types of documentation: initial evaluation, intervention plan, progress reports, daily progress notes such as SOAP (subjective, objective, assessment, plan) and RHUMBA (relevant/relates, how long, understandable, measurable, behavioral, achievable), narrative notes, and discharge reports.

KEY TERMS

Table 21-1 Key Terms

Radomski & Latham, 2008, pp. 41–48	Pendleton & Schultz-Krohn, 2006, pp. 113–122
Clinical reasoning	Assessments
Commission on Accreditation of Rehabilitation Facilities (CARF)	Client-centered goal
Evidence-based practice	Evaluation
Plan of care	Health Insurance Portability and Accountability Act (HIPAA)
The Joint Commission (JCAHO)	Intervention plan
	Occupational Therapy Practice Framework (OTPF)
	Protected health information (PHI)
	Skilled intervention

INTRODUCTION

Welcome to Day 32 of your study guide. This chapter will provide you with an in-depth review of how to document occupational therapy services. Use the outline to gather pertinent information and complete the corresponding work sheets to reinforce your understanding of the key points and application of knowledge.

OUTLINE

1. The Occupational Therapy Practice Framework

(Sames, 2005, pp. 14–20)

2. AOTA Guidelines for Documentation

(Clark & Youngstrom, 2003, pp. 646–649)

  a. Client identification: Make sure the client's full name is on all necessary documentation (including initial evaluations, reevaluations, daily notes, discharges). Abbreviations of clients' names are not appropriate when recording occupational services and are not accepted by many insurance companies.

  b. Date and type of contact: Obvious information such as the complete date (month, day, and year) as well as the type of encounter you have with the client (initial evaluation or a daily progress note) is essential information that must be present on all documentation. This information serves to show the chronological order in which events happened during treatment. The time of day may be required for inpatient acute and rehabilitation documentation.

  c. Type of document: The facility, company, or agency through which the occupational services are being rendered should appear on each piece of documentation provided as well as the type of note that is being written.

  d. Signature: The treating therapist's full name followed by professional designation (e.g., Jane Doe, MOT, OTR) should appear on each documented note to identify the person who saw the client for the corresponding treatment date.

  e. Placement of signature: All notes must have the signature line at the end of the note to prevent tampering of documentation.

  f. Countersignature: OTs must countersign the signatures of occupational therapy assistants (OTAs) and their students. This is necessary secondary to state and facility regulations when OTAs and students are assisting with treatment. The countersignature also provides documentation of the supervision that is required by law.

  g. Terminology: Facilities vary on acceptable recognized terminology, including abbreviations. Prior to completing an organization's documentation process, confirm what is considered to be acceptable terminology.

  h. Abbreviations: Abbreviations vary at each facility, therefore it is recommended to confirm the accepted abbreviations at each facility for which you are completing documentation. Table 21-2 contains a work sheet of commonly abbreviated words for you to complete.

  i. Corrections: Errors should be corrected by drawing a single line through the word(s) in error and writing your initials above or next to the line. Whiting out and erasing are not accepted on occupational therapy notes and may not be accepted by insurance carriers or be valid in courts of law.

  j. Technology: Individual facilities vary when it comes to dictating the policies and procedures of the use of technology in occupational therapy documentation.

  k. Record disposal: Federal and state laws, in combination with facility regulations, dictate appropriate disposal of occupational therapy documentation.

  l. Confidentiality: It is important to familiarize yourself with all federal, state, and individual facility rules in regards to confidentiality. According to HIPAA regulations, the therapist has a responsibility to protect confidential information from unauthorized access.

m. Record storage: Individual differences are present from facility to facility regarding record storage and retention. Obviously, you must obey all federal, state, and facility regulations when storing occupational therapy documentation. Many times charts must be kept in a locked or secure storage container if the facility is regulated by various accrediting bodies, such as CARF or The Joint Commission, also known as the Joint Commission on the Accreditation of Healthcare Organizations (JCAHO).

3. Purpose of good documentation

(Pendleton & Schultz-Krohn, 2006, pp. 111–121)

a. Basic principles
  i. Documentation acts as a permanent, legal document that is the primary method of communication used to report exactly what was done with the client.
  ii. Reimbursement for occupational therapy services is dependent upon correct, well-written documentation.
  iii. Documentation is the vehicle with which occupational therapists show others the value of the intervention.
  iv. Confidentiality is maintained throughout all documentation processes.
  v. Documentation of medical necessity may be needed to determine patient access to continued occupational therapy services.

b. According to the American Occupational Therapy Association, four main purposes of documentation exist.
  i. Articulation of the rationale for the use of occupational therapy services
  ii. Reflection of the therapist's clinical reasoning and use of professional judgment skills
  iii. Communication regarding information about the client from the occupational therapist's perspective
  iv. Documents a chronological record of the client's status, occupational therapy services provided to the client, and the client's outcomes

c. Best practices
  i. Relevant information
  ii. Concise and comprehensive
  iii. Proper grammar
  iv. Correct spelling
  v. Approved abbreviations
  vi. Signature with credentials
  vii. Reflection of the Occupational Therapy Practice Framework

d. Initial evaluation
  i. Client information
  ii. Referral information; reason for referral or physician's order
  iii. Occupational profile
    I. Occupational history and experiences
    II. Activities of daily living
    III. Interests, values, and needs
  iv. Assessments
    I. Standardized tests (e.g., grip strength)
    II. Nonstandardized tests (e.g., narrative reports)
  v. Summary and analysis
  vi. Therapy recommendations

e. The collaborative establishment of goals
  i. Short- and long-term goal or discharge goal
    I. Measurable
    II. Occupation based
    III. Functional
    IV. Client centered

        V. Time based

    ii. Another system for remembering the essential parts of goal writing is the FEAST method.

(Borcherding, 2005 p. 86)

        I. Function
        II. Expectation
        III. Action
        IV. Specific conditions
        V. Time line

f. Intervention plan

    i. Performance skills (e.g., motor, process, or communication/interaction skills)
    ii. Performance patterns (e.g., habits, routines, or roles)
    iii. Context (e.g., cultural, physical, or social)
    iv. Activity demands (e.g., space demands and social demands)
    v. Client factors/participation (e.g., body functions and structures)

g. Progress reports showing skilled intervention are needed.

    i. SOAP notes
        I. Subjective
        II. Objective
        III. Assessment
        IV. Plan
    ii. Checklist notes
    iii. Narrative notes
    iv. Descriptive notes
    v. RHUMBA
        I. Relevant
        II. How long
        III. Understandable
        IV. Measurable
        V. Behavioral
        VI. Achievable

    vi. Discharge report: A necessary piece of documentation that must include the client's progress or lack of progress from the beginning to the end of occupational therapy services. The discharge report, sometimes referred to as the discontinuation summary, serves as the final justification of OT services.

WORK SHEETS

Work Sheet 21-1

Review commonly used abbreviations and fill in the following chart.

Table 21-2 Commonly Used Abbreviations

Upper extremity	UE
Lower extremity	LE
Both upper extremities	BUEs
Left upper extremity	LUE
Right upper extremity	RUE
Both lower extremities	BLEs
Left lower extremity	LLE
Right lower extremity	RLE
Distal interphalangeal joint	DIP jt
Metacarpal phalangeal joint	MP jt
Proximal interphalangeal joint	PIP jt
Fracture	fx
Active assisted range of motion	AAROM
Active range of motion	AROM
Functional range of motion	FROM
Passive range of motion	PROM
Range of motion	ROM
Wheelchair	w/c
Within functional limits	wfl
Within normal limits	wnl
Motor vehicle accident	mva
Open reduction, internal fixation	orif
Rheumatoid arthritis	RA
Spinal cord injury	SCI
Traumatic brain injury	TBI
Total hip replacement	THR
Transient ischemic attack	TIA
Diagnosis	dx
History of	h/o
Symptoms	sx
Treatment	tx
Post operation	p/o
Short-term goal	stg
Long-term goal	ltg
As needed	prn

Source: Adapted from Borcherding, 2005, pp. 17–23; Sames, 2005, pp. 7–8

Work Sheet 21-2

Table 21-3 SOAP

	Acronym	Definition	Example
S			
O			
A			
P			

Source: Adapted from Pendleton & Schultz-Krohn, 2006, pp. 117–118

Work Sheet 21-3

Table 21-4 Definitions for Levels of Assistance Based on FIM

Level of Assistance	Definition
Complete independence	7
Modified independence	6
Supervision	5 76-100%
Minimal assistance	4 51-75%
Moderate assistance	3 26-50%
Maximum assistance	2 1-25%
Total assistance	1 0%

Source: Adapted from Radomski & Latham, 2008, p. 50

REFERENCES

Borcherding, S. (2005). *Documentation manual for writing SOAP notes in occupational therapy* (2nd ed.). Thorofare, NJ: Slack.

Clark, G. F., & Youngstrom, M. J. (2003). Guidelines for documentation of occupational therapy. *American Journal of Occupational Therapy, 57*(6), 646–649.

Pendleton, H. M., & Schultz-Krohn, W. (Eds.). (2006). *Pedretti's occupational therapy: Practice skills for physical dysfunction* (6th ed.). St. Louis, MO: Mosby.

Radomski, M. V., & Latham, C. A. T. (Eds.). (2008). *Occupational therapy for physical dysfunction* (6th ed.). Philadelphia: Lippincott Williams & Wilkins.

Sames, K. (2005). *Documenting occupational therapy practice*. Upper Saddle River, NJ: Prentice Hall.

Occupational Therapy Management and Business Fundamentals

Joseph M. Pellerito Jr., Rosanne DiZazzo-Miller, and
Fredrick D. Pociask

PART I: THE OCCUPATIONAL THERAPY MANAGER

OBJECTIVES

1. Understand and identify professional functions, including the different roles and responsibilities required of an occupational therapy (OT) manager.
2. Describe and identify the areas of competency needed to be a successful occupational therapy manager.
3. Define the occupational therapy manager's role in marketing and provide a brief description of the marketing process.
4. Identify ethical behaviors in relation to management and occupational therapy services.
5. Understand the role of the OT manager within the contexts of state and federal laws that govern the profession, including licensure, certification, accreditation, scope of practice, and client confidentiality.
6. Understand the OT manager's fiscal responsibilities, such as developing and managing an operating budget.
7. Describe the importance, process, and procedures that help ensure continuous quality improvement (CQI).

KEY TERMS

Table 22-1 Key Terms 22a

Braveman, 2006, pp. 8, 45, 179 Crepeau, Cohn, & Schell, 2009, pp. 404, 914–928, 943 McCormack, Jaffe, & Goodman-Lavey, 2003, pp. 110, 445, 516
Accreditation bodies
Administration
Continuous quality improvement (CQI)
Management
Requisite managerial authority

(continues)

Table 22-1 Key Terms 22a *(continued)*

Braveman, 2006, pp. 8, 45, 179 Crepeau, Cohn, & Schell, 2009, pp. 404, 914–928, 943 McCormack, Jaffe, & Goodman-Lavey, 2003, pp. 110, 445, 516
Risk management
Scope of practice
Supervision

INTRODUCTION

Welcome to Day 33 of your study guide. This chapter will provide you with a review of the various areas related to management of occupational therapy services and an introduction to business fundamentals and entrepreneurship. Part I covers the OT manager, and Part II outlines information relating to business fundamentals. Use these outlines as tools to direct your investigation of key points in business and management, and locate references and resources to assist in a comprehensive examination of information.

OUTLINE

1. **When searching ads for occupational therapy management positions, the job description will often include any or all of the following responsibilities or job duties:**
    a. Performing overall management of the rehabilitation department
    b. Monitoring patient admissions, treatment schedules, and discontinuance of treatment
    c. Tracking of doctors' orders and overseeing patient or client data collection
    d. Serving as a liaison between subordinates and facility administrators
    e. Ensuring effective delivery of patient care and compliance with policies and procedures
    f. Assisting with strategic planning, program development, personnel management, and fiscal planning
    g. Ensuring efficient use of personnel and facilities for optimal safety and productivity
    h. Overseeing the care and maintenance of therapy area inventory, equipment, and supplies
    i. Ensuring accurate documentation of patient care required to successfully bill for services
    j. Evaluating competence of occupational therapy personnel and provide programming for competency training and education
    k. Analyzing and maintaining records for quality assurance, safety, and infection control
    l. Continuously interacting with the interdisciplinary team members, clients, and families to help ensure optimal satisfaction and patient/client outcomes
    m. Addressing customer or stakeholder (or both) services issues
    n. Providing ongoing mentoring and support to therapy and clerical staff
    o. Having at least 3 years of therapy or management experience or both
2. **Review and understand the differences between the roles and responsibilities of administrators, managers, and supervisors.**
    a. Administrators
        i. Typically responsible for overseeing daily operations
        ii. Work to preserve the viability and positive reputation of the organization
        iii. Delegate tasks to managers (Braveman, 2006, p. 110; Crepeau, et al., 2009, p. 915; McCormack, et al., 2003, p. 8)
    b. Managers
        i. Although managers are responsible for a department or departments in a facility, supervisors mentor and supervise the individual therapists within a given department (Braveman, 2006, p. 110; Crepeau, et al., 2009, p. 915; McCormack, et al., 2003, pp. 59–60).

c. Supervisors

    i. Supervisors include titles such as senior therapists, where the more experienced therapists are empowered to mentor and facilitate day-to-day operations; however, supervisors usually do not have any of the management authority to make decisions, for example determining levels of staff compensation and recruiting, hiring, and firing personnel (Braveman, 2006, p. 110; Crepeau, et al., 2009, p. 915; McCormack, et al., 2003, pp. 59–60).

3. Functions of the occupational therapy manager

(Braveman, 2006, pp. 110–118)
(Crepeau, et al., 2009, pp. 916–918)
(McCormack, et al., 2003, pp. 18, 163, 200)

    a. Four traditional managerial functions include planning, organizing and staffing, directing, and controlling.

        i. Planning

            I. Determine goals that are congruous with the organization's mission and vision.

            II. Create and implement policies and procedures and measure their effectiveness.

        ii. Organizing and staffing

            I. Recruitment and retention of staff

            II. Salary merit, rewards, and disciplinary actions

            III. Oversee student fieldwork

        iii. Directing

            I. Staff mentoring and training

        iv. Controlling

            I. Establishing, evaluating, and correcting work performance standards

            II. Quality control (QC) and continuous quality improvement (CQI)

                a. The manager is responsible for identifying areas that require attention in terms of customer satisfaction (or dissatisfaction) and developing and implementing a plan to reinforce or ameliorate them, respectively.

                b. Evaluating and improving occupational therapy services (Braveman, 2006, pp. 274–290 [see case examples pp. 292–302]; Crepeau, et al., 2009, pp. 922, 549–550; McCormack, et al., 2003, p. 516)

                    i. Continuous quality improvement (CQI) is both a management philosophy and a method for structural problem solving.

                    ii. Key features of a CQI approach include the following:

                        1. Commitment to quality (e.g., SWOT analysis at http://www.sba.gov/idc/groups/public/documents/sba_homepage/pub_mp21.pdf)

                        2. Staff training

                        3. Methods for assessing progress

                        4. Quality or process improvement teams

                        5. Policies, procedures, and reward systems

                    iii. Deming's 14-point program to improve quality

                    iv. What is quality?

                    v. Performance characteristics that define quality

                    vi. Common CQI concepts, strategies, tools, and techniques

                    vii. Roles for a CQI team

                    viii. Stages of team development

                    ix. Tools used for analysis and display for CQI data

                    x. Determining appropriate rewards and recognition

        v. Motivation (Braveman, 2006, pp. 152–157; McCormack, et al., 2003, pp. 325–327)

        vi. Disciplinary action (Braveman, 2006, pp. 129–131; Crepeau, et al., 2009, pp. 915–916; McCormack, et al., 2003, pp. 325–327)

> **vii.** Ethics (Braveman, 2006, pp. 352–369 [see case examples pp. 360–361]; Crepeau, et al., 2009, pp. 203–204, 274–283; McCormack, et al., 2003, pp. 449, 504–505)
>> **I.** Professional ethics
>> **II.** Ethics defined
>> **III.** Ethics terminology
>> **IV.** Ethics theories and approaches
>> **V.** Ethics and management
>> **VI.** Promoting ethics within the OT department
>> **VII.** OT practice regulation
>>> **a.** State regulatory boards
>>> **b.** NBCOT
>>> **c.** AOTA and ethics
>> **VIII.** Resources
>
> **viii.** Client confidentiality
>> **I.** Health Insurance Portability and Accountability Act of 1996 (HIPAA)
>
> **ix.** Safety procedures and risk management
>> **I.** OT manager's role and responsibilities for department policies and procedures
>
> **x.** Scope and standards of occupational therapy practice (Braveman, 2006, p. 45; Crepeau, et al., 2009, pp. 242–243, 246, 279, 943–946; McCormack, et al., 2003, pp. 445–447)
>
> **xi.** Referrals (Braveman, 2006, pp. 45–46; McCormack, et al., 2003, pp. 194, 200, 378, 413)
>
> **xii.** Program evaluation (Braveman, 2006, pp. 257–259)

4. Organizational environments

(Braveman, 2006, pp. 58–59)
(McCormack, et al., 2003, pp. 279–280)

> **a.** Organizations operate within environments, and their ability to meet environmental demands and anticipate and prepare for future challenges impacts the organization's overall performance.
>
> **b.** External environments
>> **i.** Specific arenas within the external environment that should be of concern to OT managers include the following:
>>> **I.** Legislation
>>> **II.** Economics
>>> **III.** Technology
>>> **IV.** Demographics
>>> **V.** Sociocultural factors

5. Domain of knowledge, competency, and assessment of competencies

(Braveman, 2006, pp. 180–182)
(Crepeau, et al., 2009, pp. 85, 240–248)
(McCormack, et al., 2003, pp. 464–479)

> **a.** Competence
>> **i.** Definition
>> **ii.** Basic requirements
>> **iii.** Characteristics
>
> **b.** Types of competencies
>> **i.** Age-specific competencies
>> **ii.** Equipment-related competencies
>> **iii.** Specialized and advanced practice competencies
>> **iv.** Competencies related to specific skills or procedures

6. Accreditation bodies and requirements

(Braveman, 2006, pp. 179–180)
(Crepeau, et al., 2009, pp. 404, 623)
(McCormack, et al., 2003, pp. 516–547)

a. The Joint Commission

b. Commission on Accreditation of Rehabilitation Facilities (CARF)

c. Occupational Safety and Health Administration (OSHA)

7. Licensure and certification for occupational therapists

(Braveman, 2006, pp. 43–45)

(Crepeau, et al., 2009, pp. 238–259)

(McCormack, et al., 2003, pp. 440–472)

a. Types of practice regulations

b. Licensure

c. Mandatory certification

d. Mandatory registration

e. Trademark or title control legislation

f. Common components of practice acts

    i. Scope of practice

    ii. Referral requirements

    iii. Temporary license/work permit

    iv. Continuing competence

    v. The Certified Occupational Therapy Assistant (COTA) supervision requirements

8. Finances

(Braveman, 2006, pp. 118–124)

(Crepeau, et al., 2009, p. 922)

(McCormack, et al., 2003, pp. 148–150)

a. The occupational therapy manager may be required to establish and carry out a departmental budget. This responsibility includes identifying and articulating departmental priorities and needs, as well as revenue and expense projections.

b. The ability to successfully develop and follow a budget requires an understanding of healthcare reimbursement streams, human resources, and facility management in terms of supplies and maintenance.

c. The occupational therapy manager is responsible for overseeing department costs and tracking and reporting customer volume, profits, and productivity.

9. Marketing

(Braveman, 2006, pp. 333–345)

(Crepeau, et al., 2009, p. 925)

(McCormack, et al., 2003, pp. 178–189)

a. OT managers are increasingly becoming more involved with developing and implementing marketing strategies.

    i. These require managers to determine a target population or target populations to be served in addition to devising a plan that addresses and promotes services for those prospective service recipients.

b. The following four steps are identified in Braveman, 2006, pp. 333–345; Crepeau, et al., 2009, p. 925; and McCormack, et al., 2003, pp. 178–189:

    i. Organization assessment

        I. This involves the effects of the strengths and limitations within the organization that can impact the services rendered.

    ii. Environmental assessment

        I. This area focuses on analyzing data pertaining to the target audience, which informs the marketing plan.

    iii. Market analysis

        I. This includes the process of drawing conclusions as a result of analyzing target group report data.

    iv. Marketing communication

        I. Marketing communication entails presenting the service or end product to the target audience(s) with a clear and logical flow of information.

        II. Advantages and disadvantages

        III. Resources related to marketing health services

PART II: BUSINESS FUNDAMENTALS

OBJECTIVES

1. Understand what it means to be an occupational therapist entrepreneur.
2. Describe and identify the four primary resources available from the U.S. Small Business Administration (SBA) for current and prospective small business owners.
3. Define the key steps involved in planning a business.
4. Define the key steps involved in starting a business.
5. Describe the ways entrepreneurs can finance their businesses.
6. Understand the roles of the business manager in running a business.
7. Identify important resources outside of the SBA that are available to current and prospective business owners.

KEY TERMS

Table 22-2 Key Terms 22b

U.S. Small Business Administration, 2009
Breakeven analysis
Business plan
Business planning
Business resources
Business tools
Capital
Financing and accounting
SBA resources
Strategic thinking
Venture capitalist

OUTLINE

1. **Introduction to the U.S. Small Business Administration (SBA): http://www.sba.gov/aboutsba/index.html**
   a. The SBA was created in 1953 as an independent agency of the federal government to perform the following functions:
      i. Aid, counsel, assist, and protect the interests of small business concerns in the United States and throughout its territories
      ii. Preserve free and competitive enterprise
      iii. Maintain and strengthen the overall U.S. economy
   b. The SBA recognizes that small business is critical to the United States' economic recovery and strength, to building America's future, and to helping the United States compete in today's global marketplace.

2. **SBA primary resources**

   a. Planning a business: http://www.sba.gov/smallbusinessplanner/index.html

   b. Services such as financial assistance, laws and regulations, and counseling: http://www.sba.gov/services/index.html

   c. Tools such as library resources, audiovisual aids, monthly Web chats, and helpful forms: http://www.sba.gov/tools/index.html

   d. Local resources with an interactive map to find counseling, training, and business development specialists who provide free and low-cost services in any given area: http://www.sba.gov/localresources/index.html

   e. We will review the first two resources (i.e., planning a business and SBA services) next and provide links to the latter two resources (i.e., tools and local resources) for further exploration and discovery.

3. **Business planning**

   a. Careful planning is fundamental to any business's success. The Small Business Planner (http://www.sba.gov/localresources/index.html) includes information and resources that help the entrepreneur determine appropriate strategies and tactics at any stage of the business life cycle to help ensure success.

   b. The Small Business Planner is comprised of the following four steps: planning a business, starting a business, managing a business, and getting out of a business.

   c. Checklist for starting a business

      i. This is a helpful tool provided by the SBA that enables entrepreneurs to answer the following key questions to match their abilities and knowledge with attributes required of any successful business owner, irrespective of the company's size.

         I. Do you think you are ready to start a business?

         II. Have you ever worked in a business similar to what you are planning to start?

         III. Would people who know you say that you are well suited to be self-employed?

         IV. Do you have support for your business from family and friends?

         V. Have you ever taken a course or seminar designed to teach you how to start and manage a small business?

         VI. Have you discussed your business idea, business plan, or proposed business with a business coach or counselor, such as a faculty advisor, SCORE counselor, Small Business Development Center counselor, or other economic development advisor?

   d. Starting a business frequently asked questions (FAQs)

      i. Answers are provided to the following frequently asked questions:

         I. How do I get a small business loan? How do I get a small business grant? http://www.sba.gov/services/financialassistance/grants/index.html

         II. How do I get started in a business?

            a. The SBA provides a wealth of information on starting a business at the SBA home page under "Small Business Planner": http://www.sba.gov

         III. How do I get a business license?

            a. For free one-on-one counseling, please go to SBA's home page at http://www.sba.gov and select "Local Resources."

            b. The Service Corps of Retired Executives and the Small Business Development Center can assist you with your business venture.

         IV. How do I write a business plan? See the SBA's home page at http://www.sba.gov and select "Writing a Business Plan" under "Small Business Planner."

         V. What type of collateral do I need for a loan?

         VI. Is there any business assistance available in my area?

            a. Service Corps of Retired Executives (SCORE)

            b. Small Business Development Centers (SBDC)

               i. The SBDC provides a variety of management and technical assistance services to small businesses and potential entrepreneurs.

    e. A glossary of terms is provided so that entrepreneurs can get to know the specific terms of the professional business world: http://www.sba.gov/smallbusinessplanner/plan/getready/serv_sbplanner_gready_glossory.html

    f. The small business Startup Guide can help you start a successful business: http://www.sba.gov/smallbusinessplanner/plan/getready/serv_sbplanner_stguide.html

    g. Writing a business plan:
http://www.sba.gov/smallbusinessplanner/plan/writeabusinessplan/SERV_WRRITING BUSPLAN.html

        i. A written guide to starting and running your business successfully is essential.

        ii. This plan will encourage loans, promote growth, and provide a map for you to follow.

        iii. Strategic planning

        iv. Business plan workshop: An online workshop to help start and improve a business plan

        v. Using the business plan

            I. Explores ways to get the most out of a business plan

    h. Finding a niche

    i. Business planning FAQs

4. Starting a business http://web.sba.gov/faqs/

    a. Starting a business requires an entrepreneur to complete a number of steps and make some key decisions, including, but not limited to, the following:

        i. Selecting a location

        ii. Deciding on a business structure

        iii. Obtaining the necessary licenses and permits

    b. In addition, determining which financing options will meet both short-term needs and long-term goals is important.

    c. The following links provide information on these topics along with guidance on buying an existing business, copyright and trademark issues, and getting support from an outside expert: http://www.sba.gov/smallbusinessplanner/start/findamentor/index.html and http://www.sba.gov/smallbusinessplanner/start/pickalocation/signage/copyrights.html

    d. Finding a mentor

        i. Service Corps of Retired Executives (SCORE)

            I. The following is the link to retired professionals who are available to give you advice: http://www.sba.gov/smallbusinessplanner/start/findamentor/index.html

        ii. Small Business Development Centers

            I. The following is a link to organizations that can help small businesses grow and prosper: http://www.sba.gov/aboutsba/sbaprograms/sbdc/index.html

        iii. Network of training and counseling services

            I. The following link connects entrepreneurs to help with professional training and counseling: http://www.sba.gov/aboutsba/sbaprograms/ed/index.html

    e. Financing a start-up business: http://www.sba.gov/smallbusinessplanner/start/financestartup/index.html

        i. All businesses require some form of financing.

        ii. An integral component of starting a successful business is raising sufficient capital.

        iii. There are many challenges here, but numerous resources are available to help small business owners.

        iv. The SBA provides a plethora of information on numerous topics including, but certainly not limited to, the following:

            I. General financing and accounting

            II. Start-up costs: http://www.sba.gov/smallbusinessplanner/start/financestartup/SERV_SBPLANNER_MANAGE_STARTUP_.html

            III. Estimating costs: http://www.sba.gov/smallbusinessplanner/start/financestartup/SERV_ESTCOST.html

    IV. Breakeven analysis: http://www.sba.gov/smallbusinessplanner/start/finance startup/SERV_BREAKEVEN.html

    V. Finance basics: http://www.sba.gov/smallbusinessplanner/start/finance startup/SERV_FINANBASICS.html

    VI. Borrowing money: http://www.sba.gov/smallbusinessplanner/start/finance startup/SERV_BORROW.html

        a. Loan and funding information

        b. Know how to find various sources of capital to begin your business: http://www.sba.gov/smallbusinessplanner/start/financestartup/SERV_FIND CAPITAL.html

        c. The basic requirements for a business to receive an SBA loan

    VII. The process of buying a business: http://www.sba.gov/smallbusinessplanner/start/buyabusiness/index.html

    VIII. Naming a business: http://www.sba.gov/smallbusinessplanner/start/name yourbusiness/index.html

    IX. Legal requirements and implications

    X. Searching and registering business names

        a. Domain names

        b. Choosing a business structure

    XI. Protecting ideas: http://www.sba.gov/smallbusinessplanner/start/protect yourideas/SERV_SBP_PRTIDEAS.html

    XII. Understanding product basics: http://www.sba.gov/smallbusinessplanner/start/protectyourideas/SERV_SBP_S_PRODBAS.html

    XIII. Protecting ideas, copyrights, patents, and trademarks FAQs: http://www.sba.gov/smallbusinessplanner/start/protectyourideas/serv_copyrtfaq.html

        a. Intellectual property FAQs: http://www.sba.gov/smallbusinessplanner/start/protectyourideas/SERV_BP_INTFAQS.html

    XIV. Getting licenses and permits: http://www.sba.gov/smallbusinessplanner/start/getlicensesandpermits/index.html

    XV. Picking a location: http://www.sba.gov/smallbusinessplanner/start/picka location/index.html

    XVI. Leasing equipment: http://www.sba.gov/smallbusinessplanner/start/lease equipment/index.html

5. Managing a business

  a. Lead: http://www.sba.gov/smallbusinessplanner/manage/lead/index.html

  b. Make decisions: http://www.sba.gov/smallbusinessplanner/manage/makedecisions/index.html

  c. Manage employees: http://www.sba.gov/smallbusinessplanner/index.html

  d. Market and price: http://www.sba.gov/smallbusinessplanner/manage/marketandprice/index.html

  e. Market and sell: http://www.sba.gov/smallbusinessplanner/manage/MarketandSell/index.html

  f. Understand fair practice: http://www.sba.gov/smallbusinessplanner/manage/Understand FairPractice/index.html

  g. Pay taxes: http://www.sba.gov/smallbusinessplanner/manage/paytaxes/index.html

  h. Get insurance: http://www.sba.gov/smallbusinessplanner/manage/getinsurance/index.html

    i. Business insurance

      I. Workers' compensation insurance: http://www.sba.gov/smallbusinessplanner/manage/getinsurance/SERV_INSURANCEFAQS.html

      II. Surety bonds

  i. Handle legal concerns

  j. Forecast: http://www.sba.gov/smallbusinessplanner/manage/forecast/index.html

    i. Strategic thinking

        I.   Strategic vision for your business

            a. Five criteria to developing strategic vision

k. Advocate and stay informed: http://www.sba.gov/smallbusinessplanner/manage/advocate/index.html

l. Use technology: http://www.sba.gov/smallbusinessplanner/manage/technology/index.html

m. Finance growth: http://www.sba.gov/smallbusinessplanner/manage/financegrowth/index.html

    i. Finance basics: http://www.sba.gov/services/financialassistance/basics/financebasics/index.html

    ii. Two types of financing

        I.   Equity

        II.   Debt

    iii. When looking for money, you must consider your company's debt-to-equity ratio—the relation between dollars you've borrowed and dollars you've invested in your business.

        I.   Equity financing: http://www.sba.gov/smallbusinessplanner/manage/financegrowth/index.html

            a. Most small or growth-stage businesses use limited equity financing.

            b. As with debt financing, additional equity often comes from nonprofessional investors, such as friends, relatives, employees, customers, or industry colleagues.

            c. The most common source of professional equity funding comes from venture capitalists.

        II.   Debt financing

            a. There are many sources for debt financing.

                i. Banks

                ii. Savings and loans

                iii. Commercial finance companies

                iv. The SBA

            b. State and local governments have developed many programs in recent years to encourage the growth of small businesses in recognition of their positive effects on the economy.

            c. Family members, friends, and former associates are all potential sources, especially when capital requirements are smaller. See http://www.sba.gov/smallbusinessplanner/manage/financegrowth/index.html

        III. Estimating costs

            a. To determine how much seed money you will need, you must estimate the costs of your business for at least the first several months.

            b. Every business is different and has its own specific cash needs at different stages of development, so there is no universal method for estimating your start-up costs.

            c. Some businesses can be started on a shoestring budget, and others may require considerable investment in infrastructure, such as product inventory, mechanical equipment, information technology, and personnel, to name a few.

            d. It is vitally important to know that you will have enough money to launch your business venture. See http://www.sba.gov/smallbusinessplanner/manage/financegrowth/index.html

            e. The most effective way to calculate your start-up costs is to use a work sheet that lists all the various categories of costs (both one time and ongoing) that you will need to estimate prior to starting your business.

            f. The SBA provides a tool to estimate start-up costs on an affiliate's Web site: http://www.bplans.com/business_calculators/startup_costs_calculator.cfm

IV. Equity financing

    a. Most small or growth-stage businesses use equity financing in a limited way.

    b. As with debt financing, most of the time additional equity comes from nonprofessional investors, such as friends, relatives, employees, customers, or industry colleagues.

    c. Small Business Investment Company: http://www.sba.gov/aboutsba/sbaprograms/inv/index.html

    d. New Markets Venture Capital Program: http://www.sba.gov/aboutsba/sbaprograms/inv/nmvc/INV_NMVC_INDEX.html

V. Financial statements

    a. Understanding financial statements is critically important to the success of all small businesses.

    b. Balance sheet

    c. Liabilities and net worth

    d. Assets

    e. Current assets

    f. Cash

    g. Accounts receivable

    h. Inventory

    i. Notes receivable

    j. Fixed assets

    k. Intangibles

    l. Liabilities and net worth

    m. Current liabilities

    n. Notes payable

    o. Accounts payable

    p. Liabilities

    q. Equity/net worth

    r. How to prepare a loan package

VI. The SBA offers free online courses at the following URL: http://www.sba.gov/services/financialassistance/basics/statement/index.html

VII. Contract opportunities: http://www.sba.gov/contractingopportunities/index.html

    a. For small business owners

    b. For government/contracting officials

iv. Disaster assistance: http://www.sba.gov/services/disasterassistance/index.html

    I. Basics

    II. For businesses of all sizes

    III. Military reservists loans

    IV. For homeowners and renters

    V. Counseling and assistance: http://www.sba.gov/services/counseling/index.html

v. Other assistance

    I. SCORE

    II. Small Business Development Centers

    III. Women's business centers

    IV. National training events

vi. Laws/regulations: http://www.sba.gov/services/lawsandregulations/index.html

    I. Small business advocacy

    II. National ombudsman

    III. Law library

    IV. Hearings and appeals

    V. Compliance: http://www.sba.gov/services/Compliance/index.html

Exhibit 22-1 Key Research Terms

Although research and evidence-based practice are common themes throughout this book, it is important to take some time to review key research terms. This exhibit is placed in the management and business fundamentals chapter because, aside from working in academe, this area of practice is where you will likely have the most opportunity to utilize and implement research.

Research Term	Definition Depoy & Gitlin, 2005, pp. 317–325
Bias	An unintended or unavoidable effect on study outcomes. Also called *systematic error*.
Clinical trial	A controlled study involving human subjects, designed to evaluate the effectiveness of a drug or behavioral intervention.
Correlation	A method of determining the relationship between pairs of interval level variables, usually expressed from -1.00 to zero to $+1.00$.
Ethnography	A type of research concerned with description and interpretation of cultural patterns, where the observer is immersed in the culture for an extended period of time.
Experimental study	A true experiment study is one in which subjects are randomly assigned to groups that experience carefully controlled interventions manipulated by the investigator. This type of research yields numerical data for analysis.
Generalizability	The extent to which research findings and conclusions from a study conducted on a sample population can be applied to the population at large.
Guttman scale	Items are arranged in an order so that an individual who agrees with a particular item also agrees with items of lower rank order.
Hawthorne effect	The phenomenon in which research subjects experience a change simply because they are involved in a research study. Also known as *attention bias*.
Inclusion and exclusion criteria	A set of specific criteria that determine who can and who cannot be included in a research study.
Institutional review board (IRB)	A specially constituted board of experts established at each institution (e.g., university, hospital, etc.) to oversee the research conducted there and protect the welfare of human subjects.
Likert scale	A scale commonly used in questionnaires (often 5-point or 7-point scales) to measure agreement with a particular item.
Member checking	In qualitative research, this refers to the researcher checking out the facts with his or her research participants.
Nonparametric statistics	Mathematical formulas that can be used to test hypotheses using small samples and data that do not meet the assumptions of parametric statistics.
Parametric statistics	Formulas used to test hypotheses, based on three assumptions: (1) data is normally distributed; (2) the variance is homogeneous; and (3) interval level data.
Phenomenology	A qualitative research approach concerned with understanding certain individual or group experiences and behaviors from the insider's point of view.
Qualitative research	Qualitative research focuses on in-depth understanding of human behavior. Attention to social relationships and context is critical. Study findings yield narrative data that are described and interpreted.

Exhibit 22-1 Key Research Terms *(continued)*

Research Term	Definition Depoy & Gitlin, 2005, pp. 317–325
Quantitative research	Quantitative research focuses on empirical measurement with the goal of prediction of probabilistic relationships between variables. These studies yield numerical data that can be tested using statistics.
Quasi-experimental	A study that is similar to a true experimental study except that it lacks random assignment of subjects to the treatment group.
Random sample	In a true random sample, every person in the population has an equal chance of being selected for the sample.
Reliability	The consistency or stability of a measure or test from one use to the next. When repeated measurements of the same thing give identical or very similar results, the measure is said to be reliable.
Triangulation	Use of multiple methods or strategies to strengthen the research findings.
Validity	A term to describe a measurement instrument or test that measures what it is supposed to measure. A valid assessment is the extent to which the assessment is free of systematic error (bias).

Source: Work sheet courtesy of Cathy Lysack, PhD, OT(C)

WORK SHEET

Work Sheet 22-1. Occupational Therapy Manager Work Sheet
PDCA Work Sheet (Crepeau, Cohn, & Schell, 2009, p. 922) Define each step of The Plan, Do, Check, Act (PDCA) Cycle used for continuous quality improvement (CQI)

Step 1 Plan	
Step 2 Do	
Step 3 Check	
Step 4 Act	

(continues)

Work Sheet 22-1. Occupational Therapy Manager Work Sheet *(continued)*

CQI Core Concepts Work Sheet
(Crepeau, Cohn, & Schell, 2009, p. 923)

Match each core concept with its appropriate topic:

Core CQI Concepts	Topics
1. ____ Ground rules for meetings	A. Strategies
	B. Tools
2. ____ Multivoting	C. Techniques
3. ____ Process flow charts	
4. ____ Consensus	
5. ____ Balancing tasks and people	
6. ____ Icebreakers	
7. ____ Cause and effect diagram	
8. ____ Control charts	
9. ____ Roles for effective meetings	
10. ____ Brainstorming	

REFERENCES

Braveman, B. (2006). *Leading and managing occupational therapy services: An evidence-based approach.* Philadelphia: F. A. Davis.

Crepeau, E., Cohn, E., & Schell, B. (Eds.). (2009). *Willard & Spackman's occupational therapy* (11th ed.). Philadelphia: Lippincott Williams & Wilkins.

Depoy, E., & Gitlin, L. N. (2005). *Introduction to research: Understanding and applying multiple strategies* (3rd ed.). St. Louis, MO: Elsevier Science.

McCormack, G. L., Jaffe, E. G., & Goodman-Lavey, M. (Eds.). (2003). *The occupational therapy manager* (4th ed.). Bethesda, MD: AOTA Press.

U.S. Small Business Administration. (2009). *Programs for businesses to help you start, grow, and succeed.* Retrieved September 11, 2009, from http://www.sba.gov/aboutsba/index.html

WORK SHEET ANSWERS

Work Sheet 22-1. Occupational Therapy Manager Work Sheet

CQI Core Concepts Work Sheet
(Crepeau, Cohn, & Schell, 2009, p. 923)

Match each core concept with its appropriate topic:

Core CQI Concepts	Topics
1. __A__ Ground rules for meetings	D. Strategies
2. __C__ Multivoting	E. Tools
3. __B__ Process flow charts	F. Techniques
4. __A__ Consensus	
5. __C__ Balancing tasks and people	
6. __C__ Icebreakers	
7. __B__ Cause and effect diagram	
8. __B__ Control charts	
9. __A__ Roles for effective meetings	
10. __C__ Brainstorming	

Insurance and Occupational Therapy Reimbursement

Nancy Vandewiele Milligan

OBJECTIVES

1. Cite the programs and payers of medical insurance in the United States.
2. Define the structures of medical insurance coverage.
3. Describe the process for reimbursement of occupational therapy (OT) services.

KEY TERMS

Table 23-1 Key Terms

Sandstrom, Lohman, & Bramble, 2009, pp. 296–302
Access
Beneficiary
Benefit period
Capitation
Case management
Cost-based reimbursement
Dual eligibility
Fee for service
Medically necessary
Medically needy eligibility
Peer review
Predisposing factors
Spend down
Third-party payer

INTRODUCTION

Welcome to Day 34 of your study guide. In this chapter you will review the structure of healthcare payment and reimbursement in the United States. Begin this chapter by reviewing the key terms and topic areas. Then complete the work sheets to help you master the terminology and procedure of reimbursement.

OUTLINE

1. Who pays for healthcare and occupational therapy (OT) services?

(American Occupational Therapy Association [AOTA], 2002, pp. 385–418)

a. Medicare

(Sandstrom, et al., 2009, pp. 131–169)

b. Medicaid

(Sandstrom, et al., 2009, pp. 174–182)

c. Workers' compensation

(Sandstrom, et al., 2009, p. 98)

d. Rehabilitation Services Administration

(Sandstrom, et al., 2009, pp. 69–80)

e. Commercial insurance
    i. Private insurance companies

(Sandstrom, et al., 2009, p. 94)

    ii. Health maintenance organizations

(Sandstrom, et al., 2009, pp. 86–96)

    iii. Preferred provider organizations

(Sandstrom, et al., 2009, pp. 107–128)

    iv. Automobile and homeowners' casualty insurance

(Sandstrom, et al., 2009, pp. 99–100)

    v. Long-term care insurance

(Sandstrom, et al., 2009, pp. 96–97)

f. State Children's Health Insurance Program (SCHIP)

(Sandstrom, et al., 2009, p. 182)

g. Veterans Administration and military health insurance programs

(Sandstrom, et al., 2009, p. 183)

h. Self pay

(Sandstrom, et al., 2009, pp. 19–24)

2. Reimbursement structures

(AOTA, 2002, pp. 385–405)
(Sandstrom, et al., 2009, pp. 86–104)

a. Benefits
b. Benefit eligibility

   c. Benefit period
   d. Benefit package
   e. Deductible
   f. Cost-based reimbursement
   g. Defined benefit plan
   h. Prospective payment
   i. Preauthorization
   j. Capitation
   k. Utilization review
   l. Fee for service
   m. Social insurance
   n. Program eligibility
   o. Regulation

3. Reimbursement requirements

(AOTA, 2002, pp. 381–383, 405–417)

   a. Billing procedure
   b. Billing forms
      i. Uniform billing forms
         I. UB-92
         II. CMS-1450
         III. CMS-1500
   c. Diagnostic codes
   d. Procedure codes
   e. Procedural terminology
   f. Documentation
   g. Payment denials
   h. Appeal process

WORK SHEET

Work Sheet 23-1. Insurance and Reimbursement

Match the term on the left with the correct definition on the right.

Table 23.2 Insurance and Reimbursement Work Sheet

Term		Definition
A. Case management	E	Payment mechanisms for health care whereby a provider is paid an amount of money for each procedure performed.
B. Peer review organizations	G	Payment mechanism for health care whereby a provider is paid a flat fee for each covered member in a health plan per month.
C. Medically necessary	J	Persons who qualify for both Medicare and Medicaid coverage.
D. Spend down	C	The determination by a provider with physician status that a healthcare intervention is required.
E. Fee for service	H	The ability to obtain a healthcare service when you need it.
F. Beneficiary	I	A form of healthcare payment whereby providers are paid a set fee or rate prior to delivery of services.
G. Capitation	A	Process of eligibility determination and coordination of services for a person receiving multiple healthcare services.
H. Access	K	The length of time from the day of admission to the hospital to 60 days posthospital or skilled nursing facility (SNF) discharge.
I. Prospective payment	D	A process whereby a person with potential Medicaid eligibility uses up assets to a certain level to gain eligibility for the program.
J. Dual eligibility	L	A retrospective method of healthcare financing whereby a provider reports costs of providing care and is paid by an insurer.
K. Benefit period	B	Medicare-sponsored organizations that perform quality control, investigatory, and patient education functions.
L. Cost-based reimbursement	M	A state option qualification for Medicaid based on demonstrated medical need or income level.
M. Medically needy eligibility	F	The recipient of benefits from an insurance contract.

REFERENCES

American Occupational Therapy Association. (2002). *The occupational therapy manager* (4th ed.). Bethesda, MD: Author.

Hoffman, A. O. (2008). Understanding the medicare cap. *OT Practice, 13*(8), 9–14.

Robinson, M. (2007). Medicare 101: Understanding the basics. *OT Practice, 19*(3), CE-1–CE-8.

Sandstrom, R. W., Lohman, H., & Bramble, J. D. (2009). *Health services: Policy and systems for therapists* (2nd ed.). Upper Saddle River, NJ: Prentice Hall.

WORK SHEET ANSWERS

Work Sheet 23-1. Insurance and Reimbursement

Match the term on the left with the correct definition on the right.

Table 23.3 Insurance and Reimbursement Answer Sheet

Term		Definition
A. Case management	E	Payment mechanisms for health care whereby a provider is paid an amount of money for each procedure performed.
B. Peer review organizations	G	Payment mechanism for health care whereby a provider is paid a flat fee for each covered member in a health plan per month.
C. Medically necessary	J	Persons who qualify for both Medicare and Medicaid coverage.
D. Spend down	C	The determination by a provider with physician status that a healthcare intervention is required.
E. Fee for service	H	The ability to obtain a healthcare service when you need it.
F. Beneficiary	I	A form of healthcare payment whereby providers are paid a set fee or rate prior to delivery of services.
G. Capitation	A	Process of eligibility determination and coordination of services for a person receiving multiple healthcare services.
H. Access	K	The length of time from the day of admission to the hospital to 60 days posthospital or skilled nursing facility (SNF) discharge.
I. Prospective payment	D	A process whereby a person with potential Medicaid eligibility uses up assets to a certain level to gain eligibility for the program.
J. Dual eligibility	L	A retrospective method of healthcare financing whereby a provider reports costs of providing care and is paid by an insurer.
K. Benefit period	B	Medicare-sponsored organizations that perform quality control, investigatory, and patient education functions.
L. Cost-based reimbursement	M	A state option qualification for Medicaid based on demonstrated medical need or income level.
M. Medically needy eligibility	F	The recipient of benefits from an insurance contract.

APPENDIX A

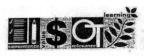 **AOTA Continuing Education Article**
Earn .1 AOTA CEU (one NBCOT PDU/one contact hour, see page CE-7 for details)

Medicare 101
Understanding the Basics

MONICA ROBINSON, MS, OTR/L
Occupational Therapy Rehabilitation Systems Consultant, HCR
   Manor Care, Toledo, Ohio
Member of the AOTA Alternatives to the Cap Committee and
   AOTA's CPT Coding Committee
AOTA Administration & Management Special Interest Section
   Communication/Reimbursement Liaison.

ABSTRACT
Medicare is the largest health care payer in the United States,
covering more than 42 million people. A high percentage of
occupational therapy practitioners provide services to Medicare
beneficiaries. The Medicare benefit is available through several
programs, each of which adheres to a different set of
rules and payment policies. Occupational therapy services
are covered in these programs at various settings under specific
criteria. Occupational therapy practitioners must understand
these rules and regulations in order to fully service
their patients and promote their profession. Congress regulates
Medicare, and when we understand the rules and regulations,
we can better advocate for occupational therapy
services or influence changes in the system.

LEARNING OBJECTIVES
After reading this article, you should be able to:
1. Differentiate between the various Medicare programs.
2. Identify basic Medicare Part B billing requirements.
3. Identify the different Medicare contractors that administer
   and manage the Medicare claims process.
4. Identify general Medicare documentation requirements.

INTRODUCTION
As the largest health care payer in the United States,
Medicare covered more than 42 million people in 2005
Approximately 35.4 million of those covered are 65 years of
age or older, with the remaining 6.6 million under 65 with a
permanent disability (Kaiser Family Foundation, 2005). A
high percentage of occupational therapy clients have medical
coverage through the Medicare program.

Funding Medicare is an ongoing federal issue. Medicare
was 13% of the federal budget in 2005, costing a staggering
$325 billion. Hospital inpatients made up 37% of those costs,
followed by physicians and other providers, including outpatient
therapy services (25%), skilled nursing facilities (5%),
and home health (4%) (Kaiser Family Foundation, 2005).
These escalating costs often result in Congress writing such
legislation as the Balanced Budget Refinement Act of 1999

(Public Law 106-113) or the Medicare Modernization Act of
2003 (Public Law 108-173) to help manage Medicare costs.
Medicare legislation significantly affects our practice settings
and service delivery. Occupational therapy practitioners provide
services in most of the Medicare-approved settings.
Certainly some clinicians work in settings that do not use
Medicare funding; however, it is important to know and
understand Medicare guidelines because many other insurance
companies follow Medicare rules and apply the same
coverage decisions when approving health care services. We
must understand the Medicare system and related legislation
so that we can optimize our opportunities to practice and
ensure reimbursement for our practice, promote occupational
therapy services, and serve our clients fully.

HISTORY OF MEDICARE
In 1965, Congress established two programs to cover the
medical costs for elderly people and persons with disabilities.
These programs, commonly referred to as Medicare, were
included in Title XVIII of the Social Security Act Amendments
of 1965 (Public Law 89-97). The "Hospital Insurance
Benefits for the Aged and Disabled," also known as Medicare
Part A, was created to provide partial funding for inpatient
hospitalization and other institutional care. The second program,
"Supplementary Medical Insurance Benefits for the
Aged and Disabled," also known as Medicare Part B, was
created to provide additional financial support for noninstitutional
costs, such as physician and other health care provider
services. The Medicare Part B benefit was created as a voluntary
program that required additional monthly premiums to
be paid by the recipient.

Medicare established a third, managed care program
option under the Balanced Budget Act of 1997 (Public Law
105-33) called "Medicare+Choice," now referred to as
"Medicare Advantage" or Medicare Part C. This program is
optional for Medicare recipients if they choose not to use the
traditional Medicare fee-for-service model (CCH Editorial
Staff Productions, 2006).

The final Medicare option is the newly developed
Medicare Part D, the "Voluntary Prescription Drug Benefit
Program." The prescription drug program became available
to Medicare recipients in January 2006 (CCH Editorial Staff
Productions, 2006).

To be eligible for any of the Medicare programs, one must
be 65 years of age or older and eligible for Social Security
benefits, survivor benefits, or railroad retirement benefits.
People under 65 are eligible for Medicare if they are entitled

AOTA Continuing Education Article

NOW AVAILABLE! CE Article, exam, and certificate are now available ONLINE.
Register at www.aota.org/cea or call toll-free 877-404-AOTA (2682).

to Social Security or railroad disability benefits or if they have end-stage renal disease or amyotrophic lateral sclerosis benefits. Those who do not meet any of the aforementioned categories and are 65 years of age or older can opt into the Medicare program by paying a monthly premium for Part A (CCH Editorial Staff Productions, 2006).

TYPES OF MEDICARE BENEFITS
Medicare Part A

The Medicare Part A benefit includes inpatient hospitalization, inpatient rehabilitation, inpatient psychiatric care, long-term-care hospitals (LTCHs), skilled nursing facilities (SNFs), home health care, and hospice. Medicare Part A is paid in these settings under a specific set of rules. Reimbursement is based on a prospective payment system (PPS), which is a comprehensive payment system that has an established rate for an episode of care based on initial diagnoses and presenting problems. A standardized set of criteria or assessments is used to determine the patient-related problems and to translate the results into a payment rate. Reimbursement fees and rates are established by Congress and may vary or be adjusted annually.

It is important for practitioners to understand how their services are paid, so they can be knowledgeable care providers. In the PPS, occupational therapy practitioners should understand the balance between patient care and the costs associated with service delivery. For example, most supplies (reachers, dressing sticks, theraputty, splints) are bundled in the PPS rate. If we understand the financial implication of our services, we can advocate for our clients from a position of knowledge and appreciation of the payment system. The following sections review the different Medicare Part A settings where occupational therapy practitioners work.

Inpatient Hospitals

In 1983, the Medicare payment system dramatically changed. President Reagan signed into law the Medicare Prospective Payment System as defined in the Social Security Act Amendments of 1983 (Public Law 98-21). Before this law, hospital services were paid by the costs, or fee for services. The new law established a per-case per diem rate based on diagnostic categories called diagnosis-related groups (DRGs). The DRG bundled rate includes room and board; nursing services; medication and supplies; diagnostic services; and other services, including occupational therapy. This flat rate also includes supplies that occupational therapy practitioners may issue to patients, such as activities of daily living (ADL) or exercise supplies.

The Medicare Part A benefit allows for 90 days of hospitalization per "spell of illness." The beneficiary pays a deductible for the first 60 days of inpatient per spell of illness, and a copayment is required for Days 61 to 90. Additionally, each beneficiary has 60 days "hospital lifetime reserve days," which can be at any time. When a beneficiary

chooses to use these days, there is a per-day copayment fee (CCH Editorial Staff Productions, 2006).

Inpatient Rehabilitation Facilities

Inpatient rehabilitation facilities (IRFs) provide intensive rehabilitation. Generally, patients receive 3 hours of combined therapy services (occupational therapy, physical therapy, speech-language pathology) a day plus other inpatient services. Beginning in January 2002, IRFs were required to follow a PPS. This program uses a per-discharge system based on case mix groups (CMGs), which are functional-related groups. A modified version of the FIM™ is used to assess the patient and assign the CMG. The Inpatient Rehabilitation Facility Patient Assessment Instrument (IRF-PAI) is used to determine the category. The instrument gathers information in nine key areas, including patient identification; demographics; medical information; patient safety; and patient functional abilities, including cognition. The IRF-PAI is completed twice during the patient's stay, once on admission and again at discharge. These two combined assessments establish the payment (CCH Editorial Staff Productions, 2006).

IRFs also are faced with adhering to the "75% rule." This rule requires that 75% of the patients in a cost-reporting year meet certain treatment categories (Medicare Program: Changes to the Medicare Claims Appeal Procedures, 2005). Some of these patients include those with stroke, spinal cord injury, amputations, multiple trauma, brain injury, and two major joints with severe osteoarthritis. Facilities had a 3-year phase-in period in which to comply with this regulation. Full implementation is expected for July 2007.

Inpatient Psychiatric Facilities

The Balanced Budget Refinement Act of 1999 created a new per diem PPS for inpatient psychiatric facilities. This system uses a standard base rate that is adjusted by various factors. This PPS uses the *International Classification of Diseases, Ninth Revision, Clinical Modification* (ICD-9-CM) diagnosis codes (Centers for Disease Control and Prevention & National Center for Health Statistics, 2006) (not *Diagnostic and Statistical Manual of Mental Disorders*, 4th ed. [American Psychiatric Association, 1994]) to establish the patient's DRG. Adjustments to the payment rate are made based on age and for patients who have 1 or more of 17 comorbidities in addition to the diagnosed psychiatric condition. Payments also are adjusted based on length of stay. The highest day rate is the first day because of the number of assessments given. Payments from Days 2 through 21 are reduced, and further reductions are made from Day 22 onward (CCH Editorial Staff Productions, 2006).

Long-Term-Care Hospitals

LTCHs treat patients who are very clinically complex and need 25 or more days of skilled service. These patients have

Earn .1 AOTA CEU (one NBCOT PDU /one contact hour, see page CE-7 for details)

very acute or chronic conditions that require extended services, including rehabilitation, respiratory therapy, pain management, traumatic brain injury treatment, and close medical management. Payment is based on a DRG system on a per-discharge basis. The LTCH PPS also considers patient demographics, discharge status, principal diagnosis, and an additional eight diagnoses and six medical procedures in order to determine the rate. These all contribute to classifying the patient in 1 of more than 500 LTCH DRGs (CCH Editorial Staff Productions, 2006).

Skilled Nursing Facilities

Medicare defines specific criteria that a beneficiary must satisfy to receive the Medicare Part A benefit in an SNF. The beneficiary must (a) be referred by a physician, (b) have a 3-day qualifying stay in a hospital, (c) be admitted to the SNF within 30 days of the qualifying stay, and (d) require daily nursing or rehabilitation services at least 5 days a week. The Medicare Part A SNF benefit allows for 100 skilled days of service per spell of illness. The first 20 days of care do not cost the beneficiary. Days 21 through 100 require a beneficiary copayment. Any days beyond 100 are covered under Medicare Part B.

This PPS was introduced into the skilled nursing setting in 1998. Payment is based on a case mix–adjusted payment system. The Minimum Data Set (MDS 2.0) is used to screen multiple aspects of data on the patient (e.g., diagnosis, time spent in therapy, functional status, complicating medical factors, medication). All these elements contribute to the overall payment category. The payment categories are called Resource Utilization Groups (RUGs). The RUGs system has 53 payment categories, and rehabilitation is defined in the highest paying RUGs levels. This payment is based on the time spent in therapy services and the number of disciplines delivering services. The MDS 2.0 is completed at specific intervals during the patient's stay in order to adjust the RUGs level and payment rate as appropriate.

Home Health Care

To qualify for the Medicare Part A home health benefit, the patient must be homebound; be under the care of a physician; and need skilled nursing or therapy services, which must be certified by a physician. The plan of care is reviewed and recertified every 60 days. The Medicare Part A home health benefit covers up to 100 visits per "spell of illness."

For occupational therapy to be involved, a nurse, physical therapist, or speech-language pathologist must open the case. After the case is opened, occupational therapy can be a stand-alone skilled service and recertify the patient. The home health PPS began in October 2000. This PPS uses the Outcomes and Assessment Information Set (OASIS) to calculate payment rates. The OASIS gathers data on the patient's discharge needs; ADL; living arrangements; support systems; equipment management; medications; diagnosed conditions;

psychosocial status; and physical status, including sensory, skin, and neurological. Based on the data submitted from the OASIS, grouper software determines the appropriate Home Health Resources Group for payment. The OASIS is completed at specific Medicare-defined intervals to establish the payment rate. The Medicare Part A benefit does not have a deductible or copayment (Centers for Medicare & Medicaid Services [CMS], 2006b).

Hospice Care

Medicare Part A hospice care is a unique program intended for beneficiaries whose physicians have certified that they have a terminal condition with a life expectancy of 6 months or less. When a patient opts into the hospice program, he or she is agreeing to palliative care. Unlike many of the other Medicare Part A services, hospice care does not limit the number of days of the benefit. At any time a patient can choose to stop the hospice benefit and return to traditional Medicare. Hospice care offers numerous benefits to the patient and caregivers, including counseling, social services, pain control, home health aide services, homemaker services, medical supplies, inpatient respite care, and therapy services. Occupational therapy services are limited and generally related to comfort, safety, quality of life issues, and caregiver education and training.

Hospice services are based on a cost-related prospective payment. Payment rates are based on four categories: routine home care, continuous home care, inpatient respite, and general inpatient care.

Medicare Part B

Medicare Part B is the supplementary medical insurance program. This voluntary program usually requires the beneficiary to pay monthly premiums and a 20% copayment based on the Medicare physician fee schedule (MPFS). Medicare Part B covers outpatient occupational therapy, physical therapy, and speech-language pathology; physician visits; durable medical equipment (e.g., wheelchairs), prosthetics, orthotics, and supplies (DMEPOS); outpatient hospital services; outpatient mental health services; and clinical laboratory (e.g., blood tests) and diagnostic tests. Payments for occupational therapy services are based on the MPFS. The MPFSs and coding are discussed later in more detail.

Outpatient occupational therapy services are provided in various settings (CMS, 2006d), including:

- Private practice: Occupational therapist private practitioners (OTPPs) are required to have a National Provider Identifier number to bill for services
- Clinic, rehabilitation, or public health agencies
- Hospital outpatient clinics
- SNFs: Services are provided for beneficiaries who have exhausted the Medicare Part A benefit or are residents of the facility who did not have a 3-day qualifying hospital stay.
- Physician office: Therapy incident to physician services or

AOTA Continuing Education Article
NOW AVAILABLE! CE Article, exam, and certificate are now available **ONLINE.**
Register at www.aota.org/cea or call toll-free 877-404-AOTA (2682).

as OTPPs in physician groups.

- Home health care: This includes visits over the 100-day Part A limit or when the patient does not meet the home health Part A benefit criterion.
- Comprehensive outpatient rehabilitation facilities (CORFs): CORFs provide a wide range of comprehensive and coordinated rehabilitation services. At a minimum, these include physician, therapy , and psychosocial services.

Medicare Part C

The Medicare Advantage Plan (also referred to as Medicare Part C) replaced the Medicare+Choice program in 2006. Medicare assigns contracts to private insurance companies to manage the beneficiary's Medicare benefits. These plans include both Medicare Part A and Medicare Part B services and many include a prescription medication benefit. Often, the copayment for services under a Medicare Part C plan are lower for the beneficiary. However, these insurance companies also are gatekeepers of service delivery and may require prior approval before services are rendered, limit the beneficiary to a specific network of providers, or both.

The new Medicare Advantage Plan includes the following options: Medicare preferred provider organizations, Medicare health maintenance organizations, Medicare private fee-for-service, Medicare Special Needs Plan, and Medicare medical savings account (CCH Editorial Staff Productions, 2006). Occupational therapy practitioners must effectively communicate with these plan providers. We need to identify the skilled services we provide and how these services will benefit the patient. Resources such as the *Medicare National Coverage Determinations* (i.e., the procedures and services Medicare will cover) (CMS, 2006e), The American Occupational Therapy Association's (AOTA's) *Scope of Practice* (2004), and the evidence-based practice resources on the AOTA Web site (www.aota.org) can be used to explain occupational therapy and the effectiveness of the services we offer.

Medicare Part D

Medicare Prescription Drug Coverage (Medicare Part D) is an optional program for beneficiaries. There are two ways to receive this benefit. First, the beneficiary can opt into a Medicare Part C program that offers a medication benefit. Second, the beneficiary can opt to enroll in the Medicare Part D program, which generally requires a monthly premium. More information on the Medicare Prescription Drug Coverage program can be found at the Medicare Web site (www.medicare.gov) or by calling 1-800-MEDICARE.

Medicare Supplemental Insurance

Medicare supplemental insurance, commonly referred to as Medigap, is additional private insurance that covers certain Medicare deductibles, copayments, and out-of-pocket expenses. This private insurance is federally regulated by Congress to avoid fraud or abuse of those beneficiaries they insure. The costs in any Medigap Plan A through L are the same for any insurance company; however, the costs to the beneficiary may vary (CMS, 2006a).

PHYSICIAN FEE SCHEDULE AND CODING

Medicare Part B occupational therapy services are reimbursed under the Medicare PFS. The PFS sets the payment for each billing code. Legislation established a payment system for services delivered across service providers based on geographic regions. The Resource Based Relative Value Scale is the system for measuring physician and provider input in medical services for the purpose of calculating a PFS. The relative value unit (RVU) is the standard for measuring the value of medical services provided by the health care provider compared with other medical services provided by other health care providers. The RVU for each service has three components: work, practice, and malpractice. The work component represents skilled time spent for setting up, preparing for, and delivering the service. For occupational therapy codes, this component represents 55% of the total code value. Considerations in defining the work component value include the technical skill and physical effort (skill, education, scope of practice intervention), mental effort and judgment (the complexity of the medical diagnosis, possible treatment options, medical urgency), and psychological stress (the risk of significant complications, morbidity, mortality). The practice component makes up approximately 40% of the total code value. The practice component includes overhead expenses of providing the service—including calculations for rent, utilities, office staffing, and equipment and supplies—that might be apportioned to the delivery of service. The malpractice component represents professional liability coverage, which is very low in therapy codes.

To establish the PFS (code value), the RVUs (for work, practice, and malpractice expenses) are each multiplied by a geographic adjustment factor (GAF) and the national uniform Medicare conversion factor (CF). The GAF makes adjustments for geographic location, and the CF converts the geographically adjusted RVUs to a dollar amount, with considerations for inflation. The Medicare PFS can be found on the CMS Web site (www.cms.hhs.gov/PhysicianFeeSched).

Occupational therapy practitioners must bill for Medicare Part B services using Current Procedural Terminology (CPT™) coding. CPT codes are used to describe the clinical contact between the patient and treating clinician. In 1983, CMS adopted CPT coding into a system called Healthcare Common Procedural Coding System (HCPCS), which contains two types of codes: Level I identifies CPT codes, and Level II represents supplies and equipment. The Level I CPT codes that CMS accepts are divided into six major categories; occupational therapy practitioners primarily use the Medicine/Physical Medicine and Rehabilitation section codes.

CPT codes are described as timed or nontimed codes. For codes calculated by time, the practitioner must consider the time spent in that procedure when billing the service. An example of timed codes includes self-care/home management and/or training (97535), neuromuscular reeducation (97112), and contrast bath (97034)*. For nontimed codes, only one unit per day can be billed by the occupational therapy practitioner, regardless of the total time spent in providing that service. An example of nontimed codes includes occupational therapy evaluation (97003), occupational therapy reevaluation (97004), and unattended electrical stimulation (G0283)*.

When billing Medicare Part B, it is essential to adhere to the billing guidelines, especially knowing and understanding the billing requirements and proper application of the "8-minute rule" (see Table 1). All the time spent delivering timed codes are aggregated. The aggregated time will establish how many units of timed codes can be billed. Units are assigned based on the codes you spent the most time providing. For examples and further instructions for assigning units, refer to Chapter 5 of the *Medicare Claims Processing Manual* (CMS, 2006c).

Medicare requires the practitioner to record the total amount of time spent providing timed codes. The units billed for timed codes must be consistent with the amount of time spent in service. Medicare also requires the practitioner to record the total amount of time spent delivering *both* timed and nontimed services. Medicare regulations do not require the therapist to record the amount of time spent delivering each CPT code, just the aggregated time (CMS, 2006b).

To avoid inappropriate billing of bundled codes, CMS implemented a policy in 1996 known as the Correct Coding Initiative (CCI). The purpose of the CCI is to develop correct coding methodologies to curtail improper "unbundling" of services for Medicare Part B claims. The CCI applies "edits" that are used to review claims and to identify potential misuse and inappropriate billing of code pairs. Beginning January 1, 2006, CCI edits applied to all providers billing Medicare Part B. CCI edits are applied to services billed by the same provider for the same beneficiary on the same date of service. If you are billing in an SNF, a CORF, or a rehabilitation agency using a single provider number for all therapies, the edits will apply among disciplines (occupational therapy, physical ther-

Table 1. Counting Minutes for Timed Codes in 15-Minute Units

Number of Units	Number of Minutes
1	≥ 8 through 22
2	≥ 23 through 37
3	≥ 38 through 52
4	≥ 53 through 67
5	≥ 68 through 82
6	≥ 83 through 97
7	≥ 98 through 112
8	≥ 113 through 127

Note. From CMS (2006b).

apy, speech-language pathology). For example, if you work in an SNF and the physical therapist provides gait training (97116) to Mrs. Smith on the same day the occupational therapist provides her with therapeutic activities (97530), these codes are edited and the physical therapist would need to modify the gait training code (97116) to get paid. Based on the CCI edit rules, a modifier ("-59") can be applied to the code when services are distinctly different and permitted to be billed together. The previous example is a good demonstration of two codes billed on the same day using the modifier -59. If you are the sole provider as an independent practitioner using your own provider number, other discipline services do not influence your coding. Therapeutic activities (97530) and self-care/home management (97535) are examples of codes that are considered bundled under the CCI edit rules. For these codes to be billed together on the same day, they need to be provided at separate time intervals that were distinctly different. For example, a patient might receive therapeutic activities (97530) for balance training from 1:00 p.m. to 1:15 p.m. and then participate in self-care/home management (97535) for lower-body dressing using adaptive equipment from 1:15 p.m. to 1:45 p.m. These services were distinctly different and can be billed together using the -59 modifier on self-care/home management (97535). It is important to know the CCI edits because some codes can never be billed together on the same day. For example, OT evaluation (97003) and OT re-evaluation (97004) can never be billed together on the same day; only one of the two codes would be paid (OT re-evaluation, 97004).

CMS updates the CCI edits code pair list every quarter. CCI edits are available at no cost by downloading them from the CMS Web site (www.cms.hhs.gov/physicians/cciedits/default.asp). Note that there are two different types of National Correct Coding Initiative (NCCI) edits based on the practice setting. OTPPs use the NCCI Edits for Physicians. Other practice settings use the NCCI Edits for Hospital Outpatient Prospective Payment System. For more information on understanding and applying CCI edits go to www.cms.hhs.gov/NationalCorrectCodInitEd.

The second type of coding used to bill for services is HCPCS Level II, which are alpha-number codes that include equipment and supply codes for dressings (A codes), DME (E codes), orthotics or prosthetics (L codes), and G codes (e.g., unattended electrical stimulation, G0283). To use the L codes for billing orthotics, the OTPP or practice setting must be a Medicare DME provider with an approved number. Recently, Medicare has required that all suppliers of DME, prosthetics, and orthotics must obtain accreditation by an approved accreditation organization to obtain reimbursement under Medicare Part B.

LIMITATIONS ON THERAPY SERVICES

The Balanced Budget Act of 1997 placed annual financial limitations on therapy services, known as the "therapy caps."

---

* *Current Procedural Terminology* (CPT) is copyright 2006 American Medical Association. All Rights Reserved. No fee schedules, basic units, relative values, or related listings are included in CPT. The AMA assumes no liability for the data contained herein. Applicable FARS/DFARS restrictions apply to government use.

AOTA Continuing Education Article

NOW AVAILABLE! CE Article, exam, and certificate are now available ONLINE.
Register at www.aota.org/cea or call toll-free 877-404-AOTA (2682).

The therapy caps were in effect in 1999, and briefly in both 2003 and 2006. The therapy caps apply to all Medicare Part B settings except outpatient hospitals, which are exempt by law. In February 2006 Congress passed the Deficit Reduction Act of 2005 (Public Law 109-171), allowing patients to receive services beyond the $1,740 limitation if they meet specific criteria. This exception process is either automatic by using a modifier (KX) on the claim when it is billed, or manual, which requires written communication with the contractor for approval.

On December 7, 2006, after significant lobbying efforts by the therapy community and other stakeholders, the therapy cap exception process was extended to apply from January 1, 2007 to December 31, 2007, through a provision in H.R. 6111, the Tax Relief and Health Care Act of 2006. As of January 1, 2007, the annual financial limitation will be $1,780 for occupational therapy services.

MEDICARE DOCUMENTATION

To qualify for occupational therapy services under the Medicare benefit, services must be medically necessary. Each of the Medicare provider settings (e.g., SNF, home health, inpatient hospitalization, outpatient) may have some unique requirements for medical necessity or for documentation; however, many of the criteria are similar. Medicare Part B has the most prescriptive requirements for documentation, which have been revised several times in the past year. For the most current requirements, refer to Chapter 15 of the *Medicare Benefit Policy Manual* (CMS, 2006b).

In all cases, the patient must have a condition that requires the skills of a therapist. The patient is under the care of a physician who certifies and recertifies the plan of care. A qualified person (e.g., a person qualified to provide occupational therapy services in that given state) must provide services. The intervention is within an accepted standard of practice for occupational therapy. Services are provided within a reasonable frequency, intensity, and duration for the condition. There is an expectation that the patient will improve in a reasonable amount of time.

It is important that as practitioners we clearly document the patient's previous level of functioning, current medical condition, functional limitations, and how skilled occupational therapy services are necessary to return the patient to his or her highest practicable level of functioning. Do not assume that the medical reviewer understands the level of sophistication of our skilled services. Use the following AOTA materials to support that the services you are providing are within the standard of practice for your profession: standards of practice for occupational therapy, practice guidelines, specialized knowledge and skills papers, and evidenced-based practice resources. Clearly document the progress the patient is making toward his or her goals and the remaining functional limitations and skilled therapy needs. Present a clear and concise picture of the patient and the occupational therapy services.

Documentation requirements may vary slightly; however, in general an evaluation and plan of care, certification and recertification, progress notes, and encounter notes are necessary (Brennan & Robinson, 2006). A treatment encounter note is written after each occupational therapy treatment session. Medicare requires documentation for every treatment day; at a minimum, this documentation identifies the skilled service provided and the identity of the qualified professional (therapist, assistant) providing the service. For more information on documentation, refer to your practice setting's chapter of the *Medicare Benefit Policy Manual*; Medicare Part B outpatient services requirements are found in Chapter 15 (CMS, 2006b).

MEDICARE CONTRACTORS AND DENIALS MANAGEMENT

Medicare has private insurance organizations that administer and pay Medicare claims. Currently, Medicare Part A claims generally are administered by fiscal intermediaries; however, home health care is managed by regional home health intermediaries. OTPPs, rehabilitation agencies, and outpatient rehabilitation facilities are billed under Medicare Part B, which is administered by a Medicare carrier. DMEPOS are billed under Medicare Part B DME regional carriers. By September 2011, Medicare administrative contractors will replace all fiscal intermediaries and carriers; once this change is completed, there no longer will be a distinction between Medicare Part A or B contractors.

Medicare contractors use Medicare program manuals to help guide medical review. In addition to these manuals, contractors use their own guidelines for medical review called local coverage determinations. To be proactive in the medical review process, know the Medicare program manual for your practice setting, *Medicare National Coverage Decisions* (CMS, 2006e), and review your Medicare contractor's local coverage determinations. Medicare redesigned the claims appeal process in 2005; now the claims process is largely the same for both Medicare Part A and Medicare Part B. There are specific time frames for response for each level of appeal; therefore, it is essential to respond immediately to an additional development request and timely to all levels of the appeals (Medicare Program: Changes to the Medicare Claims Appeal Procedures, 2005). For more information on documentation and the denial process, refer to Brennan and Robinson (2006).

FUTURE CHANGES

Medicare rules and regulations are changed or modified frequently. Some changes on the horizon include return to the therapy cap; pay for performance; competitive bidding; suppliers of DMEPOS accreditation; and therapy certification for power wheeled mobility devices. To follow these issues and other possible changes, refer to the Reimbursement page on the AOTA Web site for up-to-date information and resources (www.aota.org/members/area5/links/link01.asp).

Earn .1 **AOTA CEU** (one NBCOT PDU/one contact hour, see below for details)

CONCLUSION

Occupational therapists and occupational therapy assistants work in the majority of settings that service Medicare beneficiaries. These various Medicare programs cover more than 42 million individuals. Each of these programs has its own set of rules, regulations, and requirements. By understanding these requirements we can better serve and advocate for our patients and our profession. Legislation establishes and drives the Medicare rules, and as practitioners we must be proactive by communicating with our congressional representatives about issues and concerns regarding Medicare and other related health care legislation. In addition, we must be proactive in advocating for Medicare coverage of the full scope of occupational therapy practice with CMS and its contractors. ∎

ACKNOWLEDGMENTS

I thank the following individuals for their review and contributions to the content of this article: Cathy Brennan, MA, OTR/L, FAOTA; Sharmila Sandhu, Esq.; and Judy Thomas, MGA.

REFERENCES

American Occupational Therapy Association. (2004). Scope of practice. *American Journal of Occupational Therapy, 58*, 673–677.

American Psychiatric Association. (1994). *Diagnostic and statistical manual of mental disorders* (4th ed.). Washington, DC: Author.

Balanced Budget Act of 1997. Pub. L. 105-33, 111 Stat. 251.

Balanced Budget Refinement Act of 1999. Pub. L. 106-113, 113 Stat. 1301.

Brennan, C., & Robinson, M. (2006). Documentation: Getting it right to avoid Medicare denials. *OT Practice, 11*(14), 10–15.

CCH Editorial Staff Productions. (2006). *Medicare explained 2006: Health laws professional series.* Chicago: CCH Incorporated.

Centers for Disease Control and Prevention & National Center for Health Statistics. (2006). *International classification of diseases, ninth revision, clinical modification.* Hyattsville, MD: Author.

Centers for Medicare & Medicaid Services. (2006a). *Medicare and you 2007.* Retrieved October 20, 2006, from http://www.medicare.gov/Publications/Pubs/pdf/10050.pdf

Centers for Medicare & Medicaid Services. (2006b). *Medicare benefit policy manual* (Publication 100-02). Retrieved November 30, 2006, from http://www.cms.hhs.gov/Manuals/IOM/list.asp

Centers for Medicare & Medicaid Services. (2006c). *Medicare claims processing manual* (Publication 100-04). Retrieved November 30, 2006, from http://www.cms.hhs.gov/Manuals/IOM/list.asp

Centers for Medicare & Medicaid Services. (2006d). *Medicare general information, eligibility, and entitlement* (Publication 100-01). Retrieved October 20, 2006, from http://www.cms.hhs.gov/Manuals/IOM/list.asp

Centers for Medicare & Medicaid Services. (2006e). *Medicare national coverage determinations manual* (Publication 100-03). Retrieved December 8, 2006, from http://www.cms.hhs.gov/Manuals/IOM/list.asp

Deficit Reduction Act of 2005. Pub. L. 109-171, S. 1932.

Kaiser Family Foundation. (2005). *Briefing: Medicare basics, from (Part) A to D* [Transcript]. Retrieved October 20, 2006, from http://www.kaisernetwork.org/health_cast/hcast_index.cfm?display=detail&hc=1431

Medicare program: Changes to the Medicare claims appeal procedures: Interim final rule, 70 Fed. Reg. 11,420 (Mar. 8, 2005) (to be codified at 42 C.F.R. pt. 401 and 405).

Medicare Modernization Act of 2003. Pub. L. 108-173, 117 Stat. 2066.

Social Security Act Amendments of 1965. Pub. L. 89-97, 42 U.S.C. § 1395 *et seq.*

Social Security Act Amendments of 1983. Pub. L. 98-21, 42 U.S.C. § 1395 *et seq.*

Tax Relief and Health Care Act of 2006. H.R. 6111. Pub. L. 109-432

New Electronic Exam: Immediate Results and Certificate

How To Apply for Continuing Education Credit:

1. After reading the article Medicare 101: Understanding the Basics, answer the questions to the final exam found on p. CE-8 by registering to take them online and receive your certificate immediately upon successful completion of the exam. You can still complete the exam by darkening the appropriate boxes in Section B of the Registration and Answer Card, which is bound into this issue of *OT Practice* following the test page. In either case, each question has only one answer.

2. To register click on www.aota.org/cea or call toll-free 877-404-2682. Once you are registered, you can log on to www.aotalearning.org to take the exam online. If your are using the Registration and Answer Card, complete Sections A through D and return the card with the appropriate payment to the address indicated.

3. There is a nonrefundable processing fee to score the exam, and continuing education credit will be issued only for a passing score of at least 75%. Use the electronic exam and you can print your official certificate immediately if you achieve a passing score. If you are submitting a Registration and Answer Card, you will receive a certificate within 30 days of receipt of the processed card.

4. The electronic exam must be completed by **February 28, 2009**. The Registration and Answer Card must be received by February 28, 2009, in order to receive credit for **Medicare 101: Understanding the Basics**.

RESOURCES

Publications

American Medical Association. (2006). *AMA HCPCS Level II 2007.* Chicago: Ingenix.

American Medical Association. (2006). *AMA physician ICD-9-CM 2007* (Vol. 1 & 2). Chicago: Ingenix.

American Medical Association. (2006). *CPT® 2007 professional edition.* Chicago: Ingenix.

Centers for Medicare & Medicaid Services. (2006). *Revised long-term care facility resident assessment instrument user's manual version 2.0 (MDS).* Available: http://www.cms.hhs.gov/NursingHomeQualityInits/20_NHQIMDS20.asp

Medicare contractor: www.cms.hhs.gov/apps/contacts

CCI Edits Quarterly Updates

National Correct Coding Initiative Edits (Carrier = OTPP, PTPP, and physicians) www.cms.hhs.gov/physicians/cciedits/default.asp

National Correct Coding Initiative Edits Hospital Outpatient Prospective Payment System http://www.cms.hhs.gov/providers/hopps/cciedits/default.asp

Physician Fee Schedules (CPT codes)

http://www.cms.hhs.gov/PhysicianFeeSched/PFSFRN/list.asp#TopOfPage

Orthotics/Durable Medical Equipment Regional Carriers Fee Schedule

http//:www.cms.hhs.gov/center/dme.asp

AOTA Continuing Education Article

NOW AVAILABLE! CE Article, exam, and certificate are now available **ONLINE**.
Register at www.aota.org/cea or call toll-free 877-404-AOTA (2682).

Final Exam

MEDICARE 101: UNDERSTANDING THE BASICS
February 19, 2007

Learning Level: Intermediate
Target Audience: Occupational Therapist and Occupational Therapy Assistants
Content Focus: Category 3: Professional Issues, Legal, Legislative, & Regulatory Issues

Register for the electronic exam and certificate online at www.aota.org/cea, call toll free 877-404-2682, or use the Registration and Answer Card bound into this issue of *OT Practice* following the test page.

1. Medicare is the largest health care payer in the United States.
   A. True
   B. False

2. Congress established Medicare in Title XVIII of the Social Security Act of ___?
   A. 1941
   B. 1950
   C. 1965
   D. 1970

3. Which of the following does not follow the Medicare Part A program?
   A. Inpatient hospitals
   B. Occupational therapist private practitioners (OTPPs)
   C. Home health
   D. Inpatient rehabilitation facilities

4. OTPPs follow Medicare program
   A. Part A
   B. Part B
   C. Part D
   D. None of the above

5. The first Medicare PPS was:
   A. Inpatient (acute) hospitals (DRG)
   B. Inpatient rehabilitation facilities (IRF-PAI)
   C. Home health care (OASIS)
   D. CPT coding

6. Medicare Part B is an optional program.
   A. True
   B. False

7. Medicare Advantage Plan includes coverage for
   A. Medicare Part A
   B. Medicare Part B
   C. Medicare Parts A & B
   D. Medicare Prescription Drug Plan only

8. When billing Medicare Part B outpatient occupational therapy services, use the following to record and bill your service:
   A. CPT codes
   B. PPS categories
   C. ICD-9 codes
   D. None of the above

9. The following policy is used to prevent unbundling of CPT codes:
   A. KX modifier
   B. CCI edits
   C. ICD-9 codes
   D. None of the above

10. Which of the following describes elements of occupational therapy documentation?
    A. An evaluation/plan of care
    B. Physician involvement
    C. Encounter notes
    D. All of the above

11. Medicare contractors develop guidelines for paying services; these guidelines are:
    A. National coverage determinations
    B. Local coverage determinations
    C. Regulations
    D. None of the above

12. Federal legislation establishes Medicare rules.
    A. True
    B. False

Source: Courtesy of AOTA, *OT Practice*.

APPENDIX B

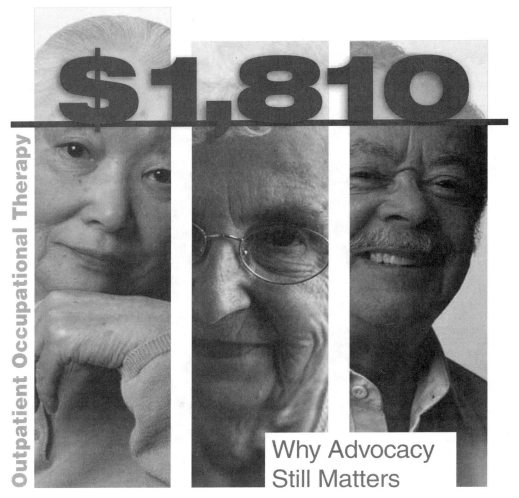

Outpatient Occupational Therapy

$1,810

Why Advocacy Still Matters

Understanding the
Medicare Cap

ASHLEY OPP HOFMANN

Why the cap was created and the implications for its continued use.

However the general public may view the role of government, very few people want it to determine how much health care their injury or illness will require, and no occupational therapy practitioner wants his or her professional judgment undermined by what the government arbitrarily deems to be appropriate care.

The current cap on outpatient therapy services reimbursable by Medicare

Part B has enormous implications for all occupational therapy practitioners. For more than 10 years, American Occupational Therapy Association (AOTA) staff, leaders, and volunteers have worked tirelessly to limit the effect this misguided public policy has on the health and well-being of clients, and they have had great success. However, the threat of the therapy cap continues to loom large. At press time, the current exceptions process was set to

expire on June 30. Every occupational therapy practitioner needs to understand the rationale behind the cap, how it came into existence, and the dangerous precedent that it sets for occupational therapy practice areas beyond those reimbursable by Medicare.

UNDERSTANDING THE MEDICARE CAP
In its simplest sense, the Medicare cap is a public policy that places limits—arbitrary limits—on Medicare

> Although the current cap might comfortably cover many beneficiaries' therapy use, it is also frighteningly easy to go beyond it.

Part B therapy services. Authorized in 1997 as part of the Balanced Budget Act (BBA),[1] the cap came into place as an effort to control escalating therapy costs. During 2008, Part B occupational therapy services have been capped at $1,810, with an exceptions process in place that is scheduled to expire on June 30. The cap limits occupational therapy, physical therapy, and speech-language pathology in any outpatient setting, except hospitals. Only occupational therapy constitutes its own category under the cap. The exceptions process allows medically necessary care to be provided.

Although the current cap might comfortably cover many beneficiaries' therapy use, it is also frighteningly easy to go beyond it. For example, rehabilitation following a typical hip replacement would exceed the therapy cap, even if the beneficiary were physically capable without any comorbidities. Under the cap, "having more than one incident within a year would have a disastrous impact on a person, particularly for a nonrelated incident," says Nancy Richman, OTR/L, FAOTA, a member of AOTA's Alternatives to the Cap advisory group.

AOTA'S POSITION

From the cap's inception AOTA has opposed it, arguing that the law puts the government squarely between the client and his or her medical provider, and that such interfering in medical decision making is the wrong direction for Medicare to take. AOTA has asked for studies and data collection to take place so that Congress and stakeholders can better understand what type of clients receive Part B therapy services and who the cap would most affect.

Throughout the ensuing legislative battles, AOTA has taken several strong positions on issues tied to the cap, such as supporting the exceptions process as a reform if the cap stays in place; maintaining the physician fee schedule as

the basis for Part B payments; keeping occupational therapy defined as a separate and distinct service under the cap; getting functional status included in the study language; and advocating for increased documentation of factors that would affect therapy use. When lobbying, the overarching message that AOTA has continually sent to Capitol Hill and the Centers for Medicare & Medicaid Services (CMS) is that occupational therapy practitioners are qualified to determine and attest to the need for therapy.

1997 TO 2008: HOW WE GOT HERE
Skyrocketing Health Care Costs

"The nineties were the glory years," says Christina Metzler, AOTA's chief public affairs officer. "There was a lot of growth in therapy and a lot of it was good, positive growth, but some of the growth was fueled by over- and inappropriate utilization."

Therapy costs escalated with therapy use, due in large part to a lack of clear Medicare guidelines for documentation and billing, among other factors. A weak, cost-based payment system allowed providers such as nursing homes, rehabilitation agencies, and hospital outpatient departments to determine what they charged Medicare. Under this payment system providers could put all of the costs associated with therapy services into the bill, and many inflated those costs to maximize their profit.

A 1996 report by the Prospective Payment Assessment Commission[2] tipped off Congress that therapy costs were getting out of hand. Within the

context of a larger effort to achieve a balanced budget and make changes in health care—efforts that eventually narrowed to Medicare reform only—the report examined the growth and use of occupational therapy in comprehensive outpatient rehabilitation facilities and in skilled nursing facilities.

At that time, outpatient therapy services provided by private practitioners and physicians were already on the physician fee schedule, which determined how much Medicare would pay for Part B services. The BBA put payment for *all* outpatient therapy on a preset basis through the physician fee schedule. Many would agree that this much-needed reform was a good way to address billing concerns and Congressional goals to save money. But legislators took cutting costs one big step further by instituting the cap.

Creating the Cap

The idea of a cap didn't come about suddenly. Since the 1970s, Medicare had capped outpatient physical therapy services provided by therapists in independent practice. When occupational therapists were allowed to enter private practice in 1987, they too were subjected to the cap. By 1997, private practitioners' therapy services were capped at $900.

At that time, the Republican Congress and Democratic President Bill Clinton had come to an agreement about the BBA. To generate revenue for Medicare's increased use and costs, reimbursement for outpatient therapy would be capped at $900 per beneficiary, across the board and to all outpatient therapy providers except hospitals.

Although the cap on private practitioners set a precedent for this therapy cap, the BBA also focused on outpatient therapy out of convenience. Congress perceived a lot of growth in therapy and decided to target cutting it to cut costs.

Right now, the most urgent concern is to extend the exceptions process beyond June 30. Go to the Legislative Action Center on AOTA's Web site at www.aota.org to find out who your representatives are and how to contact them.

The new budget might have looked good on the surface, but it put beneficiaries with greater therapy needs in an extremely difficult position. "One of the big selling points of the BBA was that you weren't cutting beneficiaries, you were cutting providers," Metzler explains. "But this was one place where they *did* cut beneficiaries." For example, legislators did not realize that before they implemented the cap, a client seeing a private practitioner (whose services were already capped) could opt to go to an outpatient facility after the cap was reached. But limiting all providers to a capped amount restricted beneficiaries' access to all outpatient services. Congress gave themselves an "out" by allowing unlimited therapy in hospital outpatient departments.

Resisting Implementation
Few may realize that the cap has been fully in effect for only 1 year (during 1999) and 3 months (during 2003) out of its 11-year history. Six bills passed by Congress have limited the effect of the cap (see "Legislative History"). Before full-blown implementation in 2003, various delays by CMS and bills that enacted moratoriums—due significantly to intense lobbying by AOTA—prevented beneficiaries from feeling much of an effect from the cap.

Although Congress eventually understood, for the most part, that the cap constituted bad policy, lifting it coincided with an unprecedented rise in therapy spending. Outpatient therapy costs shot up from $1.4 billion in 1999 (when the cap was in effect) to $3 billion in 2002 during the moratoriums.[3] What appeared to be unbridled spending made Congress nervous, and the government slapped the cap right back on in 2003.

The rise of therapy spending was due to a lot factors. In addition to many other issues, 2000–2002 saw an increase of 1 million outpatient therapy users (and a 34% increase in hip and knee replacements), due in large part to an aging population.[4] The increase also reflected a trend of beneficiaries staying in inpatient facilities for a shorter period, causing outpatient facilities to treat more acute patients. "Also contributing was a population living longer and wanting more medical care to remain independent and to stay active as they age," notes Ronnie Schein, OT/L, member of the Alternatives to the Cap advisory group.

Although the cap was fully implemented only for a little over a year, that was more than enough time to hurt beneficiaries and stymie recovery. "People were not doing good therapy," recalls Richman. Some practitioners cut back on getting clients to their maximum potential, and others provided therapy-type services with students or rehabilitation aides so clients would recover without exhausting their cap. Many clients opted to pay for therapy above the cap purely out of pocket, but, as Richman points out, "There were patients who didn't prioritize the funds or have the funds to pay for therapy."

Fortunately, the full-blown implementation was short, but that period foreshadows the devastating long-term impact that the cap would have on older adults' health, should it go into full effect again.

In December 2003, another moratorium was enacted, delaying implementation until January 1, 2006. This time, instead of another moratorium or delay in implementation, the Deficit Reduction Act[5] authorized an exceptions process, which allows clients with qualifying conditions or clinically complex medical situations to exceed the therapy cap (see "With Exception: Benefit Coverage Criteria" on p. 13). The current cap-related legislation extends the exceptions process through June 30.

Exceptions Process as Reform
AOTA considers the exceptions process to be a reform. "The exceptions process was instituted to put in place some

Legislative History

The cap was implemented and in effect in 1999, but the Balanced Budget Refinements Act[6] enacted a moratorium for 2000 and 2001, and the Benefits Improvement and Protection Act[7] extended the moratorium on the cap through December 31, 2002, totaling a 3-year moratorium. CMS then delayed implementation until July 1, 2003, and a lawsuit filed by three organizations for failing to adequately notify beneficiaries about the cap delayed implementation for an additional 2 months.[4]

On September 1, 2003, the cap was officially implemented, but it was only in effect until December 7, 2003. At that time, the Medicare Prescription Drug, Improvement, and Modernization Act[8] suspended the cap through 2005. The Deficit Reduction Act[5] authorized the exceptions process, allowing beneficiaries to receive occupational therapy beyond the cap if medically necessary. The Tax Relief and Health Care Act[9] extended the cap exceptions process through 2007. Going down to the wire, AOTA succeeded in seeing the Medicare, Medicaid, and SCHIP Extension Act[10] pass in the final hours of 2007, which extended the exceptions process for another 6 months, to June 30. ∎

kind of filter that would raise a caution flag to providers that they needed to be sure clients truly met the benefit coverage criteria," Metzler explains.

"We're strongly supportive of the exceptions process, which you can view as a fix to the cap," says Sharmila Sandhu, AOTA's regulatory counsel. "Therapists who believe it is medically necessary under Medicare rules that their clients receive care can claim and attest to this, and Medicare will pay for therapy above the cap in those circumstances."

Putting decisions back into the hands of therapists constituted a major political victory, but most immediately important was the fact that the exceptions process gave the beneficiaries with the most need a way to get occupational therapy. "The exceptions process has been remarkably helpful," Richman says. "It's smooth and it works. The process affects the therapists' time, but it doesn't affect the clients getting what they need."

LOBBYING EFFORTS—AND SUCCESSES

When the cap made its way into the BBA in 1997, AOTA had a lot of lobbying to do right away. First, AOTA lobbied to get the cap raised from $900 to $1,500—still an arbitrary number, but a higher one.

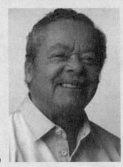

With Exception
Benefit Coverage Criteria

The exceptions process gave occupational therapists the right to use their professional judgment and allowed clients with significant therapy needs to receive services—and AOTA aimed to make sure that the reform proved successful. AOTA promoted therapists' obligation to simultaneously ensure that beneficiaries received the care they needed while recognizing when beneficiaries no longer required therapy.

The obligation to ethically determine the need for a client to receive additional therapy rested solely with the therapist, but CMS recognized that the following conditions may cause beneficiaries to exceed the cap, and their respective ICD-9 code would most likely allow exception: joint replacement; multiple fractures involving both lower limbs, lower with upper limb, and lower limbs with rib or sternum; dislocations; intracranial injury, excluding skull fracture; traumatic amputations; spinal cord injury; injury to nerve roots and spinal plexus; and head injury.[11]

In complex cases, CMS dictates that the condition causing occupational therapy services to exceed the cap must significantly affect a beneficiary's recovery rate to meet the goals of the therapy, and documentation must support the therapist's judgment. Because determining medical complexity rests with the therapist, AOTA has urged members to take great care in ensuring the appropriateness of additional treatment and to thoroughly document the entire therapeutic process. ■

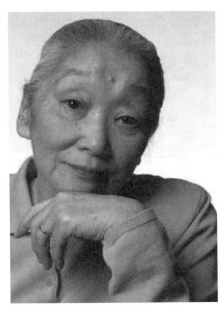

Keeping occupational therapy separate from other therapies topped the early advocacy agenda. AOTA lobbyists fended off the suggestion of putting occupational therapy, physical therapy, and speech-language pathology under one cap. "We called that idea the 'McFlurry Solution' because it really tried to blend and dissolve distinctions among the three therapies," Metzler says. "Occupational therapy is a separately covered service under Medicare, and we had to work to maintain that distinction." Although AOTA succeeded in keeping occupational therapy separate, physical therapy and speech-language pathology have the same cap as a result of a glitch in the statutory wording, which AOTA supports correcting.

In another early effort, AOTA successfully lobbied Congress to include language in bills preventing implementation of the cap to require CMS to analyze therapy use and determine better ways of controlling costs. The language endeavored to ensure that when CMS and Congress examined ways to determine how much therapy a beneficiary might need, they had to look beyond the diagnosis and consider function, comorbidities, and other factors.

As investigators carried out studies on beneficiaries' outpatient therapy use, AOTA hired various consultants who analyzed data to help develop an alternative. AOTA invested countless staff and volunteer hours into analyzing results and informing Congress and CMS of what the data did (and did not) indicate. The Association worked with CMS in multiple studies that CMS funded over the past 10 years by participating in many meetings, focus groups, data analysis sessions, and literature reviews, all in service of helping the agency understand what occupational therapy is, how people benefit from it, and what kinds of conditions and situations require significant amounts of therapy.

WHERE DO WE GO FROM HERE?

An enormous challenge to repealing the cap now is the growth in therapy. "On the policy side, we won the argument as to whether a cap was an appropriate way to control costs. Policymakers all agreed it was ham-handed, inappropriate, and that it hurt the sickest," Metzler says. "Now, though, with the continued growth in therapy, we have to struggle with the cost of getting rid of the cap."

Those who oppose the cap must now face the sheer cost difference between capping therapy and providing all beneficiaries with the care they need as use and costs rise. "Data show that perhaps 10% to 15% of beneficiaries go over the cap, but unfortunately those 10% to 15% are very expensive. Although many people are in the $3,000 to $5,000 range, there are a few outliers who go up to $8,000 or $9,000 in therapy costs," Metzler says. "When those kinds of figures come out, Congress and CMS get nervous. So every year, the cost of repeal gets higher."

Alternatives to the Cap

Nobody wants Medicare to go bankrupt, and occupational therapy practitioners have a strong interest in making sure it doesn't. Part of addressing the potential overuse of occupational therapy includes considering alternatives to the cap.

Soon after the cap became law, AOTA formed the Alternatives to the Cap advisory group to assist policy staff. The group has been mostly reactive, analyzing faulty data from CMS and reviewing and commenting on AOTA's letters and proposals. "We first looked at the figures that the Office of the Inspector General came out with, and they were almost impossible to believe," Richman says. "We analyzed why certain diagnoses had bizarre amounts of therapy." Group members carefully considered the types of conditions that would require greater amounts of therapy, pointing out, for example, that neurological conditions typically will take longer to treat than orthopedic conditions. AOTA used this information in discussions with Congress and CMS.

14

AOTA CE Article
Medicare 101:
Understanding the Basics
By M. Robinson, 2007. Bethesda, MD: American Occupational Therapy Association. (Earn .1 AOTA CEU/ 1 NBCOT PDU/1 contact hour. ($24.75 for members, $35 for nonmembers. To order, call toll free 877-404-AOTA or shop online at www.aota.org. Order #CEA0207-MI)

These practitioners and administrators also considered overuse of therapy. "I think most would agree there appeared to be overutilization in some elements of the data, but without data that accurately captured more meaningful patient information and treatment-related variables, you can't say how much utilization was appropriate, relative to a particular individual," Schein says. Among its recommendations to CMS, AOTA pointed out that to be useful, the data needed to examine better-defined and more specific characteristics that could contribute to occupational therapy need and increased use.

Why You Should Care and What You Can Do

Policies that affect Medicare can easily bleed into other arenas. Practitioners unaffected by the cap or Medicare policy are not necessarily safe from government intrusion. "The theory behind the cap could be applied in any setting," says Daniel Jones, one of AOTA's legislative representatives. "All therapists should be concerned about being able to use their education, skills, abilities, and professional judgment on the job."

Policies such as the cap do not occur in a vacuum; bad precedents lead to worse legislative and regulatory policies. "Medicare is the gold standard for all these other payers like Medicaid, private insurance, workers' compensation, and state-based types of insurance payers or health care payers," Sandhu says. "We see it all the time: When Medicare sets a policy, these other types of payers follow."

Successfully extending the exceptions process and eventually eliminating the cap depends on practitioners contacting their legislators. Yes, AOTA has asked members many, many times to contact their representatives, but such actions have significantly contributed to the multiple successes of extending the exceptions process—which thousands of clients depend on. Right now, the most urgent concern is to extend the exceptions process beyond June 30. You can go to the Legislative Action Center on AOTA's Web site at www.aota.org to find out who your representatives are and how to contact them.

Policies such as the cap affect how Congress, consumers, and other medical professionals think about occupational therapy practitioners' clinical reasoning, hindering the independence of treatment and good clinical practice. If the cap goes into effect again, clients who run out of therapy services will simply be discharged. What will happen to them? ■

References

1. Balanced Budget Act. (1997). Public Law 105-33.
2. Prospective Payment Assessment Commission. (1996). *Report and Recommendations to the Congress.* Washington, DC: Author.
3. Medicare Payment Advisory Commission. (2006). *Report to the Congress: Increasing the value of Medicare.* Washington, DC: Author.
4. Medicare Payment Advisory Commission. (2005). *Outpatient therapy services.* Retrieved February 5, 2008 from http://www.medpac.gov/publications/other_reports/Dec05_Medicare_Bascs_OPT.pdf
5. Deficit Reduction Act. (2005). Public Law 109-171.
6. Balanced Budget Refinements Act. (1999). Public Law 106-113.
7. Benefits Improvement and Protection Act. (2000). Public Law 106-554.
8. Medicare Prescription Drug, Improvement, and Modernization Act. (2003). Public Law 108-173.
9. Tax Relief and Health Care Act. (2006). Public Law 109-432.
10. Medicare, Medicaid, and SCHIP Extension Act. (2007). Public Law 110-173.
11. Centers for Medicare and Medicaid Services. (2008). *Transmittal 1414.* Retrieved February 27, 2008, from http://www.cms.hhs.gov/transmittals/downloads/R1414CP.pd

Ashley Opp Hofmann is AOTA's senior staff writer.

Source: Courtesy of AOTA, *OT Practice*.

Working with an Occupational Therapy Assistant

CHAPTER 24

Lettie M. Redley

OBJECTIVES

1. Describe the role of the occupational therapist (OT).
2. Describe the role of the occupational therapy assistant (OTA).
3. Describe the working relationship between the OT and OTA in a traditional work setting.
4. Explain methods of supervision and collaboration between the OT and OTA.
5. Explain legal and ethical considerations pertaining to the OT and OTA professional relationship.

Table 24-1 Key Terms

AOTA, 2004, p. 663
Supervision
Professional development
Legal
Ethical
Accountable
Crepeau, Cohn, & Schell, 2009, p. 942
Direct supervision
Indirect supervision
Service competency
Documentation
Practitioners
AOTA, 2005b, p. 661
Critical reasoning
Interpersonal skills
Proficiency
Code of Ethics

INTRODUCTION

Welcome to Day 35 of your study guide. This chapter reviews the working relationship between the OT and OTA in traditional work settings including hospitals, nursing homes, mental health units, and schools, to name a few. Both occupational therapists and occupational therapy assistants are OT practitioners with some similar and some different responsibilities.

OUTLINE

1. Occupational therapy practitioner roles

(American Occupational Therapy Association [AOTA], 2002, pp. 615–619)
(AOTA, 2004, pp. 663–667)

- **a.** Occupational therapist general functions
    - **i.** Performs screening
    - **ii.** Performs evaluation and interpretation of data
    - **iii.** Develops intervention plans and goals
    - **iv.** Implements intervention plans
    - **v.** Monitors and modifies intervention
    - **vi.** Evaluates outcomes, terminates service
    - **vii.** Has overall responsibility for service
    - **viii.** Maintains records and documentation
- **b.** Occupational therapy assistant general functions
    - **i.** Assists with evaluation data collection
    - **ii.** Contributes to intervention and goal planning
    - **iii.** Selects and implements intervention activities
    - **iv.** Adapts interventions as needed with OT agreement
    - **v.** Provides information on client's response to intervention
    - **vi.** Provides discharge resources
    - **vii.** Maintains records and documentation
    - **viii.** Functions under supervision

2. Competency in practice

(AOTA, 2004, pp. 663–667)
(AOTA, 2005b, pp. 661–662)

- **a.** Determines the amount of supervision needed
    - **i.** Entry level
    - **ii.** Competent level
- **b.** Means of development
    - **i.** Education and training
    - **ii.** Acquisition of skills
    - **iii.** Practice and experience
- **c.** Competency is achieved when a supervising OT and an OTA reach comparable conclusions and outcomes following assessments and interventions respectively.
- **d.** Competency includes five standards
    - **i.** Having a knowledge base in OT
    - **ii.** Using critical reasoning to make judgments
    - **iii.** Employing professional interpersonal skills
    - **iv.** Demonstrating proficiency in practice
    - **v.** Demonstrating adherence to the Code of Ethics

3. Levels and methods of supervision

(AOTA, 2004, pp. 663–667)

- **a.** Levels
    - **i.** Daily supervision on premises

  ii. Direct contact twice weekly
  iii. General monthly supervision
  iv. Minimal supervision as determined by the OT and OTA
 b. Methods
  i. Direct
   I. Face to face
   II. Observation
   III. Modeling and mentoring
   IV. Instruction
   V. Cotreatment
  ii. Indirect
   I. Telephone conversations
   II. Paperwork review
   III. Written correspondence
   IV. Electronic exchanges
 c. Collaborative supervision

(Crepeau, Cohn, & Schell, 2009, pp. 939–948)

  i. Guidance and oversight of services
   I. Level determined collaboratively
  ii. Facilitation of competence
   I. Determines changes in supervisory level
  iii. Facilitation of professional growth

4. Legal responsibilities

(AOTA, 2003)

 a. State licensure laws define supervision
  i. Vary from state to state
  ii. Definition of roles
  iii. Definition of levels of supervision
  iv. Countersigning treatment records
  v. Documentation of supervision
 b. Medicare laws and regulations provide additional rules

(Centers for Medicare and Medicaid Services, 2008)
(Crepeau, Cohn, & Schell, 2009, pp. 952–957)

  i. Definition of supervision levels
   I. Personal supervision: In the room
   II. Direct supervision: In the office suite
   III. General supervision: Available but not necessarily on premises
  ii. Definition of qualified professional (OT) and qualified personnel (OTA)
  iii. Documentation and countersigning guidelines
   I. OT must document all assessments
   II. Depending on state licensure laws, the OT may need to cosign all documentation
 c. Other reimbursement sources may have additional requirements

5. Ethical responsibilities

(AOTA, 2005a, pp. 639–642)

 a. Principles related to roles and responsibilities
  i. Delegation of duties based on competency
  ii. Appropriate supervision for level of competency
  iii. Adherence to the code by both practitioners
  iv. Accurate reporting

CASE STUDIES

Case Study 24-1. Jenny has been a certified occupational therapy assistant (COTA) for 6 months, working in an acute care hospital setting. She was asked by the OT to evaluate a new client's ADL skills, and she recorded the results on the department's ADL form. She was then asked to formulate the ADL treatment goals to be added to the rest of the intervention plan, which was developed by the OT. Were the actions of the OT and OTA appropriate?

Case Study 24-2. Harry is an OTA with 4 years of experience and now works in a prison mental health rehabilitation program. There is no OT available, but Harry is under the supervision of a certified therapeutic recreation specialist (CTRS). Harry's responsibilities include developing and implementing occupational therapy treatment plans and documenting the OT services that are rendered. Harry thinks he is supposed to have some form of supervision from an OT. Is Harry correct or incorrect?

Case Study 24-3. Becky is an OT supervising three experienced OTAs in a long-term care rehabilitation setting. She is very busy trying to keep up with new admission evaluations, discharge evaluations, documentation requirements, team meetings, and other responsibilities. Becky has trained Louise, an OTA, to perform all home evaluations prior to client's being discharged from the facility. Upon completion of the home evaluation, Louise gives her assessment information to Becky, who documents recommendations meant to optimize the client's independence and safety within her home environment. Are Becky (OT supervisor) and Louise (OTA) performing their roles appropriately?

REFERENCES

American Occupational Therapy Association. (2002). Occupational therapy practice framework: Domain and process. *American Journal of Occupational Therapy, 56*(6), 609–639.

American Occupational Therapy Association. (2003). *Occupational therapy assistant supervision requirements.* Retrieved November 27, 2007, from http://www.aota.org/Practitioners/Licensure/StateRegs/Supervision/36455.aspx

American Occupational Therapy Association. (2004). Guidelines for supervision, roles and responsibilities during the delivery of occupational therapy services. *American Journal of Occupational Therapy, 58*(6), 663–667.

American Occupational Therapy Association. (2005a). Occupational therapy code of ethics. *American Journal of Occupational Therapy, 59*(6), 639–642.

American Occupational Therapy Association (2005b). Standards for continuing competence. *American Journal of Occupational Therapy, 59*(6), 661–662.

Centers for Medicare and Medicaid Services. (2008). *Medicare benefits policy manual.* Retrieved May 30, 2008, from http://www.cms.hhs.gov/Manuals/IOM/itemdetail.asp?filterType=none&filterByDID=99&sortByDID=1&sortOrder=ascending&itemID=CMS012673&intNumPerPage=10

Crepeau, E., Cohn, E. S., & Schell, B. (Eds.). *Willard & Spackman's occupational therapy* (11th ed., pp. 952–957). Philadelphia: Lippincott Williams & Wilkins

CASE STUDY RATIONALE

Case Study 24-1. Correct Answer: The actions of the OT and OTA were appropriate in part, but not completely. Though the OTA can contribute to evaluations by collecting and reporting data, it is not appropriate for the OTA to develop treatment goals independently.

Case Study 24-2. Correct Answer: Harry is correct regarding the need for OT supervision. An OTA performing OT services always needs some form of supervision from an OT. If he were not expected to deliver OT services, he could function under the facility's policies and procedures (e.g., as a rehabilitation aide) but not document services rendered as an OTA.

Case Study 24-3. Correct Answer: Yes, Becky and Louise are performing their roles appropriately. Louise has been trained and established service competency in performing home assessments, and Becky retains her responsibility to analyze the assessment data and make recommendations.

Exhibit 1-1 Stress Vulnerability Scale

In modern society, most of us can't avoid stress. But we can learn to behave in ways that lessen its effects. Researchers have identified a number of factors that affect one's vulnerability to stress—among them are eating and sleeping habits, caffeine and alcohol intake, and how we express our emotions. The following questionnaire is designed to help you discover your vulnerability quotient and to pinpoint trouble spots. Rate each item from 1 (always) to 5 (never), according to how much of the time the statement is true of you. Be sure to mark each item, even if it does not apply to you—for example, if you don't smoke, circle 1 next to item six.

	Always	Sometimes			Never
1. I eat at least one hot, balanced meal a day.	1	2	3	4	5
2. I get 7–8 hours of sleep at least four nights a week.	1	2	3	4	5
3. I give and receive affection regularly.	1	2	3	4	5
4. I have at least one relative within 50 miles on whom I can rely.	1	2	3	4	5
5. I exercise to the point of perspiration at least twice a week.	1	2	3	4	5
6. I limit myself to less than half a pack of cigarettes a day.	1	2	3	4	5
7. I take fewer than five alcohol drinks a week.	1	2	3	4	5
8. I am the appropriate weight for my height.	1	2	3	4	5
9. I have an income adequate to meet basic expenses.	1	2	3	4	5
10. I get strength from my religious beliefs.	1	2	3	4	5
11. I regularly attend club or social activities.	1	2	3	4	5
12. I have a network of friends and acquaintances.	1	2	3	4	5
13. I have one or more friends to confide in about personal matters.	1	2	3	4	5
14. I am in good health (including eyesight, hearing, and teeth).	1	2	3	4	5
15. I am able to speak openly about my feelings when angry or worried.	1	2	3	4	5
16. I have regular conversations with the people I live with about domestic problems—for example, chores and money.	1	2	3	4	5
17. I do something for fun at least once a week.	1	2	3	4	5
18. I am able to organize my time effectively.	1	2	3	4	5
19. I drink fewer than three cups of coffee (or other caffeine-rich drinks) a day.	1	2	3	4	5
20. I take some quiet time for myself during the day.	1	2	3	4	5

(continues)

Exhibit 1-1 Stress Vulnerability Scale *(continued)*

Scoring Instructions: To calculate your score, add up the figures and subtract 20.	**Self-Care Plan:** Notice that nearly all the items describe situations and behaviors over which you have a great deal of control. Review the items on which you scored three or higher. List those items in your self-care plan. Concentrate first on those that are easiest to change—for example, eating a hot, balanced meal daily and having fun at least once a week—before tackling those that seem difficult.
Score Interpretation: A score below 10 indicates excellent resistance to stress. A score over 30 indicates some vulnerability to stress. A score over 50 indicates serious vulnerability to stress.	

Source: Exhibit courtesy Copyright 2009 Stress Directions, Inc., Lyle H. Miller and Alma Dell Smith, Boston, MA www.stressdirections.com

Exhibit 5-1 Reflection Question Journal

1. What? (What have I accomplished? What have I learned?)

2. So what? (What difference did it make? Why should I do it? How is it important? How do I feel about it?)

3. Now what? (What's next? Where do we go from here?)

Source: Exhibit courtesy of Live Wire Media.

Wrapping Up the Review (Days 36–45)

Ten Days and Counting

CHAPTER 25

Rosanne DiZazzo-Miller, Joseph M. Pellerito Jr., and Fredrick D. Pociask

INTRODUCTION

Welcome to Days 36 through 45 of your study guide. It is now time for you to insert the CD-ROM into your computer and begin the practice examinations. You will begin the practice test section of exam preparation, calculate domain areas, and identify and review challenging areas of study. The following time line presents an example of a potential time frame to complete the two interactive practice examinations:

Table 25-1 Time Frame

Day 36	Review all materials. Try to get at least 8 hours of uninterrupted sleep every night if you can! Remember, there are 170 questions including three clinical simulation test (CST) questions, and you have 4 hours to take the examination. This averages out to approximately one multiple choice question per minute, to allow for approximately 20 minutes to answer each CST question. Make sure to frequently refer back to the question that is presented and focus on exactly what the question is asking. Is it asking what's best for the caregiver, OT, client, or OTA? Is it asking about best practices related to intervention or assessment or both? Students report that this is the most common mistake they make when taking the NBCOT exam (i.e., students become distracted by the amount of information presented instead of focusing on the sentence containing the specific question).
Day 37	Locate a quiet room with computer access to mimic (as closely as possible) the description of the real testing environment and take test #1.
Day 38	Calculate the domain areas and review the area(s) that are the most challenging to you. Remember to make sure to focus on answering exactly what the question asks, and don't get sidetracked by options that sound good or additional information presented in the questions.
Day 39	Continue review work from exam #1.
Day 40	Locate a quiet room with computer access to mimic (as closely as possible) the description of the real testing environment and take test #2.
Day 41	Calculate the domain areas and review the area(s) that are the most challenging to you.
Day 42	Continue review work from exam #2.

(continues)

Table 25-1 Time Frame *(continued)*

Day 43	Review any chapters and/or areas that you think you need more work on. Continue this review process until you feel confident with the reviewed areas.
Day 44	Congratulations, you have completed a rigorous 45 days of test preparation! Rest assured in your knowledge and ability. We recommend the following steps be taken to optimize your success: (1) Get a good night's sleep and wake up rested and confident that you are ready to take the exam! Studies have shown that it is not enough to simply get one good night's sleep the night before an exam. Remember to get several nights of restorative sleep heading up to the exam (i.e., at least 8 hours of uninterrupted sleep). (2) Maintain a positive attitude, especially in the days leading up to the exam. In other words, think positive, and stay calm, cool, and collected. (3) Maintain good nutritional habits throughout your exam preparation, especially in the days leading up to, and the day of, the exam. Proper nutrition and being well hydrated can make a big difference in recall and test performance. (4) Stop studying 1 to 2 days prior to taking the exam. Cramming will not help you, and spending a day or two decompressing and relaxing will go a long way to help you get mentally prepared for the big day. Identify activities that you enjoy and that help you to relax, and do them without feeling guilty! (5) Lastly, we recommend taking the exam shortly after you have completed your test preparation, keeping in mind the importance of feeling confident in your knowledge and ability prior to taking the exam. In other words, if you need more time to review questions and answers or specific domains or chapter content, it is important that you take that time. As stated in Chapter 1, the typical application turnaround after you send NBCOT your transcripts is approximately 1 week before receiving your Authorization to Test (ATT) letter, and then you can typically schedule your exam right away. When you complete or come close to completing the 45 days, you will have a better idea of when you should schedule your examination.
Day 45	Down time! Think of one or two relaxing activities and do them.

OUTLINE

1. **Life after the NBCOT exam: What's next**
   a. Passing the examination
      i. State licensure
         I. Contact your state regulatory board immediately after passing the examination to apply for state licensure. This is crucial!
         II. Send your application and payment as soon as possible.
      ii. NBCOT certification
         I. Professional development units (PDU) are required for all practicing occupational therapists who are registered with the NBCOT. There is an online source called "Professional Development Log Portal" located on the NBCOT home page where you can keep track of your PDU to facilitate the renewal process that occurs approximately every 3 years.
      iii. Renewal process
         I. On both your state license and NBCOT registration cards, there will be an expiration date. Approximately 2 months prior to expiration, each agency will send you a notification to renew your license and registration. Make sure to follow up with them if you do not receive anything; also make certain your contact information is always current with both agencies, including address, phone, and name changes. Make a habit of keeping verification of payment and application receipts.
   b. Retaking the examination
      i. If you don't pass the exam on your first attempt, follow these steps:
         I. First, keep your chin up, be strong, and learn as much from this experience as you can. It's okay to feel sad, but don't be discouraged. There are many great occupational therapists who have had to repeat this exam. The most common

reason for performing poorly on the exam is test-taking strategies that result in confusion while attempting to answer the questions being asked. Pick yourself up again, hold your head up high, and begin again. Each day you work toward retaking your exam puts you one day closer to becoming an OT.

II. Next, review your letter (i.e., if you haven't burned it already) and take note of the domain areas that presented the most challenge to you.

III. Make sure that your new study plan focuses specifically on those areas. If you need more explanations on what those areas cover, make sure to read pages 9–22 of the NBCOT Practice Analysis located on their home page.

IV. Go to http://www.nbcot.org/candidates/index.html.

V. Locate and click on the "Score Reports" link.

VI. Follow the "Steps for Re-Applying to Take the NBCOT Certification Examination for Candidates" link.

VII. You need to wait 45 days before retaking the examination. Map out a new study plan with a calendar and give yourself enough time to practice and feel confident in your review before scheduling your retake. Remember that at this point if you're confident with your knowledge, your focus should be on reading and answering questions. Make certain you are confident with test-taking strategies (see Chapters 2 and 3) before retaking the exam.

We hope you enjoyed your 45-day journey through this book. It is our hope that we have provided you with the guidance and materials needed to successfully pass the NBCOT examination to become an OTR. Now, GO GET 'EM!

REFERENCE

National Board for Certification in Occupational Therapy, Inc. (2009). *Welcome, exam candidates.* Retrieved March 27, 2009, from http://www.nbcot.org/candidates/index.html

Index

pages followed by t, f, or ex denote tables, figures, and exhibits respectively